Bolivia

WORLD BIBLIOGRAPHICAL SERIES

General Editors:
Robert G. Neville (Executive Editor)
John J. Horton

Robert A. Myers   Hans H. Wellisch
Ian Wallace   Ralph Lee Woodward, Jr.

John J. Horton is Deputy Librarian of the University of Bradford and was formerly Chairman of its Academic Board of Studies in Social Sciences. He has maintained a longstanding interest in the discipline of area studies and its associated bibliographical problems, with special reference to European Studies. In particular he has published in the field of Icelandic and of Yugoslav studies, including the two relevant volumes in the World Bibliographical Series.

Robert A. Myers is Associate Professor of Anthropology in the Division of Social Sciences and Director of Study Abroad Programs at Alfred University, Alfred, New York. He has studied post-colonial island nations of the Caribbean and has spent two years in Nigeria on a Fulbright Lectureship. His interests include international public health, historical anthropology and developing societies. In addition to *Amerindians of the Lesser Antilles: a bibliography* (1981), *A Resource Guide to Dominica, 1493-1986* (1987) and numerous articles, he has compiled the World Bibliographical Series volumes on *Dominica* (1987), *Nigeria* (1989) and *Ghana* (1991).

Ian Wallace is Professor of German at the University of Bath. A graduate of Oxford in French and German, he also studied in Tübingen, Heidelberg and Lausanne before taking teaching posts at universities in the USA, Scotland and England. He specializes in contemporary German affairs, especially literature and culture, on which he has published numerous articles and books. In 1979 he founded the journal *GDR Monitor*, which he continues to edit under its new title *German Monitor*.

Hans H. Wellisch is Professor emeritus at the College of Library and Information Services, University of Maryland. He was President of the American Society of Indexers and was a member of the International Federation for Documentation. He is the author of numerous articles and several books on indexing and abstracting, and has published *The Conversion of Scripts and Indexing and Abstracting: an International Bibliography*, and *Indexing from A to Z*. He also contributes frequently to *Journal of the American Society for Information Science*, *The Indexer* and other professional journals.

Ralph Lee Woodward, Jr. is Director of Graduate Studies at Tulane University, New Orleans. He is the author of *Central America, a Nation Divided*, 2nd ed. (1985), as well as several monographs and more than seventy scholarly articles on modern Latin America. He has also compiled volumes in the World Bibliographical Series on *Belize* (1980), *El Salvador* (1988), *Guatemala* (Rev. Ed.) (1992) and *Nicaragua* (Rev. Ed.) (1994). Dr. Woodward edited the Central American section of the *Research Guide to Central America and the Caribbean* (1985) and is currently associate editor of Scribner's *Encyclopedia of Latin American History*.

VOLUME 89

Bolivia

New Edition

J. Valerie Fifer

Compiler

CLIO PRESS

OXFORD, ENGLAND · SANTA BARBARA, CALIFORNIA

DENVER, COLORADO

British Library Cataloguing in Publication Data

Fifer, J. Valerie
Bolivia. – New ed. – (World bibliographical series; v. 89)
1. Bolivia – Bibliography
I. Title
016.9′84

ISBN 1–85109–300–1

ABC-CLIO,
Old Clarendon Ironworks,
35A Great Clarendon Street,
Oxford OX2 6AT, England.

_____

ABC-CLIO Inc.,
130 Cremona Drive,
Santa Barbara,
CA 93117, USA

Designed by Bernard Crossland.
Typeset by ABC-CLIO, Oxford, England.
Printed and bound in Great Britain by print in black, Midsomer Norton.

THE WORLD BIBLIOGRAPHICAL SERIES

This series, which is principally designed for the English speaker, will eventually cover every country (and some of the world's principal regions and cities), each in a separate volume comprising annotated entries on works dealing with its history, geography, economy and politics; and with its people, their culture, customs, religion and social organization. Attention will also be paid to current living conditions – housing, education, newspapers, clothing, etc. – that are all too often ignored in standard bibliographies; and to those particular aspects relevant to individual countries. Each volume seeks to achieve, by use of careful selectivity and critical assessment of the literature, an expression of the country and an appreciation of its nature and national aspirations, to guide the reader towards an understanding of its importance. The keynote of the series is to provide, in a uniform format, an interpretation of each country that will express its culture, its place in the world, and the qualities and background that make it unique. The views expressed in individual volumes, however, are not necessarily those of the publisher.

VOLUMES IN THE SERIES

Contents

Contents

Contents

Introduction

Bolivia is known throughout the world as a poor, landlocked country in the heart of South America, rich in resources but with a long-standing reputation for political instability, military dictatorship, and rampant inflation. The last few years, however, have seen dramatic changes as the country has returned to democracy, and introduced bold new measures to rescue the economy, and to raise living standards in this multi-ethnic society.

Whatever the changes, Bolivia remains a land of spectacular contrasts in its landscapes and its history. Here, the Andes are at their widest and most complex, a mountain world of soaring peaks, high plateaux, and deep valleys that plunge eastwards to the vast plains known as the Oriente. Bolivia covers an area of 1,098,581 sq. km (424,164 sq. miles), but although less than one-third of the country lies in the mountains, Bolivia is widely regarded as an Andean country because the most densely populated and economically developed part of its territory is located within the Andes or close to its foothills.

The mountainous western region is dominated by two great parallel ranges. The Western Cordillera (Cordillera Occidental) runs along the border with Chile; it is crowned by Mount Sajama at 6,542 metres (21,463 feet), Bolivia's highest peak. To the east is the Cordillera Oriental. Although the name Eastern Cordillera is often loosely applied to the first great mountain escarpment, in reality the Cordillera Oriental de los Andes in Bolivia is a huge jumble of three major cordilleras, high sierras and isolated valleys tilting eastwards towards the plains. The spectacular edge of the Eastern Cordillera is known as the Cordillera Real (Royal Range), where the mountain front forms a dazzling rampart of snow-capped peaks exceeding 6,000 metres. Two of the most dramatic are Mount Illampú at 6,485 metres (21,276 feet), and Mount Illimani at 6,457 metres (21,184 feet) which towers above La Paz.

Between these two bounding ranges lies the altiplano (high plateau), averaging some 3,800 metres (12,500 feet), and one of the highest inhabited areas in the world. The surface of this great plateau, composed mostly of water- and wind-borne deposits, slopes gently southwards, its evenness occasionally broken by protruding ridges and volcanic cones or by mountain spurs and alluvial fans. The altiplano breaks many geographical records; its drainage system is the largest area of inland drainage in South America, while Lake Titicaca is the highest commercially navigated lake in the world. Its outlet, the River Desaguadero, flows into Lake Poopó, which, unlike Titicaca, is shallow and very salty. Farther south again are the great salt flats (*salares*), some of them seasonally flooded but generally visible as shimmering white sheets on a barren land. Soils in the southern altiplano are also highly saline, but in the north, rich silts border Lake Titicaca.

This huge lake, which is shared with Peru, also has an important moderating influence on the local climate, and in bright winter sunshine temperatures may reach 70°F (21°C). Cloudless skies and astonishingly clear air bring distant peaks sharply into focus, providing hauntingly beautiful views across the altiplano. But cold winds sweep the area and rainfall is slight, coming mostly in the form of summer thunderstorms during December and January. In these harsh conditions it is easy to see how the combination of richer soils and milder climate in the Titicaca Basin were of crucial importance in prehistory since they were to attract increasing numbers of Aymara Indian farmers and llama and alpaca herders to settle around the lake, and in time to lay the foundations of the great Andean agricultural civilizations – the Tiwanaku and subsequently the Inca empires.

Beyond the high, snow-capped slopes of the Cordillera Real, the descent northeastwards to the plains is sudden and often terrifying. The rivers pour through the heavily forested belt of rugged terrain known as the Yungas – an Indian word roughly meaning 'warm lands'. Clouds of moist air from Amazonia fill the valleys and make the atmosphere rich with the smell of vegetation. The Yungas' luxuriant mountain jungle (*montaña*) contains an enormous variety of tropical hardwoods, dyewoods, medicinal and aromatic plants, citrus fruits, bananas, cacao and coffee. The cinchona tree (for quinine) and the coca shrub are both indigenous to this region.

South of the Yungas, the Andes widen to about 450 km (over 400 miles) and are dominated by a high, tilted block called the puna, with west-facing escarpments and gentler eastward slopes down to the plains. The puna contains a system of mountain basins and valleys known simply as the Valles which are larger and more open than those farther north. Lying mostly at heights of 1,830-3,000 metres (6,000-9,800 feet), the Valles contain the 'garden cities' of Cochabamba, Sucre, and Tarija. Soils are deeper here, and have long been noted for their fertility and varied agriculture, although high productivity depends on irrigation.

Beyond the Andes to the north and east, the Oriente sprawls across more than two-thirds of Bolivia. This vast area presents many contrasts – low alluvial plains (*llanos*), great swamps, scrub, open savannahs, jungle, and rain forest (*selva*). In the extreme south, the Chaco becomes flooded and marshy in the summer, but it is a hot, semi-desert during the remaining seven or eight months of the year. Northwards, the relief of the Santa Cruz area is more varied, with a narrow arc of sierras swinging eastwards to form a low watershed between the Amazon and Paraguay river basins. North again, in the Departments of Beni and Pando, the savannahs gradually merge into the Amazonian rainforest, with its wild rubber, Brazil nuts, and a rich variety of tropical hardwoods such as mahogany and walnut, but much of the Beni suffers from extensive flooding, which begins in March or April, towards the end of the summer rainy season. As the water levels rise, thousands of cattle retreat to patches of higher ground, while the scattered villages and ranches isolated by the floods rely on local airstrips or small boats to bring in their supplies. Soils over much of the Oriente are poor, lacking in nutrients, and alternately parched or waterlogged.

Spain's main assault on South America early in the 16th century was launched from the Pacific coast into the high Andes. In 1532-33, the heart of the Inca empire fell to Francisco Pizarro and a small band of Spanish *conquistadores*, who found over the next few years that they had captured a large, well-organized, densely populated Indian civilization, as well as a wealth of golden treasure beyond their wildest dreams. The discovery of Cerro Rico, the 'silver mountain' at Potosí in 1545 was one of the greatest mineral strikes of all time, and Chuquisaca (now Sucre) became the administrative centre of Upper Peru, as Bolivia was known during the colonial period. The region was governed from the Viceroyalty in Lima for nearly 250 years, and from Buenos Aires in the new Viceroyalty of the Río de la Plata during the final years of empire, but Upper Peru was remote from both centres and its extreme isolation encouraged Bolivia's determination to become separate from both Peru and Argentina when independence from Spain was finally achieved in 1825 by a liberating army led by Antonio José de Sucre. The new state was named República Bolívar (soon amended to Bolivia) in honour of the Liberator and in part to please him, since Bolívar did not at first support Sucre's role in legitimizing this breakaway movement by Upper Peru, favouring instead the retention of the legal, and larger, viceregal political units in the newly independent Hispanic America.

Independence brought no peace. Bolivia fell into chaos. The country's independence marked the beginning of a long period of civil and military turmoil dominated by *caudillo* dictatorship. The country's poor internal communications intensified the strong sense of regionalism and rivalry within Bolivia, while its weakness externally was revealed by the progressive loss of territory to each of its five neighbours. Indeed, over the years, Bolivia was to lose half the territory it had claimed at the time of independence. The country's remote borderlands remained empty or at best sparsely populated, distant from the cities and villages clustered in the high Andes, and for most Bolivians merely unknown frontiers that remained out of sight and out of mind. But Bolivia's lost lands included its Litoral Department and with it, the country's independent outlet to the sea, along with rich copper and nitrate resources, following Chile's victory in the War of the Pacific (1879-84). Bolivia had never been able to acquire the port of Arica from Peru, or later from Chile, despite the fact that it had been Upper Peru's official port during colonial times. Bolivia's lost lands were also to include a large portion of the Chaco to Paraguay after the devastating Chaco War (1932-35). In their different ways, both these humiliating defeats were to have lasting effects on Bolivia – politically, psychologically, and socially.

After 1880, a more settled period of government began with the formation of political parties and the introduction of a parliamentary system in the bi-cameral Bolivian Congress. Greater stability attracted inward investment. New railways were built into the Bolivian Andes from Pacific ports in Chile and Peru, tin mining expanded and tin export quickly dominated the Bolivian economy. In 1898, the seat of government and administration was transferred from Sucre (Chuquisaca) to the more accessible city of La Paz which now became the *de facto* capital of Bolivia, although Sucre remained the legal capital and retained Bolivia's Supreme Court. But whether the government was led by Conservatives or Liberals, power remained exclusively in the hands of a small mine-owning, land-owning, and military élite.

At the other extreme, the Indians, who numbered about 60-70 per cent of the total population, remained mostly landless, illiterate or semi-illiterate, and without a vote. Bolivia's population consisted of three groups: the Indians; the *mestizos* (of mixed Indian and mainly Spanish descent, c. 30-35 per cent); and those of unmixed Spanish and other European ancestry, c. 5-10 per cent), although, as the generalized figures indicate, it has never been possible to measure accurately the percentage of each group, while the percentages themselves vary greatly in urban and rural areas, and in the different regions of Bolivia.

Bolivia's crushing defeat in the Chaco War proved a turning-point in the country's history. Shock and anger after a war that Bolivia had assumed it could not lose triggered deep disillusionment with Bolivia as it still was after more than 100 years of independence. The new 'Chaco Generation' had emerged, groups of mostly middle-class intellectuals, civilian and military, who demanded a radical rethinking of politics, land reform, the nationalization of industry, and improvement to the status of the Indian in society. This new struggle against Bolivia's traditional élites eventually culminated in the National and Social Revolution of 1952, led by the Movimiento Nacional Revolucionario (MNR). Víctor Paz Estenssoro was installed as Bolivia's new President, soon demonstrating that this revolution was no superficial palace coup like so many others before it, but a process of fundamental reform which included the break-up of the large landed estates (*haciendas, fincas*), nationalization of the tin mines, universal suffrage without literacy and property requirements, and a new education programme.

The new land reform policies also encouraged poor, formerly landless Andean farmers to migrate eastwards and colonize zones in the Alto Beni, the Chapare, and around the city of Santa Cruz. Foreign immigrants, including Japanese, Okinawans, Mennonites, and a few Russian, German, and Italian families, also arrived to establish new agricultural colonies around Santa Cruz (de la Sierra), which in 1954 was linked for the first time by a paved road to Cochabamba, and thus to other highways linking the major cities in the Andes. The early 1950s marked the first serious step to end Santa Cruz' isolation overland, and the start of dramatic new population growth, agriculture and agro-industry that has continued to the present day.

For the moment, the MNR's 1952 revolution had clipped the wings of the military and built a broad base of political support which included miners, small rural farmers (now known as *campesinos*, not *indios*), and initially the urban middle class. Changes were forced through quickly and often violently. In the 1956 and 1960 elections the MNR consolidated its power, but the Bolivian economy was now in decline, world tin prices were falling, unions were restless, and the party was losing support in the cities. Soon after his re-election in 1964, Paz Estenssoro was overthrown in a military coup, the start of nearly two decades of military rule by both the right and left wing. Democratic government was restored in 1982 under President Siles Zuazo, but by now the Bolivian economy was nearing total collapse. World tin prices were plummeting and crashed in 1985, mass strikes and demonstrations were commonplace, the illegal coca/cocaine trade was out of control, and by 1984-85, Bolivia's hyperinflation had reached one of the highest levels ever in world history.

What happened next was again revolutionary – drastic change driven by dire circumstance. In July 1985, Víctor Paz Estenssoro was elected President of Bolivia for the fourth time and in conjunction with the International Monetary Fund, immediately introduced a New Economic Policy that comprised a stabilization programme, the reduction of state subsidies for nationalized industries, huge cuts in government spending, and free-market reforms. The combination of the international tin market crash coupled with the collapse of Bolivia's own internal economy (apart from the illegal coca/cocaine trade), led to sudden and widespread unemployment; while hyperinflation was rapidly brought under control, the severity of the measures needed to rescue the Bolivian economy caused great hardship, especially among miners and their families.

Introduction

Violent opposition and a general strike called by union leaders quickly followed, but Paz Estenssoro's government held firm. In a closely fought election in 1989, and an eventual left–right party alliance, Jaime Paz Zamora of the Movimiento de la Izquierda Revolucionaria (MIR) became President, despite having come third in the elections. Coalition with the former right-wing military dictator Hugo Banzer Suárez of the Acción Democrática Nacionalista (ADN), had resulted in Paz Zamora's success, but it had also ensured that the fundamental economic reforms continued in place.

In 1993, Gonzalo Sánchez de Lozada (MNR), formerly the economic planning minister in Paz Estenssoro's 1985-89 administration and winner of the most votes in 1989, became President. He immediately began to extend Bolivia's economic reform policies with proposals to privatize Bolivia's major state-owned industries in a type of privatization to be known as capitalization. Under this innovative programme, capitalization's distinguishing feature was that following competitive bidding, private investors would purchase 50 per cent of the shares in the enterprise, and contract to provide new capital and new management skills to modernize the company and raise productivity. The other 50 per cent of the shares were to be allocated to the Bolivian people by placing them into a trust fund, and then transferring them into privately managed individual pension accounts which started operating in the late 1990s, after the passage of the Pension Reform Law in November 1996.

The Capitalization Law was approved by Congress in March 1994. This Bolivian model of privatization avoided internal opposition to the idea of a wholesale sell-off of the nationalized companies while at the same time it addressed the need for massive new investment and new technology in Bolivia's basic industries, public utilities, and national infrastructure. The policy has continued unabated (though not without localized opposition), and by the end of the year 2000, sales of the last twenty-one public companies remaining to be capitalized are scheduled for completion. Both the New Economic Policy of 1985 and the Capitalization programme of the 1990s attracted widespread analysis and comment by both Bolivian and international economists, who produced a literature of their own on the immediate and long-term prospects for such fundamental reform.

This was not all. The reform programme was extended still further under President Sánchez de Lozada by the Popular Participation Law (April 1994) and the Education Reform Law (July 1994), both of which aimed to decentralize much government administration and bring responsibility closer to the people, e.g. in the areas of education, health, housing, infrastructure, and development projects. This involved the creation of 198 new municipalities, making 314 in all. The pressing need for educational reform and the alleviation of poverty, especially rural poverty, has been acknowledged for over half a century, but progress on these two daunting problems is painfully slow. Although Aymara and Quechua have joined

Spanish as Bolivia's official languages, and bilingual education has been introduced locally in Spanish, Aymara, Quechua, and Guaraní, about 35 per cent of the total population remain functionally illiterate. Some advances have been made; health provision in rural areas is becoming more accessible and there is new priority given to the educational reform programme, although the people's demands on the government, all governments, for more schools and higher standards in primary and secondary education never cease.

The 1997 national election brought Hugo Banzer to power once again for a newly extended term of five years, this time as the democratically elected President heading a coalition of the Acción Democrática Nacionalista (ADN) with three other parties. There were renewed pledges to fight corruption at all levels, and to consolidate the basic reform programme. President Banzer also announced drastic new measures in the fight against the illegal coca/cocaine trade, in association with United States requirements for 'certification' in the war against drugs. The cultivation of coca on a small scale in certain areas is traditional and legal, but the five-year 'Dignity Plan' for 1997-2002 aims to eradicate all illegal coca cultivation, and to put further pressure on *campesinos* to raise alternative crops. International investigation into coca cultivation, cocaine trafficking, and Bolivia's dependence on the revenue that the illegal trade pumps into the economy has soared since the late 1980s, as evidenced in the selected books and articles included here. Crop substitution will at best provide a limited solution. Commentators are generally pessimistic about the prospects for total eradication of illegally grown coca, but the Banzer administration's determination to do so persists, and is showing results.

Bolivia's total population is now just over 8 million. La Paz remains the country's largest city with 1,573,200, while its metropolitan region is expanded by the explosive growth of the city of El Alto (446,189), which sprawls across the altiplano immediately above La Paz. Cochabamba (448,756), long Bolivia's second city, has been overtaken by the phenomenal growth of Santa Cruz with c. 900,000 people, but within a region now approaching 2 million – the fastest-growing region in Bolivia. Since the late 1980s, more rural immigrants have moved into these four largest cities in Bolivia than into any other areas, putting huge pressure on existing urban services as new immigrant communities join the earlier arrivals.

As noted above, the growth of the Santa Cruz region was triggered in the 1950s by colonization and new highway links sponsored by the MNR's revolution and land reform programme. By the 1980s, however, the government had begun to reduce its support for small farm colonization schemes in favour of providing more public land, with title, to large commercial farmers engaged in expanding Bolivia's agro-industries, and food and fibre export (particularly of soya and sunflower products, and more recently cotton). Wheat, rice, and sugar-cane are other major crops produced on a large scale. The policies embodied in the New National Agrarian Reform of 1996, favouring large-scale production, proved to be a highly contentious issue, with many indigenous and small peasant families fearing that their land rights would be undermined, or lost altogether. Some concessions were won from the government following a well-publicized protest march from the Oriente up to La Paz. But many of these new agro-industrial entrepreneurs in the Santa Cruz region are not new to Bolivia; they include the second and third generations of the original Mennonite, Japanese, Brazilian, and Russian pioneers of the 1950s and 1960s.

Mineral wealth, overall, continues to dominate Bolivia's legal export economy, including zinc, tin, gold, silver, and natural gas, while the country contains further important sources of lead, copper, iron, platinum, tungsten, antimony, and lithium. After at least six centuries, what is now Bolivia remains a rich storehouse of minerals, many still to be exploited.

One vital ingredient in the success of Santa Cruz' regional economy has been the spectacular growth of the oil and natural gas industries. The existence of petroleum deposits along the Andean mountain front in southeast Bolivia had been known since the 1870s, and in 1920 the Standard Oil Company of New Jersey acquired a concession for exploration and development. Indeed, oil was to be one of many factors which led to the devastating land struggle between Bolivia and Paraguay in the Chaco War of 1932-35.

Loans from Argentina for new railway extensions into Bolivia, to be repaid with Bolivian oil and natural gas, were a feature of the 1950s and 1960s, but following major new gas discoveries in southeast Bolivia, coupled with the insatiable demand for energy in southern Brazil, planning began in 1992 on the construction of a gas pipeline eastwards from the city of Santa Cruz, across the edge of the Chaco, to Corumbá in Brazil. It was built and feeding natural gas into the São Paulo manufacturing region by the end of the 1990s. More rich reserves of natural gas were confirmed in the Department of Tarija in March 2000, prompting new discussions between Bolivia and Brazil on the feasibility of constructing another pipeline to supply Rio Grande do Sul.

A significant reinterpretation of Bolivia's geographical location has occurred. Today, the country claims a role as the natural bridge between the huge southern common market of MERCOSUR and the Andean Community. And although still an unwillingly landlocked state, Bolivia also now emphasizes the *advantages* of its location, seeing itself as the potential hub of South America in terms of energy resources, and of long-range transport between the countries on the Atlantic and Pacific coasts. This would demand massive improvement of Bolivia's transport infrastructure, especially new paved highways and new bridges, as well as modernization and connection of the country's separate western and eastern rail systems. Meanwhile, increasing use of the Paraguay-Paraná river for barge transport of non-perishable products from Puerto Suárez/Corumbá to the Atlantic, via ports in Argentina and Uruguay, is being encouraged as part of Bolivia's associate membership of MERCOSUR.

Bolivia has been called the 'Land of Tomorrow' ever since its independence in 1825 – great natural wealth forever awaiting development in order to bring stability, economic growth, and higher living standards to the vast majority of the population. But Bolivia remains the poorest country in South America, one of the Highly Indebted Poor Countries of the world in receipt of major IMF/World Bank debt-relief packages and loans. Even now, no sudden changes are likely to occur, but important and far-reaching structural reforms have been introduced since 1985, and it is fair to say that the last few years have seen Bolivia's elusive 'Land of Tomorrow' gradually coming a little closer to what Bolivians mean by that well-worn phrase: success in the struggle for better health, education, and individual opportunity; release from abject poverty and instead, a fair and tangible share in the benefits to be derived from the development of Bolivia's rich physical and human resources.

Content and arrangement of the bibliography

In line with editorial policy, the works cited are mainly in English, although foreign-language items are included where they are an important source of information, and where there is no English equivalent. The entries are in chronological order within their sections and subsections; works published in the same year are placed alphabetically by title. The entries include books, periodicals, doctoral theses, and research reports from government, university, business, and other sources. The items range widely and should be readily accessible, either in the reference libraries of university or government departments, or in large public libraries, where they will be available to readers directly or through inter-library loan. General studies on Latin America are included where they contain substantial material on Bolivia or helpful background for an understanding of the Bolivian experience. Newspaper articles, reviews, and master's theses are omitted.

Selected entries, with their original annotation, have been carried forward from the first edition of the bibliography compiled by G. M. Yeager. Earlier works have also been included where they retain permanent reference value, where they enable the reader to follow the development of an idea or a policy over time, or where they have become classic accounts of their period. Aside from some basic texts (grammars, etc.), included again for the most part within the 'Languages' section, nearly ninety per cent of the entries in this edition are new.

Introduction

Some titles are relevant to more than one section, but no title is entered twice. Cross-references are few. Each title is placed in the section which the compiler considers to be the most appropriate; the indexes will help readers to locate what they need. All works which are primarily for reference only, or are exclusively bibliographical, are placed in the 'Encyclopaedias' or 'Bibliographies' sections respectively, even when they deal specifically with subjects for which there is a separate section in this book.

Acknowledgement

I am most grateful to Dr Juan de Dios Yapita in La Paz for his valuable assistance in updating part of the 'Languages' section.

J. Valerie Fifer
London
July 2000

The Country and Its People

General

1 Bolivia: the central highway of South America, a land of rich resources and varied interest.
Marie Robinson Wright.   Philadelphia: G. Barrie; London; Paris:
C. D. Cazenove, 1907. 450p. map.

A major survey of Bolivia at the start of the 20th century, remarkable for its range and thoroughness. Well-illustrated chapters cover the country's history and constitution, archaeology, population, transport, mining, commerce, and the major regions, including the Beni and the Chaco. Wright herself made a thousand-mile muleback trip into the interior. She presents a positive image of Bolivia and its future, without ignoring the political problems and the deep gulf present in society.

2 Bolivia.
Encyclopedia Britannica.   New York: Encyclopedia Britannica Co.,
1910. 11th ed. vol. 4, p. 166-77. map. bibliog.

This landmark 11th edition of the *Encyclopedia Britannica* provides one of the rare systematic English-language descriptions of Bolivia published in the first decade of the 20th century. It presents an informative record of the country's early and recent history, its geography, geology, flora and fauna, population, government, finance, trade, industry, communications, and social conditions, thereby offering a balanced and accessible account of Bolivia well suited to both the general reader and the business visitor.

3 Bolivia: its people and its resources; its railways, mines, and rubber-forests.
Paul Walle, translated by Bernard Miall.   London: T. Fisher Unwin,
1914. 407p. maps.

Walle's long and detailed study was commissioned in 1911 by the French Ministry of Commerce in order to assess Bolivia's potential for increased trade and investment,

1

particularly since at this time, France trailed well behind Britain, Germany, and the United States in the value of its exports to Bolivia. The book provides a well-rounded, methodical account of the country's geography, population, government, finance, education, mining, agriculture, forestry, and major cities. Great emphasis is given to the improved accessibility, externally and internally, that recently completed and projected railways will bring. On this basis, and without disguising the problems, Walle is reasonably hopeful that Bolivia is about to enter a period of greater prosperity and technological progress.

4 Bolivia: the heart of a continent. A few facts about the country and its activities.
William Alfred Reid.   Washington, DC: Pan American Union, 1916. 2nd ed. 1919. 70p. maps.

A good example of the Pan American Union's determination in the early 20th century to tackle widespread ignorance in the United States about Latin America, and to promote business by providing a wide range of information about the region through books, pictures, statistics, study kits, and other material. Reid had travelled extensively in Latin America and was appointed head of the Union's publications department, where the skill and variety of his work were outstanding. New series appeared in rapid succession, and this illustrated booklet on Bolivia in the 'Nations' set gives a typically readable, reliable account of the country at that time.

5 Bolivia: a land divided.
Harold Osborne.   London: Oxford University Press; Royal Institute of International Affairs, 1964. 3rd ed. 181p. maps. bibliog. (Reprinted, Westport, Connecticut: Greenwood Press, 1985. maps. bibliog.).

This well-written introduction to Bolivia by a British diplomat was originally published in 1954. It was the first general survey of modern Bolivia to be published in England and, as part of a series on Latin America, was designed to present a concise, comprehensive picture of the physical, historical, political, and social conditions for the non-specialist. This third edition was fully revised by the author, and included new assessments of the 1952 revolution and its subsequent reforms.

6 Bolivia: a country study.
Edited by Rex A. Hudson, Dennis Michael Hanratty.   Washington, DC: Federal Research Division, Library of Congress, 1991. 3rd ed. 354p. maps. bibliog. (Area Handbook Series).

One of a continuing series prepared under the Country Studies–Area Handbooks worldwide programme. It contains basic facts and background information on a wide range of topics, including Bolivia's history, politics, social and economic conditions, national security systems and institutions, the armed forces and the police. The book is well organized, objective, and clear.

7 Bolivia: land of struggle.
Waltraud Queisner Morales. Boulder, Colorado: Westview Press,
1992. 234p. map. bibliog. (Westview Profiles/Nations of
Contemporary Latin America).
A good introduction for the general reader, with concise summaries on Bolivia's regions,
peoples, history, politics, and trade.

8 Bolivia: a guide to the people, politics and culture.
Paul van Lindert, Otto Verkoren. London: Latin America Bureau,
1994. 74p. maps. bibliog. (In Focus Series).
A brief introduction to Bolivia, with emphasis on political and economic events in the
1980s and early 1990s.

9 Bolivia update.
London: Bolivian Embassy. 4p. 1999- . monthly.
Published monthly since August 1999, this bulletin reports the most important current
events in Bolivia, and covers news in the political, economic, social, and cultural fields.
Government policies, goals, progress to date, new legislation, new infrastructure,
privatization/capitalization projects, business and finance, trade figures, foreign affairs,
international exhibitions, and cultural events are among the items summarized and
supported with statistics and illustrations. The bulletin's main purpose is to widen
knowledge about Bolivia in the United Kingdom, an aim clearly achieved by this
informative publication.

Children's books

10 Bolivia in pictures.
Bernardine Bailey. New York: Sterling Publishing; London;
Sydney: Oak Tree Press, 1974. 64p. maps. (Visual Geography Series).
This is a book for young people in the 12-15 age group which, if updated, would be
equally useful for class work or private study. It provides a concise, well-organized
introduction to Bolivia's geography, history, government, people, cities and rural areas,
and economic development, based on more than 100 informative black-and-white
photographs, all well supported by captions and a crisp text. The book's structure is
sound, with a good balance of word and picture. Editing of the existing material and
expansion to cover events in recent decades would enable the most to be made of this
interesting and adaptable schoolbook. A revised edition of Bailey's book (*Bolivia in
pictures*, Minneapolis, Minnesota: Lerner Publications Co., Geography Department,
1998. 64p. maps) expands the text and reduces the number of photographs to eighty-six,
many of them new and in colour. Still in the Visual Geography Series, the book is
attractive and often informative although, unfortunately, it lacks some updating, and also
includes a number of errors.

11 Bolivia, Paraguay and Uruguay.

Harvey Radcliffe. Melbourne; London: Macmillan, 1988. 30p.
maps. (Clifford Education in association with H. Radcliffe).

Profusely illustrated with coloured photographs, the book provides a pleasing short introduction for children to the lands and people in these three states.

12 Bolivia.

Edited by Michael Martin, photographs by Yoshiyuki Ikuhara.
London; Milwaukee: Gareth Stevens Children's Books, 1989. 64p.
maps. (Children of the World Series).

The story is developed around the life of a Bolivian boy living by Lake Titicaca, and describes his everyday life at home, in school, and at work in the fields. Short text and captions for young children are set alongside large, coloured photographs. Simple follow-up projects and more background on the country are added at the end to complete a bright, informative book that provides an excellent starting-point for individual or classroom work about life on the Bolivian altiplano.

13 Ecuador, Peru, Bolivia.

Edward Parker. Hove, England: Macdonald Young Books; Austin, Texas: Raintree Steck-Vaughn Press, 1998. 47p. maps. bibliog.
(World Fact Files Series).

A colourful introduction for children to the landscapes, climates, natural resources, and culture of these three Andean states. The book is organized by topic, with the three countries distinguished, but grouped under such headings as daily life, food and farming, trade and industry, transport, and the environment. The text, and a variety of attractive photographs, maps, graphs and diagrams, provide the basis for further work by children at different levels, mainly within the 10-14 age range.

14 Bolivia: a portrait of the country through its festivals and traditions.

Hannah Beardon, Héctor Fernandes. Danbury, Connecticut: Grolier Educational, 1999. 31p. map.

A delightful book for young children, with colourful pictures and little nuggets of information not only on festivals and costumes but also on everyday life, with simple phrases in Spanish, and examples of traditional music, food, recipes, and crafts. In addition, several appropriate activities are included in this stimulating first introduction to Bolivia.

Geography

General

15 Bolivia: land, location, and politics since 1825.
J. Valerie Fifer.   Cambridge, England: Cambridge University Press,
1972. 301p. maps. bibliog.
The best English-language work available about Bolivia. It combines a discussion of
historical development with geography, and stresses the relationship between geography,
economic development, territorial losses and history. This work should be read by any
scholar, diplomat or tourist who is interested in Bolivia.

**16 South America: international river basins, including a section on
rivers and lakes forming international boundaries.**
New York: United Nations, 1977. [not paginated]. map. bibliog.
Discusses international rivers, boundaries and watersheds, and considers Lake Titicaca
and various rivers in eastern Bolivia.

17 The Central Andes.
Clifford T. Smith.   In: *Latin America: geographical perspectives.*
Edited by Harold Blakemore, Clifford T. Smith.   London; New
York: Methuen, 1983. 2nd ed., p. 253-324. maps. bibliog.
This perceptive geographical essay on Peru, Bolivia and Ecuador begins by considering
the physical and human features they have in common. The stark contrasts in relief,
climate, and vegetation that occur between the Pacific coast, the high Andes, and the
eastern plains are clearly presented, as are the shared social characteristics. Then follows
a detailed examination of each of these three countries – their agriculture, mining, trade,
industry, population and urbanization, as well as the impact of internal migration and
agrarian reform. In all, Smith provides a concise, scholarly analysis of the geographical
distinctiveness of these three central Andean states within Latin America as a whole.

18 Latin America.

Preston Everett James, Clarence W. Minkel. New York: Wiley, 1986. 5th ed. 578p. maps. bibliog.

Preston James's classic geography of Latin America has been an invaluable comprehensive text ever since it was first published more than half a century ago. This fifth and final edition, updated and restyled in collaboration with Minkel, maintains an excellent standard, with a wealth of information expressed with ease and clarity in a most readable text, which covers all the major aspects of the physical, historical, economic, and social geography of the region. As with the other chapters, that on Bolivia is discerning, fluent, and jargon-free, while the whole volume is supported by more than 100 high-quality maps and nearly as many photographs.

19 The Latin American city.

Alan Gilbert. London: Latin American Bureau, 1994. 190p. maps. bibliog.

Although there is very little specifically on Bolivia in this volume, it provides useful background on the major features and modern trends that characterize many of the most important cities of Latin America, including, for example, urban primacy, the effects of migration from the rural areas, housing, employment opportunities, the informal economic sector, and the problems of urban management. Students and general readers will find several points for discussion that are relevant to the largest cities of Bolivia.

20 Latin American development: geographical perspectives.

Edited by David Preston. Harlow, England: Longman, 1996. 2nd ed. 313p. maps. bibliog.

A well-illustrated text designed for undergraduates engaged in Latin American and Third World studies. The approach is by theme, not by country, with individual chapters by different authors devoted, for example, to the colonial background, environmental issues, rural development, migration, industry, culture, health, education, and urban growth. There are only passing references to Bolivia, but students will find portions of the material presented for other regions applicable to the Bolivian experience, whether directly or for comparative purposes.

21 Geografía y recursos naturales de Bolivia. (Geography and natural resources of Bolivia.)

Ismael Montes de Oca. La Paz: 'EDOBOL', 1997. 3rd ed. 614p. maps.

An excellent general reference volume by a noted Bolivian scholar on the country's human and physical geography. Among a wide range of other topics, there are sections on energy, the richness of Bolivia's natural resources, the environment and the problems of pollution, and on the diversity of population and of linguistic groups. Many coloured illustrations and diagrams accompany the text in this elegant, informative study, which is also clearly indexed.

Earthquakes

22 Bolivian quake gives a rare glimpse of Earth's interior.
Ray Ladbury. *Physics Today*, vol. 47 (October 1994), p. 17-19. bibliog.

Bolivia's deep earthquake in June 1994 excited the scientific world, and Ladbury conveys this excitement most vividly to the general reader, defining the terms used, summarizing existing theories, and explaining with admirable clarity the significance of these deep-focus quakes in the constant search to understand the Earth's complex inner structure.

23 Great quake in Bolivia rings Earth's bell.
R. Monastersky. *Science News*, vol. 145, no. 25 (June 1994), p. 391.

This is a succinct but informative preliminary report on earthquake activity in Bolivia. In the 1970s, seismologists strung detectors round the world to record earthquakes deep within the planet. On 8-9 June 1994 came their first result, an earthquake in Bolivia of 8.2 magnitude originating 600 kilometres (nearly 400 miles) below the surface, and estimated to be the biggest deep-focus earthquake this century. Less damaging to life and property because few surface seismic waves are produced, deep earthquakes are of major interest to scientists studying the structure of the inner earth.

24 Biggest deep quakes may need help.
Richard A. Kerr. *Science*, vol. 267 (January 1995), p. 329-30.

Reports the proceedings of the latest meeting of the American Geophysical Union held in December 1994 which debated whether fractures at great depth, the cause of rupture, really are the result of changes in crystal form. It was generally agreed that research into the causes of deep quakes should include the possibility of other factors and mechanisms.

25 Deep earthquakes: a fault too big?
Seth Stein. *Science*, vol. 268 (7 April 1995), p. 49-50. bibliog.

Emphasizes that the causes of large earthquakes at great depth will remain open for some time because of the rarity of their occurrence. The Bolivian example in June 1994, 630 km down, is the largest deep earthquake ever recorded on instruments, and Stein concentrates here on the possibility of complex and variable deep-slab thermal processes being of major significance.

26 The good earthquake.
Tim Appenzeller. *Discover*, vol. 16 (January 1995), p. 65-66.

The deep earthquake of 8-9 June 1994, nearly 400 miles (some 600 kilometres) below the surface of Bolivia and confirmed as the biggest deep earthquake ever recorded, was near the bottom of the zone where the Nazca Plate, the floor of the eastern Pacific, is plunging beneath the South American continent. Research so far suggests that rock fracture at such depths probably involves mineral changes produced by greatly increased temperature and pressure, and that these changes can result in deep faults liable to sudden slip.

27 Rupture characteristics of the deep Bolivian earthquake of 9 June 1994 and the mechanisms of deep-focus earthquakes.
Paul G. Silver, Susan L. Beck, Terry C. Wallace, Charles Meade, Stephen C. Myers, David James, Randy Kuchnel. *Science*, vol. 268 (7 April 1995), p. 69-73. maps. bibliog.

This is a detailed report for the specialist. The team of seven scientists conclude that so far their findings do not support the theory of change in the crystal structure at depth as the cause of the Bolivian earthquake. Instead, they suggest that deep earthquakes may represent slip along pre-existing faults which were formed when the zone was near the Earth's surface.

28 Geometry and state of stress of the Nazca Plate beneath Bolivia and its implication for the evolution of the Bolivian orocline.
Mark Andrew Tinker, Terry C. Wallace, Susan L. Beck, Stephen C. Myers, Andrew Papanikolas. *Geology*, vol. 24 (May 1996), p. 387-90. map. bibliog.

Crustal shortening in South America has been most marked in Bolivia, and deep earthquakes of moderate magnitude have occurred regularly in association with the Nazca Plate. Until 1994, however, the plate's geometry under Bolivia was extremely speculative. The authors examine the geometrical evolution of the Nazca Plate, including the critical different geometries of its upper and deeper slabs that together form one plate. This is an important contribution to the subject, well explained both in the text and in the supporting diagrams.

29 Another look at great South American deep earthquakes; results from body wave inversion.
Charles H. Estabrook. *Eos* (American Geophysical Union), vol. 78, no. 46, Suppl. fall meeting (1997), p. 450-51.

The author examines the great earthquakes of 15 August 1963 (Peru-Bolivia) and 31 July 1970 (Colombia), and compares them with the Bolivian earthquake of 8-9 June 1994. These three were the largest deep events of the 20th century ever recorded in South America, but while the 1963 and 1970 quakes probably ruptured on a steeply dipping surface at depths from 540 to 630 km, the 1994 quake ruptured on a nearly horizontal surface at a depth of about 650 km. Estabrook's findings support earlier research by Creager *et al.* in 1995 that high horizontal strain rates occur under Bolivia where the great continental bend occurs in the deep-sea trench and volcano-earthquake zone edging the Pacific.

30 Does rupture in deep earthquakes propagate preferentially towards the bottom of the subducting lithosphere?
Heidi Houston. *Eos* (American Geophysical Union), vol. 78, no. 46, Suppl. fall meeting (1997), p. 449.

Houston notes that studies of more than forty large deep and intermediate earthquakes since the 1950s suggest that rupture occurs towards the base of the subducting (underthrusting) lithosphere. But the earthquakes of 1963, 1970, and 1994 were propagated towards the top of the slab, suggesting that there is a different mechanism at work in triggering the greatest of the deep earthquakes.

31 Frictional melting during faulting.
Hiroo Kanamori, Don L. Anderson, Thomas H. Heaton. *Eos*
(American Geophysical Union), vol. 78, no. 46, Suppl. fall meeting
(1997), p. 464.

The authors speculate on the possibility of frictional melting during fault movement in the
1994 deep earthquake in Bolivia, since the amount of non-radiated energy released was
comparable to, or larger than, the thermal energy of the Mount St Helens volcanic
eruption in the United States in 1980, and would have been sufficient to melt a layer in
the fault zone of up to thirty-one centimetres thick. But could such a thin layer have had
a significant effect on sliding friction? They draw attention to an interesting piece of
research on skiing carried out in the 1930s by Bowden and Hughes which showed that
even a very thin melt layer can reduce friction and promote rapid sliding of the skis. Here,
the authors conclude that once rupture is initiated, melting appears to be unavoidable and
is likely to encourage the extensive sliding associated with large, deep-focus earthquakes.
See also the same authors' article, 'Frictional melting during the rupture of the 1994
Bolivian earthquake' (*Science*, vol. 279 [6 February 1998], p. 839-42. bibliog.).

32 Sliding skis and slipping faults.
Douglas A. Wiens. *Science*, vol. 279 (6 February 1998), p. 824-25.
bibliog.

Clarity and direct appeal distinguish this informative article. Given the huge pressures
involved, Wiens considers why deep earthquakes as much as 670 km (420 miles) below
the Earth's surface occur along deep faults that would be expected to remain locked tight.
His account is valuable in its succinct analysis of all the major explanations put forward
in recent years, including that by Kanamori *et al.* of deep melting, which can produce a
thin fluid layer that reduces friction in much the same way as a thin layer of water reduces
friction between a ski and the underlying snow. But what type of instability creates the
initial slip? Wiens' commentary is well measured, his scholarly survey full of ideas for
specialist and non-specialist alike.

Volcanoes

**33 The Soledad Caldera, Bolivia: a Miocene caldera with associated
epithermal Au-Ag-Cu-Pb-Zn mineralization.**
Stewart D. Redwood. *Geological Society of America Bulletin*,
vol. 99 (September 1987), p. 395-404. maps. bibliog.

This paper describes the Soledad Caldera and its associated mineralization for the first
time, discussing its origins and the evolution of the Soledad volcanic field. The caldera
(wide crater) lies on the eastern side of the Bolivian altiplano, northwest of Oruro, its rich
complex having been mined for gold and silver since the 16th century, and for copper,
lead, and zinc in the 19th and 20th centuries. The author presents the results of a detailed,
scholarly investigation, which is well supported by maps and photographs.

34 Volcanoes of the Central Andes.
Shanaka L. de Silva, Peter W. Francis. Berlin; Heidelburg,
Germany; New York: Springer-Verlag, 1991. 216p. maps. bibliog.

This stylish book provides a valuable source of reference for vulcanologists. Forty-four potentially active volcanoes are studied in Bolivia, Chile and Peru. Each entry includes the volcano's evolution and structure, its type, dimensions, flow lengths, and hazard factor. The study is ably supported by 219 figures, 90 of them in colour.

35 Volcanic rocks from the Bolivian Altiplano: insights into crustal structure, contamination, and magma genesis in the central Andes.
Jon P. Davidson, Shanaka L. de Silva. *Geology*, vol. 20 (December 1992), p. 1127-30. maps. bibliog.

An examination of selected minor volcanoes on the Bolivian altiplano in the region of the Salar de Uyuni, Salar de Coipasa, and Lake Poopó. Minor volcanoes normally comprise only one or two lava flows, and here the authors report on the magma compositions, patterns of eruption, and the evidence of magma accumulation in sub-volcanic chambers. See also a discussion of the paper in *Geology*, vol. 21 (December 1993), p. 1147-49.

36 Compositional characteristics of Middle-to-Upper Tertiary volcanic rocks of the Bolivian Altiplano.
Edward A. du Bray, Steve Ludington, William E. Brooks, Bruce M.
Gamble, James C. Ratté, Donald H. Richter, Eduardo Soría-Escalante.
Washington, DC: US Government Printing Office, 1995. 30p. maps.
bibliog. (US Geological Survey Bulletin, No. 2119).

The US Geological Survey and the Servicio Geológico de Bolivia conducted a joint mineral resource assessment of the altiplano and the Cordillera Occidental in southwest Bolivia during 1990-91. This region forms part of the Pacific's continental volcanic arc, whose origin is related to the subduction (underthrusting) of the Nazca Plate beneath the western edge of the South American Continental Plate. The team examined Middle-to-Upper Tertiary lava flows, hypabyssal flow domes, and ash-flow tuffs, obtaining major oxide and trace element data which are presented here. The discussion of the geochemistry and petrography is accompanied by the team's conclusions on both the altered and unaltered rocks. This is a detailed and well-organized monograph, which also draws in earlier research.

Palaeoclimatology: ice cores and climate change

Ice cores

37 Pre-Incan agricultural activity recorded in dust layers in two tropical ice cores.
L. G. Thompson, M. E. Davies, E. Mosley-Thompson, K-b Liu.
Nature, vol. 336 (22-29 December 1988), p. 763-65. map. bibliog.

The authors record and interpret their research findings, based on ice cores obtained from the Quelccaya ice cap in the Lake Titicaca region of southern Peru. Among the cores' other contents, Thompson's party discerned two unusually intense dust episodes before AD 1000, each lasting about 130 years, the first c. AD 490-AD 620, the second c. AD 830-AD 960. Although volcanic activity was a secondary source of dust, the primary source appears to have been periods of prolonged drought, when lower water levels in Lake Titicaca exposed sediments on the lake floor. Dust blow may also have been aggravated by local agricultural activity and over-grazing, leading the team to suggest that 'the dust peaks from before AD 1000 probably reflect a combination of agricultural and grazing activity, and climatic change'. The peak period of Tiwanaku raised-field construction and maintenance occurred mainly between AD 400 and AD 900, with most of the fields abandoned by AD 1100. The Quelccaya ice cores also revealed the onset of more prolonged severe drought conditions after AD 1000, which intensified between c. AD 1245-AD 1300. The series of ice core studies on the Quelccaya icecap carried out by Thompson *et al.* have had an important influence on archaeological interpretations of pre-Incan history.

38 Hot air, big chill.
Philip Newton. *Nature*, vol. 387 (26 June 1997), p. 854.

Describes the ingenious method originally devised to solve the problem of transporting the ice cores from the Sajama glacier down through the warmer air at lower tropical elevations without melting. Indeed, temperatures of less than -15°C were to be maintained in order to preserve the tiny air bubbles trapped within the ice. To meet this challenge, sections of a hot-air balloon were backpacked up the mountain by the research team and assembled at the summit, from where the cores would be flown down to the base camp freezers and then on to the United States. [In the event, exceptionally high winds around the summit prevented the use of the hot-air balloon and the cores had to be carried down to base camp, an arduous journey lasting six hours. Even so, the temperatures of some of the cores went no higher than -10°C, and valuable data were obtained.]

39 Ice cores.
Kimbra Cutlip. *Weatherwise*, vol. 50 (October-November 1997), p. 10.

Reports the US-based research project into climate variation over the last 20,000 years which involves drilling ice cores through the glacier covering the summit of Mount Sajama, part of the great western chain of the Andes southwest of La Paz. At more than

6,500 metres (over 21,000 feet), these ice cores are significant as the highest ever recovered; as such, they can provide unique evidence concerning earlier atmospheric conditions and climate based on trapped gases, pollen, and dust particles within the ice. See also J. O. Childress, 'Coring a tropical glacier' (*Geotimes*, vol. 42 [October 1997], p. 6-7).

40   Thompson's ice corps.
Mark Bowen.   *Natural History*, vol. 107 (February 1998), p. 28-41. map.

This is a fascinating, well-illustrated report on the expedition to the Mount Sajama glacier, led by palaeoclimatologist Lonnie Thompson, which concentrates on the detailed planning and the extremely difficult working conditions involved. Using the team's experience in Bolivia, Thompson moved on to Tibet to obtain ice cores at a height of over 7,100 metres (23,500 feet), thus breaking the record for the highest samples ever recovered that he had only just set at Sajama.

41   A 25,000-year tropical climate history from Bolivian ice cores.
L. G. Thompson, M. E. Davies, E. Mosley-Thompson, T. A. Sowers, K. A. Henderson, V. S. Zagorodnov, P.-N. Lin, V. N. Mikhalenko, R. K. Campen, J. F. Bolzan, J. Cole-Dai, B. Francou.   *Science*, vol. 282 (4 December 1998), p. 1858-64. map. bibliog.

This important paper analyses the cumulative evidence provided by ice cores drilled in the Central Andes during the 1980s and 1990s by teams led by Lonnie Thompson. Cores from the Quelccaya ice cap (5,670 metres), the Huascarán col ice cap (6,048 metres), and the Sajama ice cap (6,542 metres/21,463 feet) have enabled Thompson *et al.* to present an ice-core record from Bolivia, based on ^{14}C dating, that now extends the tropical palaeoclimate history from the Late Glacial Maximum, through deglaciation and the whole of the Holocene period. The cores contain insects, insect and bark fragments, and an abundance of plant material; the cores also allow the team to reconstruct accumulation rates on Sajama and Huascarán as moisture swept in from the Amazon basin. At times during the Late Glacial Stage, much of the altiplano was covered with large palaeolakes which retreated during the warmer, drier Holocene period. Indeed, the waxing and waning of these palaeolakes becomes a dominant feature of the altiplano's climate history. The team's procedures and conclusions are well set out. They are also placed in the context of other interdisciplinary findings and present a stimulating study of value to all scholars researching palaeoclimatology in general, and the climate history of the Central Andes in particular.

Other evidence of climate change

42 **Century-scale shifts in the precipitation–evaporation balance of
the Bolivian Andes as identified from lake records.**
M. B. Abbott, G. O. Seltzer, A. P. Wolfe. *Eos* (American
Geophysical Union), vol. 77, no. 46, Suppl. fall meeting (1996),
p. 117.

Core analysis is extended here from Lake Titicaca to include Lake Taypi Chaka Kkota (on
the western slopes of the Cordillera Real), and Lake Viscachani (on the eastern slopes of
the Cordillera Real). Between them, a nearly complete history of environmental change
in the Holocene period is represented. The analysis includes investigation into the
lithology, sediment geochemistry, smear-slide mineralogy, magnetic properties, and
diatom content of the cores, and again indicates that the altiplano was significantly drier
during the mid-Holocene, with the lake-level changes relatively abrupt.

43 **High-resolution seismic reflection records from Lake Titicaca,
Peru/Bolivia.**
Geoffrey O. Seltzer, Scott L. Cross, David Mucciarone, Paul A.
Baker, Sherilyn C. Fritz, Robert B. Dunbar. *Eos* (American
Geophysical Union), vol. 77, no. 46, Suppl. fall meeting (1996),
p. 30.

The authors present the first high-resolution seismic reflection profiles from Lake
Titicaca which suggest that the lake was considerably lower in the geologically recent
past. The information obtained includes the lake's erosional record, pelagic
sedimentation, and incised channels extending to depths of 85 metres (nearly 280 feet)
below the modern lake level in the deltas of the in-flowing rivers. Earlier analysis of
sediment cores from Lake Titicaca indicates that the low level of the lake associated with
these erosional features began either in Late Glacial or Early Holocene times. The lowest
lake level recorded is dated in the mid-Holocene during warmer, drier conditions lasting
at least several thousand years. These findings, although prepared for the specialist, also
afford the general reader another good example of the wide range of disciplinary, and
interdisciplinary, work that is gradually uncovering the past in the Lake Titicaca region.
See also G. O. Seltzer, P. A. Baker, S. L. Cross, R. Dunbar, S. C. Fritz, 'High resolution
seismic reflection profiles from Lake Titicaca, Peru-Bolivia; evidence for Holocene
aridity in the tropical Andes' (*Geology*, vol. 26, no. 2 [1998], p. 167-70. map. bibliog.).

44 **Holocene paleohydrology of Lake Titicaca.**
Scott L. Cross, Paul A. Baker, Geoffrey O. Seltzer, Sherilyn C. Fritz,
Robert B. Dunbar. *Eos* (American Geophysical Union), vol. 77,
no. 46, Suppl. fall meeting (1996), p. 30.

Piston cores taken from Lake Titicaca show strong evidence of substantially lower lake
levels in the early to mid-Holocene period, indeed as much as 100 metres lower, a level
tentatively dated at about 3600 ^{14}C BP. The magnitude of this lake-level drop is much
greater than previously suggested, and is based on the authors' delimitation of old lake
shorelines from the relative contributions of littoral versus pelagic organisms in the cores.
Lake levels are related to the westward movement of moisture from the Amazon basin,

and the authors contend that lake-level changes recorded in the lake's sediments have palaeoclimatic implications that extend well beyond Lake Titicaca's watershed.

45 Annual and daily meteorological cycles at high altitude on a tropical mountain.
Douglas R. Hardy, Mathias Vuille, Carsten Braun, Frank Keimig, Raymond S. Bradley. *Bulletin of the American Meteorological Society*, vol. 79, no. 9 (1998), p. 1899-1913. bibliog.

An automated weather station was installed in October 1996 at the summit of Mount Sajama. This paper analyses the first annual cycle measurement and day-to-day variability that have been recorded, including pressure, incoming solar radiation, air temperature, humidity, wind, and snow accumulation. Already there is evidence that snowfall events and periods of evaporation are more episodic that previously believed. Results over time will make a valuable contribution to current research into the dramatic changes in climate, and in the hydrological cycle, that are occurring at high altitudes in the tropics, as well as being of value in ice-core analysis. The article is clear and well organized, describing in detail the preparation, design, and operation of the new Sajama weather station, and presenting material of interest to a wide range of professional meteorologists.

46 Climate and lake-level history of the northern Altiplano, Bolivia, as recorded in Holocene sediments of the Río Desaguadero.
Pattie C. Baucom, Catherine A. Rigsby. *Journal of Sedimentary Research*, vol. 69, no. 3 (1999), p. 597-611. maps. bibliog.

Another important piece in the jigsaw of reconstructing the palaeoclimatic history of the altiplano, this time through detailed investigation of the strata exposed in the Desaguadero's banks and river terraces. The depth, composition, and particle size of the gravel, sand, and mud deposits are found to correlate closely in the north with both the seasonal and longer-term water-level fluctuations of Lake Titicaca during the Holocene period, while farther south they are linked to base-level changes and sediment input from the Río Mauri. The paper will be of value to regional palaeoclimatologists; it is clearly developed and well supported with annotated photographs.

Geomorphology

47 Glacial history and climate change in the Peruvian-Bolivian Andes.
Geoffrey Owen Seltzer. PhD thesis, University of Minnesota, Minneapolis, Minnesota, 1991. 202p. bibliog.

The Late Pleistocene glacial maximum in Peru and Bolivia was followed by periods of retreat, stillstand, readvance, and further retreat well into the Late Holocene period, with associated climatic changes. This glacial history of the central Andes is based, among other evidence, on radio-carbon dating of ancient lake sediments and peat on the altiplano.

48 Snowline altitude and climate in the Central Andes (5°S-28°S) at present and during the Late Pleistocene glacial maximum. (Peru, Bolivia, Chile, Argentina.)
Andrew Norman Fox.   PhD thesis, Cornell University, Ithaca, New York, 1993. 527p. bibliog.

A comparative investigation into snowline altitude in the Central Andes in Late Pleistocene and modern times. The methods and findings of the research are clearly presented in detail. Both the present and the lowest Late Pleistocene snowlines rise from east to west, indicating that moisture at both times was derived principally from tropical easterly winds.

49 Modern and Late Pleistocene glacial studies in the central Andes of Peru and Bolivia: application of satellite remote sensing and digital terrain analysis.
Andrew George Klein.   PhD thesis, Cornell University, Ithaca, New York, 1997. 204p. bibliog.

This is an investigation into short-term and long-term climate changes that have occurred in the Central Andes. Satellite remote sensing was used to map the current extent of glaciers (now rapidly retreating) and snow cover, as well as the maximum extent of Late Pleistocene glaciation by plotting the position of moraines. Among other findings, reconstruction suggested that the Late Pleistocene snowline was 500 to over 1,200 metres lower than today.

50 A multivariate analysis of clast displacement rates on stone-banked sheets, Cordillera Real, Bolivia.
Bernard Francou, Pascal Bertran.   *Permafrost and Periglacial Processes*, vol. 8, no. 4 (1997), p. 371-82. bibliog.

Clast is clutter – individual rock fragments and other material produced by mechanical or chemical disintegration of a larger rock mass. In periglacial environments, the slipping and sliding movements promoted by regular freeze–thaw produce stone pavements, stone banks, and scree such as those found at the ski resort of Chacaltaya in the Cordillera Real. The authors record the results of investigations made over five years at this site, where clast movement is relatively rapid. Geomorphologists will find the comparative study made between tropical and alpine periglaciation a useful one.

51 Erosion rates on the northeast escarpment of the Eastern Cordillera, Bolivia derived from aerial photographs and thematic mapper images.
Troy Alexander Blodgett.   PhD thesis, Cornell University, Ithaca, New York, 1998. 149p. bibliog.

A geomorphological study centred on the eastern slope of Bolivia's Cordillera Real which plots and measures visible landslide scars along the steep slopes just below the treeline, using aerial photographs and Landsat Thematic Mapper images. From this information, supplemented by field surveys, erosion rates over the previous 10-35 years are estimated at selected sites.

52   Glaciers in South America.
G. Casassa, L. E. Espizua, B. Francou, P. Ribstein, A. Ames.
In: *Into the second century of worldwide glacier monitoring: prospects and strategies.*   Paris: UNESCO, 1998, p. 125-46. maps. bibliog. (Studies and Reports in Hydrology, no. 56).

A strong, scholarly contribution to the global study of glaciers, which surveys the large number of mountain glaciers throughout the Andes before concentrating on those in Argentina, Bolivia, Chile, and Peru. The glacierized area of South America at the start of the 21st century is estimated to be about 26,000 sq. km (10,000 sq. miles), the bulk of it in the Patagonian Ice Fields and Tierra del Fuego. Farther north, the glaciers form a distinctive and important group, i.e. mountain glaciers which exist under tropical climatic conditions. Indeed, those in the Central Andes represent more than 95 per cent of the surface area of all glaciers found in the tropics. The Cordillera Real in Bolivia has been part of a continuous programme of glacial monitoring and hydrology since 1991, and records are presented here in meticulous detail, including the patterns of local glacial advance and retreat in the Andes during the 19th and 20th centuries. Two significant general points are also emphasized: (1) Recent studies (including those by L. Thompson *et al.*) suggest that the effects of global warming could be more pronounced in the short term for tropical glaciers like these than for glaciers in medium and high latitudes; and (2) Tropical glaciers are excellent indicators of short-term climatic variations, including those resulting from El Niño phenomena, and they are well suited, following the first point, as indicators in the current research on global warming. This authoritative study is essential reading for specialists in this field.

53   Characterisation of river bed and suspended sediments in the Río Madeira drainage basin (Bolivian Amazonia).
Jean-Loup Guyot, Jean Marie Jouanneau, Jean Gabriel Wasson.
Journal of South American Earth Sciences, vol. 12, no. 4 (1999), p. 401-10. maps. bibliog.

Reports the findings of research into the gradation of river-bed and suspended sediments which occurs between the Andean and the plains section of the Beni and the Mamoré, notably the abrupt transition in gradation at the junction of the mountain front and the Llanos de Mojos. Attention is also given to the differing patterns of sedimentation found within the vast floodplains of the Beni and Mamoré rivers, which unite in northern Bolivia to form the source of the Madeira, the greatest southern tributary of the Amazon.

54   NASA pictures of Earth: Parapetí River fan, southern Bolivia.
Justin Wilkinson, Kamlesh Lulla, Mike Slattery.   *Geography Review*, vol. 12, no. 5 (1999), p. 26-27.

An interesting geomorphological case-study of alluvial deposition at the mountain–plains junction in the Department of Santa Cruz. The River Parapetí rises in the Andes and spills on to the surface of the Chaco, where it has laid down a large, almost horizontal fan of river sediments. The article presents, with diagrammatic analysis, pictures taken by NASA which show the present morphology of the fan, the ancient courses of the River Parapetí, and the effects of wind on dune patterns in the area.

Maps, atlases, and gazetteers

Maps

55 Bolivia: topographical maps.

La Paz: Instituto Geográfico Militar.

Sheets on the scales of 1:50,000 and 1:250,000 provide the two basic topographical map sets of Bolivia. The 1:50,000 series includes contours at 20-metre intervals, the 1:250,000 series at 100-metre intervals. Both also plot spot heights, and employ colour tints and symbols to record settlement, landmarks, road categories, railways, airports, and river systems. Details of the vegetation-cover differentiate cultivated areas, forest types, grassland, scrub, flood zones, and swamp. The 1:250,000 sheets also include the key and glossary of terms in English, among other languages. Both sets are distinguished by a high standard of cartography and of aesthetic design.

56 Mapa geológico de Bolivia. (Geological map of Bolivia.)

La Paz: Yacimientos Petrolíferos Fiscales Bolivianos y Servicio Geológico de Bolivia, 1978.

This early, but still serviceable, geological map is on four sheets on a scale of 1:1,000,000. A 27-page text accompanies the map, together with a bibliography.

57 Mapas campesinos en Bolivia. (Bolivian rural maps.)

Nadia Carnero Albarrán.   Lima: Universidad Nacional Mayor de San Marcos, Dirreción de Proyección Social, Seminario de Historia Rural Andina, 1980. 57 leaves.

Property maps of the Chaquí region, Department of Potosí.

58 Bolivia: mapa geológico del área del Proyecto Precambrio (1976-1983). (Geological map of the study area of the Precambrian Project in Bolivia, 1976-83.)

Santa Cruz de la Sierra: Servicio Geológico Británico, Servicio Geológico de Bolivia, 1984.

On a scale of 1:1,000,000, this is the Project's summarizing map, one of many produced by the team of geologists investigating a zone along the edge of the ancient Precambrian Brazilian Shield in eastern Bolivia with the aim of locating new commercially exploitable mineral resources in the area. The findings were to prove extremely promising, initially with regard to gold, silver, copper, and polymetallics. Indeed, by the late 1990s, over forty foreign companies were working in this new, non-traditional mining region of Bolivia.

59 Mapa de communicaciones de la República de Bolivia.
(Communications map of Bolivia.)
La Paz: Instituto Geográfico Militar, Departamento Cartográfico,
1990.

Comprises one map, in colour, on a scale of 1:3,000,000. This is a most useful and
comprehensive sheet which shows roads, railways, waterways, airports and airstrips, as
well as river and lake ports. In addition, the map locates radio and telegraph stations, and
petrol service points. Distance charts also give the distances by road and by river between
the main centres of population.

60 Mapa hidrográfico de Bolivia. (Hydrological map of Bolivia.)
La Paz: Instituto Geográfico Militar, Departamento de Geografía y
Recursos Naturales in collaboration with the Servicio Geodésico
Interamericano, 1990. 2nd ed.

Consists of one map of Bolivia, on nine sheets, on a scale of 1:1,000,000. This detailed
record of Bolivia's lakes and waterways also includes coloured pictures of river scenes,
and of river and lake transport, around the margins of each sheet.

61 Fauna silvestre de Bolivia. (Forest animals of Bolivia.)
La Paz: Instituto Geográfico Militar, Departamento de Geografía y
Recursos Naturales; Centro de Datos para la Conservación in
collaboration with the Servicio Geodésico Interamericano, 1991.

Comprises one map on two sheets on a scale of 1:1,500,000. Both sheets contain
distribution patterns and illustrations of the forest fauna in colour. The map is
accompanied by an informative 98-page booklet of notes on the animals, as well as a
glossary and bibliography.

62 Mapa de provincias fisiográficas de Bolivia. (Map of the
physiographic provinces of Bolivia.)
La Paz: Instituto Federal de Geociencias y Recursos Naturales, y
Servicio Geológico de Bolivia, 1994.

This map of Bolivia's physical features, particularly its regional landforms, is on four
sheets on a scale of 1:1,000,000, plus a fifth summary sheet on a scale of 1:2,500,000. Its
detailed landscape analysis, in colour, provides a most valuable source of reference for
geomorphologists, geologists and geographers. The relief shown on the summary sheet is
produced by satellite imagery, while a 75-page explanatory text accompanies the set.

Atlases

63 Latin American history: a teaching atlas.
Edited by Cathryn L. Lombardi, John V. Lombardi, K. Lynn Stoner.
Madison, Wisconsin: University of Wisconsin Press, 1983.

A sound reference tool which comprises 104 pages of maps and a 40-page index.
Although basically a history atlas, the contents extend into other fields also and include

Latin America's physical environment, the Iberian background, the Amerindian background, discovery and conquest, colonial governments, national boundary changes, resources, and (up to the late 1970s) trade, population, and the economy. The maps are well drawn and well annotated.

64   Atlas de los ayllus de Chayanta. (Atlas of the *ayllus* [indigenous rural communities] of Chayanta.)
Fernando Mendoza, Willer Flores, Catherine Letourneux.   Potosí: Programa de Autodesarrollo Campesino, 1994. 61p.
This is the first volume in an ambitious geographical and anthropological study. After mapping the *ayllus* in the Department of Potosí, special attention is given to those in Chayanta province. Using maps, text, and illustrations, some of them in colour, the authors record landscape features, transport, and the local economy, as well as community organization, ceremony and ritual. This is an atlas that provides a unique glimpse of the lives and livelihoods of Chayanta's peasant population.

65   Bolivia: atlas y geografía. (Atlas and geography of Bolivia.)
Mario Murillo P., Ahmed Restrepo Enciso.   La Paz: Transcontinental de Ediciones, 1995. 175p.
A volume that skilfully combines maps and text to produce a well-balanced geography of Bolivia. The authors provide comprehensive coverage of the country's physical and human aspects, with liberal use of colour in the maps and illustrations. The geographical analysis also includes a study of the characteristic features of each of Bolivia's nine departments.

66   Atlas de Bolivia. (Atlas of Bolivia.)
La Paz: Instituto Geográfico Militar, 1997. 2nd ed. 272p.
This national atlas of Bolivia maintains a consistently high standard and provides an excellent source of reference. It contains large, clear maps showing relief, landforms, climate, geology, soils, vegetation, natural resources, history, political divisions, and transport, as well as the country's population distribution, composition, and language. Colonization zones and patterns of internal migration are also well shown. Colour is effectively used throughout, in the maps and in the numerous pictures and diagrams.

67   Bolivia: un mundo de potencialidades. Atlas estadístico de municipios. (Bolivia: a world of potential opportunities. A statistical atlas of the municipalities.)
La Paz: Centro de Información para Desarrollo/CID; Ministerio de Participación Popular y Fortalecimiento Municipal; Instituto Nacional de Estadística, 1999. 485p.
This latest official atlas of Bolivia provides a detailed record of the country's new 314 municipalities which have become the framework for Bolivia's decentralizing, Popular Participation legislation of the mid-1990s. In addition to the introductory maps in colour of Bolivia's physical and human geography, its resources, municipality boundaries, poverty incidence, indigenous territories and protected areas, there are also preliminary maps on soil erosion and desertification. Then follow analyses of each department by province and municipality, including population, health, education, and other socio-

19

economic data, with accompanying text. This excellent, well-produced atlas is a key reference for administrators, and a valuable new source of information for researchers.

Gazetteers

68 Gazetteer of Bolivia. Names approved by the United States Board on Geographic Names.
Washington, DC: Defense Mapping Agency, 1992. 2nd ed. 719p. maps.

An indispensable source of reference that contains a total of 24,900 places and features in Bolivia. The entries include approved standard names, unapproved variant names, and unverified names. In fact, 33,300 names are listed to include these alternative names or spellings. Information is organized by name, designation (e.g. town, station, lake, etc.), latitude and longitude, administrative division, and location reference. This volume remains in a class of its own. Among general gazetteers, the best and most detailed is *The Columbia Gazetteer of the World*, edited by Saul B. Cohen (New York; Chichester, England: Columbia University Press, 1998. 3 vols.).

Geology

Palaeontology: plant and animal fossils

69 Fossils flesh out early vertebrates.
B. Bower. *Science News*, vol. 133, no. 2 (January 1988), p. 21.
Reports an exciting discovery made at the beginning of January 1988 of a collection of the oldest known vertebrates, the remarkably preserved remains of thirty jawless fish in the mountains of southern Bolivia. An international team of palaeontologists found the fossils embedded in large stone slabs dating to about 470 million years ago, with at least ten of the specimens virtually complete. These primitive fish appear to represent a new genus, named by the team *Sacabambaspis*, and thus extend the history of the vertebrates much farther back in time.

70 A new carnivorous marsupial from the Palaeocene of Bolivia and the problem of marsupial monophyly.
Christian de Muizon. *Nature*, vol. 370 (21 July 1994), p. 208-11. bibliog.
In a specialized report, the author discusses his discovery of new marsupial fossils in Bolivia and the problems they raise when attempting to confirm marsupials as a unique group within the class Mammalia.

71 A quantitative review of the horse *Equus* from South America.
José L. Prado, María T. Alberdi. *Palaeontology*, vol. 37, no. 2 (1994), p. 459-81. map. bibliog.
One of the decisive factors in the Spanish Conquest of the New World was the horse. So much drama is attached to the shock and fear experienced by the Indian population when they saw horses for the first time with the arrival of the *conquistadores*, that it is interesting to recall that the horse had once been widespread throughout the American continent. It became extinct in the New World and was reintroduced by Spain. This paper concentrates on the rich fossil record of *Equus* (*Amerihippus*) across South America dating from the Middle and Upper Pleistocene. All parts of the skeleton of all the species

can be found in various collections, including fossils that have been found in Bolivia near Tarija. The authors examine the varying adaptations by *Equus* both to open grasslands and to mountain habitats. The text is well illustrated and will be of particular interest to those engaged in comparative evolutionary studies of *Equus* on a global scale.

72 The first record of *Cooksonia* from South America in Silurian rocks of Bolivia.

E. Morel, D. Edwards, M. Iñigez Rodriguez. *Geological Magazine*, vol. 132, no. 4 (1995), p. 449-52. map. bibliog.

Large fossils of Silurian land plants are rare, and usually found in the northern hemisphere. Bolivia now provides fresh insights into land vegetation on the western edge of the largest early landmass, the palaeocontinent of Gondwana, in late Silurian times. The authors report their discovery of *Cooksonia*, initially near Tarija, the first record of a Silurian land plant in South America, and only the fourth Silurian record from Gondwana as a whole. Indeed, the team suggests that Bolivia may well contribute significant evidence in the future for learning more about the global pattern of land vegetation in the Silurian period.

73 Letters home from the bone camps: annals of a field museum paleontologist, Argentina and Bolivia, 1926-27; original letters and photos by Robert C. Thorne.

Robert Coin Thorne, edited by Robert Neil Thorne. Silver City, New Mexico: R. N. Thorne, 1995. 201p. maps.

An illuminating account of the life of a fossil-hunter in Argentina and Bolivia in the mid-1920s. It is based on the correspondence and photographs taken in the field by R. C. Thorne and edited by his son. Thorne Snr was a palaeontologist from Utah employed by the Field Museum of Natural History in Chicago to lead a fossil-collecting expedition to South America; the team returned with more than 300 specimens, many of them from Bolivia's Tarija and Padcaya regions. The letters and photographs record much more than camp life, and the huge difficulties of collecting and moving the specimens using primitive local transport, valuable though these descriptions are. Thorne's letters also contain vivid impressions of the countryside and the people, including life in some of the most remote towns and villages in northern Argentina and southern Bolivia.

74 *Pucadelphys andinus* (Marsupialia, Mammalia) from the early Paleocene of Bolivia.

Larry G. Marshall, Christian de Muizon, Denise Sigogneau-Russell. Paris: Editions du Muséum, 1995. 164p. bibliog. (Mémoires du Muséum National d'Histoire Naturelle, Vol. 165, Paléontologie).

A detailed report on *Pucadelphys andinus* specimens first discovered in 1982 in the early Palaeocene beds of the Santa Lucía Formation at Tiupampa, in the Mizque province of Cochabamba. This is one of the earliest complete dentition and skull assemblages of a metatherian mammal to be found, a rich and taxonomically diverse vertebrate fauna where the majority of the bones are still articulated, with little or no postmortem dismemberment – the result, it is thought, of flash floods which trapped the animals in their burrows. This is a substantial and scholarly monograph, with clear diagrams and photographs, and with an excellent reconstruction of the habits, locomotion and environment of these marsupials.

75 **The origin of the dog-like borhyaenoid marsupials of South America.**
Christian de Muizon, Richard L. Cifelli, Ricardo Céspedes Paz.
Nature, vol. 389 (2 October 1997), p. 486-89. map. bibliog.
This is an important paper for the specialist. Dog-like marsupials were the largest predatory mammals in South America during the Tertiary period. The authors report the discovery of exceptionally well-preserved skulls and skeletons in Bolivia which shed new light on the origins of these marsupials, since they are the oldest remains found to date in South America. The discussion includes the timing of the arrival of the higher mammals in South America, and the dispersal patterns between North and South throughout the American continent.

76 **Pleistocene horses from Tarija, Bolivia, and the validity of the genus *Onohippidium* (Mammalia: Equidae).**
Bruce J. MacFadden. *Journal of Vertebrate Paleontology* (Chicago), vol. 17, no. 1 (1997), p. 199-218. map. bibliog.
The rich Pleistocene mammalian fauna from Tarija contains abundant fossil horses. This detailed, well-illustrated paper by a leading scholar in the field traces the development and diversification of the horse in North America during the Late Miocene, prior to its dispersal into South America after the formation of the Panamanian Land Bridge, and the Great American Interchange which followed. MacFadden argues that the hippidiform horses *Hippidion* and *Onohippidium* are both valid genera. They shared a common ancestry with *Equus*, which arrived later in South America. All co-existed there during the Pleistocene period. The Tarija fossil horses are a crucial element in the evolutionary evidence; they contain either two or three genera, and between three and five valid species of horse in the local Pleistocene deposits – without doubt, a palaeontologist's El Dorado. See also the discussion between M. T. Alberdi, J. L. Prado, B. J. MacFadden, 'Pleistocene horses from Tarija, Bolivia, and the validity of the genus *Onohippidium*' (*Journal of Vertebrate Paleontology*, vol. 18, no. 3 [1998], p. 669-75).

77 **Toxodontia of Salla, Bolivia (late Oligocene): taxonomy, systematics, and functional morphology.**
Bruce J. Shockey. PhD thesis, University of Florida, Gainesville, Florida, 1997. 279p. bibliog.
The Salla fossil-bearing beds of Bolivia, which include a diverse sample of mammals, are of Late Oligocene age and provide a snapshot of life during the early period of mountain-building in the Andes. The author's research has identified four new species (two notohippids and two leontiniids) which are described here in detail. They provide evidence that the fauna of the Salla beds is more diverse, both in terms of species richness and morphological adaptation, than was previously known.

78 **Bolivia's Jurassic tracks.**
Mike Ceaser. *Américas*, vol. 51, no. 4 (1999), p. 3.
Palaeontologists are excited by the discovery of thousands of perfectly preserved dinosaur tracks in a quarry wall near Sucre, where an old lake floor, tipped vertically, provides an excellent display of what is the longest dinosaur trackway ever found. Detailed scientific

study by an international team is recent, but already an application to UNESCO for World Heritage Site status has been made.

Tectonics and stratigraphy

79 Granite petrogenesis in the Cordillera Real, Bolivia and crustal evolution in the central Andes.
J. F. Miller. PhD thesis, Open University, UK, 1988.

Two periods of granitoid intrusion have been identified in the geochronology of the Cordillera Real, the first in Carboniferous-to-Early Permian times, the second in Mid-Miocene, both of them periods of crustal thickening. This study examines and models the different characteristics of these granitoids, and considers their relationships to the Hercynian and the Andean mountain-building phases.

80 Late Oligocene-Early Miocene major tectonic crisis and related basins in Bolivia.
Thierry Sempere, Gerard Hérail, Jaime Oller, Michel G. Bonhomme. *Geology*, vol. 18 (October 1990), p. 946-49. maps. bibliog.

Basing their conclusions on recent advances in structural geology, biochronology, and basin analysis, the authors challenge existing tectonic interpretations on a point of dating, and argue that the first major Andean-type deformational episode in Bolivia was not in the Middle Eocene period (as defined in central Peru) but in Late Oligocene-Early Miocene times, which were highly active in Bolivia.

81 Lower bound on the amount of crustal shortening in the central Bolivian Andes.
Barbara Moths Sheffels. *Geology*, vol. 18 (September 1990), p. 812-15. maps. bibliog.

From her study area across the Cordillera Oriental and sub-Andean zone in central Bolivia, Sheffels examines the relative importance of two different factors in the formation of the Bolivian Andes. She concludes that, in this region, mountain-building is largely the result of a shortening of the earth's crust rather than the result of an addition of magmatic (molten rock) material, which here contributes at most no more than one-third to the thickening of the earth's crust. This is a concise, carefully argued paper, and recommended reading for any specialist in this field.

82 Cambridge Geological Project Bolivia, 11th July-26th September 1991.
Beatrice Gibbs, Stephen Thornley, Heather Green. Cambridge: The authors, December 1991. 29p. maps. bibliog.

A report on an undergraduate geological mapping expedition to the Ubina region of southern Bolivia. Of interest to others planning a similar project, the account includes information on financing, transport, and essential equipment as well as the environmental hazards and health problems experienced by the team.

83 Tectonics and geomorphology of the eastern flank of the Central Andes, 18° to 23° South latitude in Bolivia.
Timothy Louis Gubbels.   PhD thesis, Cornell University, Ithaca, New York, 1993. 224p. bibliog.

The Central Andes in Bolivia contain an old and extensive plateau known as the San Juan del Oro surface. Spectacular remnants of this composite surface are found throughout Bolivia's Eastern Cordillera between 18°S and 23°S. This study discusses the complex geological and tectonic processes involved in the formation of the San Juan del Oro high-level surface, and its subsequent dissection.

84 Composition and thickness of the southern Altiplano crust, Bolivia.
George Zandt, Aaron A. Velasco, Susan L. Beck.   *Geology*, vol. 22 (November 1994), p. 1003-06. maps. bibliog.

From fieldwork in 1993, the authors support models that explain the uplift of the Andes as predominantly the result of crustal shortening as opposed to magmatic addition. The construction of the Andes mountains is clearly associated with the subduction (underthrusting) of the Nazca Plate beneath western South America, and with specific reference to the altiplano, three models have already been proposed for its formation and uplift. Here, the authors present new estimates of the altiplano's crustal thickness and composition, and discuss the implications for the formation of this high plateau.

85 Upper Devonian and Carboniferous of the Altiplano of Bolivia: stratigraphy, sedimentology and paleogeographic evolution.
Enrique Diaz Martinez.   PhD thesis, University of Idaho, Moscow, Idaho, 1994. 221p. bibliog.

This study presents a palaeogeographic and palaeoclimatic chronology of the Upper Devonian and Carboniferous sedimentary rocks in the Bolivian Altiplano Basin, whose evolution during this geological period records important climatic changes that were related to the latitudinal shift of this part of the ancient landmass of Gondwana towards lower latitudes.

86 Geodynamics of the Central Andes.
J. Toth.   PhD thesis, University of Liverpool, England, 1995.

A study of subduction (underthrusting) dynamics, tectonic stress, mountain-building, and sedimentary basin formation in the Central Andes, including northern Chile, southern Bolivia, and northwest Argentina. These lie at a convergent plate boundary, and a numerical model is developed to analyse crustal shortening, crustal thickness, and foreland stratigraphy.

87 Cenozoic tectonics of the central Bolivian Andes.

L. J. G. Kennan.   DPhil thesis, University of Oxford, England, 1996.

The author investigates the complex geochronology of the Central Andes in the Cochabamba region of the Cordillera Oriental, including crustal shortening, patterns of folding, uplift, tear-faulting, magmatic addition, and erosion during the Cenozoic (Cainozoic) epoch; indeed, faulting around the Punata and Cochabamba Basins continued into Pleistocene times.

88 The problem of crustal thickening and the nature of Moho in the Central Andes.

Peter Giese.   *Eos* (American Geophysical Union), vol. 77, no. 46, Suppl. fall meeting (1996), p. 646-47.

Many problems related to mountain-building in the Andes remain unsolved. Giese reports the launching of a new research project at institutions in Berlin and Potsdam into the highly complex and anomalous structure of the Central Andes, where crustal thickening in the Eastern Cordillera reaches up to 80 km (50 miles). Crustal thickening in the Eastern Cordillera is thought to be explained by different processes from those in the western part of the altiplano, comprising overall an extremely complicated Andean convergence system involving a number of different Mohos (i.e. discontinuities that separate the Earth's crust from the subjacent mantle).

89 Interseismic strain accumulation on the northern Bolivian crustal ramp (Central Andes).

R. Ayala, J. P. Avouac, G. Wittlinger.   *Eos* (American Geophysical Union), vol. 78, no. 46, Suppl. fall meeting (1997), p. 451.

The intense microseismicity located in northern Bolivia tends to cluster beneath the mountain front of the Cordillera Real, and continues to attract major international research. The authors investigate seismic activity at a depth of 10-30 km (c. 6-19 miles), noting the accumulation of both stress and strain during the interseismic periods which is associated with the underthrust of the Brazilian Shield beneath the sub-Andean zone and the Eastern Cordillera.

90 Neogene shortening contribution to crustal thickening in the back arc of the Central Andes.

Patrice Baby, Philippe Rochat, Georges Mascle, Gérard Hérail.

Geology, vol. 25, no. 10 (1997), p. 883-86. map. bibliog.

Studies of the relationship between crustal shortening and crustal thickening in the Central Andes continue to focus on the great Andean orocline (elbow bend) in Bolivia. The authors examine the shortening–thickening tectonic processes that took place during the Neogene (i.e. the Miocene and Pliocene periods of the Tertiary era), and also discuss their relationship to the uplift of the altiplano. This is a concise, well-written paper of interest to both the specialist and the general reader, and is well supported with clear diagrams.

91   Origin of the high plateau in the Central Andes, Bolivia, South America.
Simon Lamb, Leonore Hoke.   *Tectonics*, vol. 16, no. 4 (1997), p. 623-49. maps. bibliog.

One of the major problems in structural geology is the origin of high plateaux within mountain chains. Here, the authors examine the altiplano and puna in Bolivia, a complex plateau system second only in the world, in height and size, to the plateau of Tibet. The study is divided into four parts: (1) The structure and stratigraphy of critical sections; (2) The geological evolution of this region within the wider context of the Cenozoic (Cainozoic) development of the Central Andes, which involved the separate development of the Western and Eastern Cordilleras; (3) The mechanisms of crustal thickening and surface uplift; and (4) The overall controlling processes which resulted in the creation of Bolivia's high plateau region of the altiplano and puna. This is a carefully prepared paper for the specialist, well supported with maps, diagrams, and cross-sections.

92   Seismic topography of the shallow mantle in the Bolivian Andes: tectonic implications.
Stephen C. Myers, Susan Beck, George Zandt, Terry Wallace.
Eos (American Geophysical Union), vol. 78, no. 46, Suppl. fall meeting (1997), p. 446.

In this interesting correlation of events, the authors contend that in their study area, volcanic activity in the Bolivian Andes during Tertiary times was confined to a relatively narrow band some 50 km (c. 30 miles) wide beneath the altiplano and the Eastern Cordillera. Given the dramatic crustal shortening that occurred in this section of the Bolivian Andes, they conclude that volcanic activity and seismic processes continued during the crustal shortening of the South American Plate, keeping open a window in the lithosphere mantle that would otherwise have been closed.

93   Climatic and tectonic implications of the late Miocene Jakokkota flora, Bolivian Altiplano.
Kathryn M. Gregory-Wodzicki, W. C. McIntosh, Kattia Velásquez.
Journal of South American Earth Sciences, vol. 11, no. 6 (1998), p. 533-60. maps. bibliog.

This is a significant application of palaeobotany to the history of mountain-building in the Central Andes. The authors examine Late Miocene fossil flora from the Jakokkota area, southwest of La Paz, and compare their findings with Potosí fossil flora from the Early to Mid-Miocene period. They find evidence that both groups of flora grew at estimated palaeo-elevations considerably lower than their present sites, even when the effects of latitudinal continental drift and global climate change are taken into account. This leads them to conclude that the complex uplift history revealed by the Jakokkota fossil flora of Late Miocene times reinforces the two-stage tectonic models that have been developed to explain the formation of the Andes.

94 **Heat-flow density across the Central Andean subduction zone.**
Michael Springer, Andrea Förster. *Tectonophysics*, vol. 291,
nos. 1-4 (1998), p. 123-39. maps. bibliog.

The authors present fresh insights into the Central Andes great ocean–continent collision zone. The underthrusting of the Nazca Plate beneath the advancing South American Plate is relatively fast in geological terms, while crustal thickening in the Eastern Cordillera is affected by the underplating of the Brazilian Shield. Complex crustal stacking in this region has been going on since Miocene (Tertiary) times. Springer and Förster set out their fieldwork methods in southern Peru, Bolivia, northern Chile and northwest Argentina, and present new and revised heat-flow density determinants for the Central Andes between 15°S-30°S and 60°W-75°W. This is a valuable addition to the specialist literature. The paper is clearly written and well supported with maps, diagrams, and statistics. It also correlates its findings with other research, and notes the uncertainties that remain.

95 **Space geodetic observations of Nazca–South America convergence across the Central Andes.**
Edmundo Norabueno, Lisa Leffler-Griffin, Ailin Mao, Timothy Dixon, Seth Stein, Selwyn Sacks, Leonidas Ocala, Michael Ellis. *Science*, vol. 279 (16 January 1998), p. 358-62. maps. bibliog.

The Andes mountains continue to build. The authors analyse the recorded rates and directions of motion across the convergent boundary zone between the oceanic Nazca Plate and the continental South American Plate in Bolivia and Peru, and conclude that the convergence is about 30-40 millimetres a year. About 10-15 millimetres a year of crustal shortening also occurs in the sub-Andean fold-and-thrust belt of the Eastern Cordillera region. They present estimates of the shortening, sliding and partial locking involved which can be released in future earthquakes. This is a succinct, informative article, well annotated and usefully linked to other research work in this field.

Mineralogy

96 **Precious-metals districts and resources of Bolivia.**
Bertrand Heuschmidt, Raúl Miranda M.   La Paz: Bolinvest, 1993.
127p. maps. bibliog.

An excellent synopsis of more than thirty precious-metals districts in Bolivia. The survey includes areas of the Precambrian Shield, the Eastern Cordillera Palaeozoic Belt, the altiplano and Western Cordillera Volcanic Belt, and the Northern Piedmont and floodplain basins. The text is well supported by a summary of Bolivia's geology, by clear geological maps in colour, and by a detailed index of additional deposits found at the study sites.

97 The Bolivian death switch.
Rock H. Currier. *The Mineralogical Record*, vol. 26, no. 3 (1995), p. 195-200.
Records a professional collector's trip to Bolivia to obtain mineral and crystal specimens, several of them beautifully photographed here in colour. Currier travels through the major Andean mining centres, sprinkling his tale with lively anecdotes and droll observation.

98 Influences of parent material and time on soil properties in a perudic area of the Bolivian Amazon basin.
Steven Eugene Monteith. PhD thesis, North Carolina State University, Raleigh, North Carolina, 1995. 169p. bibliog.
An analysis of the properties of alluvial soils found on the floodplains and river terraces in part of the Bolivian Amazon basin, with particular reference to their varying correlation with the rock minerals of their headwater regions.

99 Supergene mineralisation in gold-rich Bolivian polymetallic vein deposits.
K. E. Darke. PhD thesis, University of Aberdeen, Scotland, 1996.
An investigation into the geology of Bolivia's gold-rich vein deposits at four sites in the Cordilleras and the altiplano – Kori Kollo, Kiska, La Riviera, and Escala. Particular attention is given to the acidic, oxidizing conditions that favoured gold mobilization, and the mechanisms leading to its subsequent precipitation.

100 Gemstones and ornamental stones from Bolivia.
Jaroslav Hyrsl, Alfred Petrov. *Journal of Gemmology* (London), vol. 26, no. 1 (1998), p. 41-47. map. bibliog.
Notes the growing international awareness of Bolivia as a source of gemstones, including beryl, aquamarine, amethyst, ametrine, and chalcedony. The authors map the principal sources both in the Andes and in the Precambrian Shield, where mines are located in the eastern region of Santa Cruz Department. This is a concise, informative article, well illustrated in colour.

101 Tungsten-bearing rutile from the Kori Kollo gold mine, Bolivia.
C. M. Rice, K. E. Darke, J. W. Still, E. E. Lachowski.
Mineralogical Magazine, vol. 62, no. 3 (1998), p. 421-29. bibliog.
Tungsten (wolfram)-bearing rutile is a rare occurrence but it is well represented at Kori Kollo, Bolivia's largest gold mine. The authors' discussion of the nature and origin of this mineralization expands into a wider analysis of the Kori Kollo complex. Tungsten-bearing rutile is a relatively late hydrothermal event at Kori Kollo, and may be connected with the formation of the gold veins. The paper emphasizes the importance of accessory minerals in petrogenetic studies, and offers a useful case in point.

102 Chrome chalcedony: a review. Zimbabwe and Bolivia.
Jaroslav Hyrsl. *Journal of Gemmology* (London), vol. 26, no. 6 (1999), p. 364-70. bibliog.

With reference to Bolivia, the paper expands upon the recent discoveries and mining of chalcedony in eastern Bolivia, where the best stones are facetable and of gem quality. Most of the rough material is exported directly to Brazil. Detailed chemical analysis is provided, along with excellent photographs in colour.

103 Trace element geochemistry in the Upper Amazon drainage basin (Bolivia).
Françoise Elbaz-Poulichet, Patrick Seyler, Laurence Maurice-Bourgoin, Jean-Loup Guyot, Claude Dupuy. *Chemical Geology*, vol. 157, nos. 3-4 (1999), p. 319-34. map. bibliog.

A detailed investigation into the trace elements found in the dissolved and suspended material in the headwaters of the Mamoré and Beni rivers; they included barium, cadmium, copper, manganese, molybdenum, nickel, rubidium, strontium, uranium, and zinc. The Mamoré and Beni's highly turbid and turbulent headwaters flowing from the Andes provide a well-chosen location for the study of trace element transport, allowing the authors to discuss the varied geology of the two catchment areas, the differing patterns of chemical weathering, and the contribution of vegetation to the water chemistry. The team's sampling stations are clearly mapped, their methods and findings well recorded. This is an excellent case-study for the specialist.

Tourism and Travel Guides

104 South America: river trips.
George N. Bradt. Cambridge, Massachusetts; Chalfont St. Peter, Buckinghamshire, England: Bradt Enterprises, 1981. 103p. maps. bibliog.

A travel guide to boating and river trips in South America which is still of value as background reading because of its unique approach and organization of material for both the tourist and the naturalist.

105 New altitudes, old attitudes.
Heidi Hughes. *Travel Holiday*, vol. 169 (March 1988), p. 14, 18.

The author records with pleasure a visit to La Paz, with its churches, shops and street markets, and then describes her excursions to Moon Valley, Lake Titicaca, Chacaltaya ski resort, and Tiwanaku. Emphasis is on the astonishing contrasts to be found among the people and the landscapes in and around the city, but part of the appeal of this article is the way in which Hughes captures the wonder and excitement of seeing Bolivia for the first time.

106 Oh, linda La Paz! Oh, beautiful La Paz! Oh, schönes La Paz!
Oscar Eduardo Ruiz C. La Paz: Libreria Editorial 'Popular', 1990. 88p. map.

Ruiz gets his message across with a good written introduction to the city, and with his fine colour photographs of La Paz and its surroundings. There are striking shots of the Andes, condors, vicuñas, and other wildlife. This is La Paz for the tourist, and comes with appropriate helpful information on getting the best from a quiet exploration of the city and the magnificence around it. The text throughout is in Spanish, English and German.

107 Santa Cruz: la otra cara de Bolivia. (Santa Cruz: the other face of Bolivia.)
Willy Kenning.   Santa Cruz de la Sierra: Willy Kenning, 1991. 138p. maps.

This appealing study is probably the best book devoted entirely to the city and Department of Santa Cruz. With over 100 excellent colour illustrations by Kenning, some historic prints, and a text by Oscar Zambrano (in Spanish and English), the book includes many features not depicted elsewhere in the tourist literature. There are views of the city and its region, colonial and modern architecture, farms and ranches, El Palmar sand-dune country, Amboró National Park, rock-paintings, Jesuit missions, the remote Inca fort at Semaipata, and much more. Readers are drawn out of the city into the Chaco, the Valles, and across Chiquitania to the Otuquis swamps at the edge of the Pantanal on the River Paraguay, one of the largest freshwater wildlife refuges in the world. This is certainly a secret, very beautiful 'other face' of Bolivia.

108 The Titicaca tonic.
The Economist, vol. 320 (31 August 1991), p. 36.

Announces the opening in October 1991 of a hotel and health spa on Lake Titicaca, a development by the tour operator who already runs a hydrofoil service across the lake between Bolivia and Peru.

109 An insider's guide to Bolivia.
Edited by Peter McFarren.   La Paz: Fundación Cultural 'Quipus', 1992. 2nd ed. 412p. maps.

This well-illustrated volume, enhanced by the addition of several new chapters, concentrates on the strong links between 'Bolivia's cultural past and traditional present', the age-old customs and rituals that add such flavour and variety to the modern scene. There are lively entries on art, music, literature, cuisine, and many other aspects of life in the Andes. The book offers sparkling, often rare, gems of information for the tourist, although today it is best used as a back-up, rather than as an up-to-date guide to the country.

110 Bolivia, Peru.
Edited by Michael Shichor.   Tel Aviv: Inbal Travel Information, revised and updated 1993. 259p. maps.

This well-illustrated guide offers practical advice for tourists of all ages. It provides clear, concise entries on Bolivia's major cities and regions, details on short side-trips and longer excursions, and an outline of the country's history, geography, and economy.

111 Bolivia: a travel survival kit.
Deanna Swaney.   Hawthorn, Victoria, Australia: Lonely Planet Publications, 1996. 3rd ed. 488p. maps. bibliog.

A wholly inappropriate title for what is in fact a general guidebook to Bolivia, where the emphasis is neither on survival nor on roughing it. Detailed entries on the cities, regions, general background, and local information are designed to meet the needs and interests of a wide range of tourists, from those travelling first class to others having to make a little go a long way. The text is comprehensive, well written, and well illustrated.

112   Central and South America by road.

Pam Ascanio, Robb Annable.   Chalfont St. Peter, Buckinghamshire,
England: Bradt Publications; Old Saybrook, Connecticut: Globe
Pequot Press, 1996, 244p. maps.

A useful manual for those driving cars, trucks, recreational vehicles, motor-cycles and
mountain bikes. The section on Bolivia provides information on roads, road conditions,
camp sites, and points of entry, while a substantial general introduction offers practical
advice on the preparation and outfitting required for touring South America by road.

113   Culture shock! Bolivia.

Mark Cramer.   Portland, Oregon: Graphic Arts Center Publishing
Co., 1996. 244p. map.

This is not a systematic guidebook to the country but a personal view by a US journalist
based in Bolivia that offers, in his own words, a guide to customs and etiquette. The result
is a series of descriptions, conversations, and impressions on a wide range of Bolivian
events and personalities which provides light, back-up reading for the intending traveller.

114   Bolivia handbook.

Alan Murphy.   Bath, England: Footprint Handbooks; Chicago:
Passport Books, 1997. 367p. maps. bibliog. (2nd enlarged ed., 2000).

This handbook expands the information on Bolivia in the *South American Handbook*
(item no. 121), adding new material throughout and including extra maps and
illustrations. It is an excellent guide for those concentrating their travels in Bolivia, and
intending to spend considerable time there.

115   Riding the Che-chic route.

The Economist, vol. 345 (11 October 1997), p. 36.

Sensing that there is money to be squeezed from the Che Guevara episode, Bolivia has
launched the first 'Che Guevara Week' on the thirtieth anniversary of his death in 1967.
A new tourist trail has been organized through the jungles on the western edge of Santa
Cruz Department, including the town of Vallegrande, where Che's body was located in
1995. Che Guevara has become a cult figure in several foreign states, and the 'Che Route'
along his campaign trail of 1966-67 is now being promoted by Bolivia's tourist board and
several tour companies. The failed, dead revolutionary is big business, and local
inhabitants are ready to exploit what they regard as Che Guevara's only useful legacy to
this remote area of Bolivia.

116   South America.

Emily Hatchwell, Simon Calder, Adam Lechmere.   Oxford:
Vacation Work Publications, 1997. 2nd ed. 799p. maps. (Travellers
Survival Kit).

Tailored to those seeking cheap, comfortable accommodation, and good value for money
in other areas also, e.g. in transport, sightseeing, shopping, and so forth. The section on
Bolivia (p. 339-405) includes practical tips and succinct entries on the country's history,
geography, culture, major cities, Lake Titicaca and the altiplano, the Yungas, and on river
trips down the Beni and the Mamoré. The guidebook's layout is particularly clear and
well designed for rapid reference.

117   Trekking in Bolivia: a traveler's guide.
Yossi Brain, Andrew North, Isobel Stoddart.   Seattle, Washington:
The Mountaineers, 1997. 221p. maps. bibliog.

An authoritative guidebook full of ideas, information, and advice in concise form on
trekking in Bolivia. Twenty-three treks are included, twenty-two of them around Lake
Titicaca and in the Eastern Cordilleras, and one in the Amboró National Park, west of
Santa Cruz. After brief notes on the local geology and natural history, the guide provides
detailed recommendations on organization, clothing, equipment, personal security, and
health and safety.

118   Bolivia: a climbing guide.
Yossi Brain.   Seattle, Washington: The Mountaineers, 1999. 221p.
maps.

A superb mountaineering guidebook for specialists climbing in the high Andean
cordilleras of Bolivia. It provides information both on the major and the alternative routes
to thirty-seven peaks, accompanied by detailed maps and photographs, as well as advice
on sources of supplies, local transport, health, and safety. An interesting history of
mountaineering in Bolivia is also included, starting with the first ascent of Mount Illimani
in 1877, then the highest point reached anywhere in the world. This is a comprehensive,
indispensable climbing guide to the mountains of Bolivia, and the only one in the English
language.

119   Insight guide to South America.
Edited by Natalie Minnis, Huw Hennessy, Brian Bell.   Singapore:
APA Publications GmbH & Co./Verlag KG, 1999. 4th ed. 421p.
maps.

The sections on Bolivia (p. 173-93, 365-67) concentrate on the country's history and
culture – its customs, fiestas, churches and museums, particularly those on the altiplano
and in the Andean valleys. The Mamoré river region of the Beni is included, but no more
than a note on the city and Department of Santa Cruz. The text is lavishly illustrated by
excellent colour photographs which together succeed in capturing much of the spirit and
diversity of Bolivia and its people.

120   Peru and Bolivia: backpacking and trekking.
Hilary Bradt.   Chalfont St. Peter, Buckinghamshire, England: Bradt
Publications; Old Saybrook, Connecticut: Globe Pequot Press, 1999.
7th ed. 358p. maps. bibliog.

A splendid guidebook for backpackers, whether they seek gentle hiking or strenuous
trekking in some of the contrasted regions of central South America. The section on
Bolivia (p. 244-347) includes independent trips or, where advisable, guided tours lasting
anything from one to ten days in both the Andean and lowland areas, and comes with
information on routes of varying difficulty, timing, equipment, and points of interest. A
joint introduction to both Peru and Bolivia presents additional advice on preparation for
the trip before departure, as well as much general wisdom for walkers and nature lovers.

121 South American handbook 2000.

Edited by Ben Box. Bath, England: Footprint Handbooks; Chicago: Passport Books, 1999. 76th ed. 1648p. maps.

Published annually since 1924, this is the best known guidebook to South America, and remains unsurpassed in its detail and coverage of the region. The Bolivian section (p. 243-348) includes general background to the country, followed by practical information on cities, towns, transport, accommodation, dining, shopping, excursions, travel tips, and much more besides.

122 Adventure travellers South America.

Basingstoke, Hampshire, England: AA Publishing, 2000. 320p. maps. (AA World Travel Guides).

An imaginative publication written to encourage readers 'to plan your own adventure'. Twenty-five adventures in all are included, with the two on Bolivia presented by Simon Richmond. The first describes trekking and climbing in the Sorata region of the Cordillera Real, as well as the ascent of Mount Huayna Potosí, 6,088 metres (19,973 feet). The second involves hiking or mountain-biking in the Yungas, and rafting down the River Coroico ('not for the faint-hearted'). Throughout, the well-illustrated text offers sensible advice on planning and preparation, solo or group activity, equipment, accommodation, health, personal safety, and where necessary, essential previous experience. This is no wild, gung-ho approach to adventure. The guide lists useful contacts for cultural tours and conservation projects, as well as the best months for each trip. It will appeal to those who wish to make their entire journey a series of adventures in the different countries of South America, as well as to those who want to sample all or part of a particular adventure within a more broadly based trip. There is much here to fascinate travellers to Bolivia, but the volume is not a substitute for either a general or a mountaineering guidebook, nor is it intended to be.

123 Ecuador, Peru and Bolivia: the backpacker's manual.

Kathy Jarvis. Chalfont St. Peter, Buckinghamshire, England: Bradt Publications; Old Saybrook, Connecticut: Globe Pequot Press, 2000. 376p. maps.

A guide written specifically for first-time backpackers in the Central Andes. In addition to the necessary detail on the selected routes, the section on Bolivia (p. 295-368) includes basic, up-to-date advice on preparation, health, local transport, and reasonably priced accommodation, along with suggested detours to outstanding cultural sites not to be missed along the way.

124 Fodor's South America.

Edited by Melisse Gelula, Natasha Lesser, Laura M. Kidder, Holly S. Smith. New York: Fodor's Travel Publications, 2000. 4th ed. 653p. maps.

An attractive guidebook which focuses on the main essentials in concise, manageable form. After a general introduction to the country, the Bolivian section (p. 121-58) concentrates on the Andean region – La Paz and Lake Titicaca, Cochabamba, Potosí, and Sucre, with the addition of Santa Cruz. The text provides well-arranged information on the cities' main features and cultural centres, selected side-trips, shopping, dining and accommodation, and also includes the necessary practical travel advice.

125   South America on a shoestring.
Edited by James Lyon.   Hawthorn, Victoria, Australia: Lonely Planet Publications, 2000. 7th ed. 1120p. maps.

This popular guide is designed for those travelling on a tight budget but still determined to visit the major points of interest both on and off the beaten track, particularly the country's cultural treasures. The section on Bolivia (p. 223-305) is clear and well organized; it suggests ways of economizing wherever possible, lists only moderately priced accommodation, and conveys a lively sense of safe and adventurous travel throughout.

Travellers' Accounts

126 Travels from Buenos Ayres, by Potosí, to Lima.
Anthony Zachariah Helms. London: Richard Phillips, 1806, 1807.
292p. maps. (First published in Dresden, 1798.)

Helms was an experienced German mining engineer and metallurgist who, at the invitation of Spain, accompanied Baron von Nordenflicht, a Swedish mineralogist, on a mission in the 1790s to modernize Upper and Lower Peru's silver-mining and refining industry. Helms built a laboratory in Potosí's Royal Mint, gave lectures, and with a team of German miners demonstrated improved techniques of refining and flood control. He was an outspoken critic of the existing conditions: 'All the operations at the mines of Potosí, the stamping, sifting, wasting, quickening and roasting the ore are conducted in so slovenly, wasteful, and unscientific a matter.' Helms aroused much local hostility among the mine owners, who were as glad to see him go as he was to leave. For a more comprehensive account of the Nordenflicht mission, see Rose Marie Buechler, 'Technical aid to Upper Peru' (item no. 211); also *Report on Bolivia, 1827, by Joseph Barclay Pentland* (item no. 247).

127 Journey from Buenos Ayres, through the provinces of Córdova, Tucumán, and Salta, to Potosí, thence by the deserts of Caranja to Arica, and subsequently, to Santiago de Chili and Coquimbo, undertaken on behalf of the Chilian and Peruvian Mining Association, in the years 1825-1826.
Joseph Andrews. London: John Murray, 1827. 2 vols.

Volume 2 (321p.) contains a long and graphic account of Bolivia's Andean region in the immediate aftermath of the War for Independence. Andrews is an observant traveller and skilfully captures the local atmosphere of place and people. He records his meetings with Bolívar and General Sucre, and reports in detail on the state of the mines and the methods of mining at Potosí.

128 Travels in various parts of Peru, including a year's residence in Potosí.

Edmond Temple.   London: Henry Colburn, Richard Bentley, 1830.
2 vols; Philadelphia: E. L. Carey, A. Hart; Boston: Lilly, Wait, 1833.
2 vols. (Reprinted, New York: AMS Press, 1971).

Speculative ventures in South American mining by foreign investors grew rapidly after the wars of independence were over. Temple travelled from London in 1825-26 as secretary of the newly formed Potosí, La Paz, and Peruvian Mining Association but was shocked to discover the extent of the damage done to the mines during the revolutionary wars, and the widespread flooding of the workings. He provides valuable detail on the condition of the mines and the existing methods of mining and extraction. Not surprisingly, Temple recommended that the Association should be dissolved immediately. The volumes reflect a keen eye, and contain striking engravings.

129 Three years in the Pacific; including notices of Brazil, Chile, Bolivia, and Peru.

William Samuel Waithman Ruschenberger.   Philadelphia: Carey, Lea & Blanchard, 1834. 441p.

Among its other merits, this book provides the best description of Bolivia's Pacific port of Cobija in the early 1830s. Ruschenberger, a US Naval Surgeon, records the approach to the port, the appearance and layout of the town (population 600-700), its isolation in the Atacama desert, severe water shortage, and virtual total dependence on imported food and timber supplies. He also includes details of Cobija's trade, and an account of his visit to a local copper mine.

130 Exploration of the Valley of the Amazon.

Lardner Gibbon, USN.   Washington, DC: United States Senate, 1854, vol. 2. 339p. map.

This is one of the great classic accounts of 19th-century travel and exploration in Bolivia. Lieutenant Gibbon and his colleague, Lieutenant William Herndon, were among a small group of US naval officers commissioned by Congress in the early 1850s to explore large parts of South America, and to record both their existing condition and their estimated potential. Herndon and Gibbon were assigned the entire Amazon basin, with orders to report on: 'the navigability of its streams; the number and condition, both industrial and social, of its inhabitants, their trade and products; its climate, soil, and productions; also its capacities for cultivation, and the character and extent of its undeveloped commercial resources, whether of the field, the forest, the river, or the mine.' Gibbon was responsible for the Bolivian portion of the survey. He and his few assistants travelled widely over the altiplano, and through the cities and mining areas of the high Andes, before descending the Mamoré river to a point below the Madeira-Mamoré Falls. The lieutenant's meticulous eye for detail was happily matched by a polished and effective writing style, so that his report acquired that rare added distinction of becoming a highly readable book. Unlike Herndon, busily engaged farther north, Gibbon was also an accomplished artist, and his record includes thirty-six of his own finely lithographed sketches of the land, the rivers, and the local inhabitants encountered on his travels throughout Bolivia.

131 Explorations made in the valley of the River Madeira from 1749 to 1868.
George Earl Church.   London: The National Bolivian Navigation Company, 1875. 355p.

Colonel Church, a Massachusetts railway engineer and American Civil War veteran, was recruited by the Bolivian government in the late 1860s (immediately after Brazil had opened the Amazon and its tributaries as an international waterway) to assess the feasibility of a navigable outlet for Bolivia via the Mamoré, Madeira and Amazon rivers to the Atlantic. It became an enterprise he was to pursue with fanatical zeal. To widen knowledge of this isolated interior, Church published an account of his own exploration, together with this collection of seven earlier expeditions to the region, on behalf of the National Bolivian Navigation Company, a newly formed Bolivian enterprise with Church as its London agent.

132 The route to Bolivia via the River Amazon. A report to the governments of Bolivia and Brazil.
George Earl Church.   London: Waterlow & Sons, 1877. 216p. maps.

Church's official report presented an optimistic picture of the river route destined to link Bolivia to the Atlantic, calculating that it would reduce the journey of 180 days to the northern markets via Cape Horn to 30 days, and cut freight charges to one-quarter of existing rates. The only obstacles to navigation, it was argued, were the Madeira-Mamoré Falls, and these could be bypassed by a railway. But the attempt to construct the railway at this stage failed completely, with Church having underestimated the enormous problems involved. His conviction, however, that navigable waterways held the key to stimulating the development of the South American interior should be placed in the context of the United States official mid-19th century 'waterway school' of development, a continental strategy originally based on the Mississippi system and extended by the US planners of the period to the Amazon and Paraguay-Paraná rivers also. See also J. V. Fifer, *United States perceptions of Latin America, 1850-1930* (Manchester, England: Manchester University Press; New York: St Martin's Press, 1991. 203p. maps. bibliog.).

133 Up the Amazon and Madeira Rivers, through Bolivia and Peru.
Edward Davis Mathews.   London: S. Low, Marston, Searle & Rivington, 1879. 402p. map.

Mathews had been employed in the early 1870s as the resident engineer on George Earl Church's disastrous venture to build the Madeira-Mamoré Railway. This volume provides an excellent account of Mathews's subsequent journey up the Amazon, Madeira and Mamoré rivers and into the Andes, including his impressions of Trinidad, Cochabamba, Sucre, Potosí, and Oruro. His readable style and forthright comment offer insights into life along the rivers, as well as on transport in the mountains, politics, commerce, and the general state of the country's economy. This is the most comprehensive travel report on Bolivia at this period.

134 Bolivia: sept années d'explorations, de voyages, et de séjours dans l'Amérique Australe. (Bolivia: seven years of exploration, travel, and residence in South America.)
André Bresson. Paris: Challemel Ainé, 1886. 639p. maps.

Bresson was the French Consul in Bolivia for seven years during the 1870s-1880s and his book provides a lucid, first-hand account of the country at this period, including descriptions of the major towns, and of Bolivia's desert ports of Cobija and Mejillones in the Litoral Department before the War of the Pacific. The book is well illustrated with engravings, and filled with evidence of Bresson's energy and enthusiasm for travel, and for gaining a better understanding of the land and its people.

135 Papers from the notes of an engineer.
Frederick Gleason Corning. New York: Scientific Publishing, 1889. 103p. maps.

This concise report on the Lake Titicaca region and the Tipuani gold deposits is well illustrated with sketches, soil profiles and geological sections, along with Corning's general impressions of Bolivia.

136 The Bolivian Andes; a record of climbing and exploration in the Cordillera Real in the years 1898 and 1900.
Sir (William) Martin Conway. London; New York: Harper Brothers, 1901. 403p. maps. bibliog.

A fascinating account of mountaineering in Bolivia, including Conway's ascent of Mount Illimani, and his near-ascent of Mount Illampú, better known then as Mount Sorata. The book is much more than this, however. Conway was a prolific writer with a readable style, and his record includes numerous photographs and useful observations on mining, the rubber industry, transport, and the region around La Paz.

137 Recollections of an ill-fated expedition to the headwaters of the Madeira River in Brazil.
Neville B. Craig. Philadelphia: J. B. Lippincott, 1907. 479p. maps.

After George Earl Church's failure in the early 1870s, the firm of Philip and Thomas Collins in Philadelphia undertook the commission to build the Madeira-Mamoré Railway. Craig was one of the company's engineers, and later he wrote this vivid account of the proposed terminus at San Antonio, the rivers and jungle surroundings, and the deplorable conditions suffered throughout by the workforce. Only just over two miles of 'permanent' track were laid before the company withdrew in 1878-79, beaten by death, sickness, lack of food, and exhausted funds.

138 A search for the apex of America. High mountain climbing in Peru and Bolivia, including the conquest of Huascarán, with some observations on the country and the people below.
Annie Smith Peck. New York: Dodd, Mead, 1911; London: T. Fisher Unwin, 1912. 370p. map.

Annie Peck was an accomplished American mountaineer who had been one of the first women alpinists to scale the Matterhorn, and who undertook a series of expeditions to the high Andes between 1903 and 1908. Her first objective was to climb Mount Illampú at 6,485 metres (21,276 feet) but, like Sir Martin Conway in the same period, she was forced to abandon the ascent when close to the peak – 'almost to the summit but not quite'. She scaled Huascarán, 6,768 metres (over 22,000 feet) in Peru, and records her climbing experiences in this well-written book, practical and conversational in style, illustrated with many of her own photographs, and peppered with shrewd observations. Peck returned to South America many times during the next thirty years, and through her lecturing, photography and travel writing did much to bring knowledge about the region to a wide audience in the United States.

139 **Across the Andes: a tale of wandering days among the mountains of Bolivia and the jungles of the upper Amazon.**
Charles Johnson Post. New York: Outing Publishing, 1912. 362p. maps.

An absorbing account of Post's journey across Bolivia by pack-mule and river-boat from La Paz and Sorata, through the Yungas and the Beni rubber country, to the Madeira-Mamoré Falls. His detailed observations include notes on the Aymara settlements and Aymara music. As his travels continue, the book becomes a most interesting, extended cross-section of the varied landscapes and peoples of Bolivia.

140 **The sea and the jungle.**
Henry Major Tomlinson. London: Duckworth & Co., 1912. 354p. (Reprinted, Evanston, Illinois: Marlboro Press/Northwestern, 1996).

This is a masterpiece of travel literature. Tomlinson, a Londoner bored by a routine desk job, on impulse joined the crew of a small cargo steamer preparing to journey up the Amazon and Madeira towards Bolivia in 1909-10. Perceptive and witty, his account of the voyage is packed with easy anecdote and sharp observation of life along the great rivers. The extraordinarily detailed narrative is suffused with the colours, moods, sounds and silences of the sea and the jungle, and provides captivating reading from beginning to end.

141 **South America: observations and impressions.**
James Bryce. London: Macmillan. 1912. 512p. maps. (rev. ed., New York: Macmillan, 1914. 611p. maps).

Bryce, a brilliant scholar whose long career included that of historian, lawyer, parliamentarian, and diplomat, published his impressions of a four-month journey through parts of South America. The section on Bolivia (p. 119-204) recorded a series of reflections on life in and around La Paz, Oruro, Uyuni, and much of the altiplano. Although this volume does not possess the range or the insights of Bryce's masterly *The American Commonwealth*, first published in 1888, and one of the 19th century's two best books on the people, institutions, and spirit of the United States, Bryce's impressions of Bolivia offer objective comments on the differences, where he found them, between preconceived images and visible reality. The impact of the physical landscape is also well conveyed.

142 **Adventures in Bolivia.**
Cecil Herbert Prodgers. London: John Lane, 1922. 232p.

The story of an English expedition to the remote, and previously isolated, Challana Indians. The expedition took place during the rubber boom, in 1903, when the author was employed by the Challana and Tongo Rubber Company. The volume includes lists of items of equipment needed on such an expedition, which still make interesting reading for travellers a century later.

143 Six years in Bolivia. The adventures of a mining engineer.
Anselm Verner Lee Guise. London: T. F. Unwin; New York: E. P. Dutton, 1922. 246p. map.

Recounts the experiences of a young mining engineer, who was the assistant manager of a tin mine in the Oruro area. The work contains numerous references to flora and fauna, as well as descriptions of native life and local customs.

144 Three asses in Bolivia.
Lionel Portman. London: Grant Richards, 1922; Boston; New York: Houghton Mifflin, 1922. 236p. map.

Three asses, according to their friends, go chasing rainbows in Bolivia. Portman's breezy account avoids giving any impression that they took the unusual in their stride; instead, he wrings every last bit of adventure, oddity and discomfort out of his travels, which are concentrated along the altiplano and around Potosí. Despite his theme, however, here is an ass who clearly enjoyed it all.

145 The land of tomorrow: a mule-back trek through the swamps and forests of eastern Bolivia.
Henry M. Grey. London: H. F. & G. Witherby, 1927. 224p. map.

One advantage of this detailed and readable travel account is the graphic observations it provides of some of the places and regions in eastern Bolivia that are not included in other English books of this date. Thus, there are memorable pictures of the Brazilian Paraguay river port of Corumbá and of Bolivia's Puerto Suárez, impressions of mission sites and villages well to the north and northeast of the city of Santa Cruz, such as San Javier, Concepción, and San Ignacio; and a lively record of the author's experiences on the isolated trail south from Santa Cruz through the Andean foothills to the Bolivian border settlement of Yacuiba, and on into Argentina.

146 Green hell: a chronicle of travel in the forests of eastern Bolivia.
Julian Duguid. London: Jonathan Cape, 1931. 344p. maps.

Duguid was a British freelance journalist who joined a small, official expedition to eastern Bolivia in the late 1920s that was designed to explore the Lake Gaíba region of the River Paraguay, to assess its possibilities for colonization, and to judge the feasibility of a new route along the edge of the Chaco from the lake to the city of Santa Cruz. His colourful description of the journey is well written; it skilfully captured the atmosphere of the times and the landscape, and quickly became a popular travel book on both sides of the Atlantic.

147 Exploration Fawcett.
Percy Harrison Fawcett. London: Hutchinson, 1953. 312p. maps. (Reprinted, London: Century, 1988).

Lieutenant-Colonel Fawcett became famous only after his mysterious disappearance in 1925 while leading an expedition to find a legendary 'lost city' in the Mato Grosso jungles of Brazil. His professional introduction to South America, however, was as a British Army surveyor invited by the Royal Geographical Society in London to survey sections of the Bolivia–Brazil and Bolivia–Peru boundaries, on Bolivia's behalf, between 1906 and 1913. After his disappearance and presumed death at the hands of local Indians, Fawcett's manuscripts, letters and log-books were edited and published by his son Brian, and *Exploration Fawcett* became a best-seller. It is indeed an exciting record of Fawcett's boundary work and endless adventure in the rubber forests and river wilderness of central South America, and is also well illustrated with his own photographs. The book was published in the USA under the title *Lost Trails, Lost Cities* (New York: Funk & Wagnall, 1953).

148 In Bolivia.
Eric Lawlor. New York: Vintage Books, 1989. 226p.

A joyless picture of Bolivia in the late 1980s by an Irish journalist who concentrates his observations and interviews on the poorest in society, including miners, subsistence farmers, and the most deprived urban dwellers – 'the victims of power'. Lawlor emphasizes the harsh conditions and destitution that so many suffered after the collapse of the world tin market and the introduction of the government's New Economic Policy. His mood does not lift, and during his rapid reconnaissance he remains depressed about the future of Bolivia.

149 Sons of the Moon.
Henry Shukman. London: Weidenfeld and Nicolson, 1990. 151p. map.

Describes a few months' travel as a young man through the central Andes, which in Bolivia includes impressions of La Paz, Oruro, and the altiplano. Although one of many similar travel accounts, this has a freshness and a fluency that should interest the general reader.

150 Bushmaster fall.
Carl A. Posey. New York: Donald I. Fine, 1992. 311p.

A heady tale of adventure in the Beni jungle region. Posey keeps the action going with good descriptive passages on the forests and the wildlife, the need for environmental protection, and on how to cope with the unexpected.

151 Journey to the Island of the Sun.
Alberto Villoldo. San Francisco, California: HarperSan Francisco, 1992. 210p. maps.

This is a personal odyssey, a pilgrimage along the old Inca trails of Peru and Bolivia to reach Lake Titicaca. As the author approaches the Island of the Sun, the tension heightens as he feels drawn into the centre of a great drama – its myths, its power, and its legacy. Villoldo records his experiences along the trails and on the Island, where he spent several days, capturing and conveying the atmosphere well in simple, unaffected prose.

152   Back from Tuichi: the harrowing life-and-death story of survival in the Amazon rainforest.
Yossi Ghinsberg, translated by Yael Politis, Stanley Young.
New York: Random House, 1993. 239p.

A colourful, gripping account of Ghinsberg's adventures while lost and alone in the Beni and Tuichi river jungles. Originally visiting Bolivia as an Israeli tourist, he was later to return to assist in setting up the Chalalán Project in Bolivia's Madidi National Park, which was created in 1995, and where Chalalán was designed to pioneer ecotourism along the Tuichi with the help of the local indigenous community of San José de Uchupiamonas.

153   Land without evil: utopian journeys across the South American watershed.
Richard Gott.   London; New York: Verso, 1993. 211p. maps. bibliog.

Records his journey across central South America through parts of Brazil, Paraguay and Bolivia, broadly following the watershed between the Amazon and Paraguay river systems. The account of his own travel is greatly expanded by the accounts of earlier expeditions across the same region, or parts of it, during the Spanish and Portuguese colonial period as well as in the 19th and 20th centuries, many of them already well-known classic studies by government officials, missionaries, scientists, explorers, and pioneering settlers. As his title indicates, Gott's unqualified theme throughout, with reference to the Indian communities, is of a lost utopia, a debatable viewpoint, but in devoting the larger part of his travel book to the early Jesuit and Franciscan missions dotted across this region, the author provides an interesting account of their present condition set against the selected historical anthology of past events.

154   Digging up Butch and Sundance.
Anne Meadows.   New York: St Martin's Press, 1994. 388p. maps. bibliog. (rev. ed., Lincoln, Nebraska: University of Nebraska Press, 1996. 390p. maps. bibliog.).

Never mind the cliché, this really is the stuff of legend. Meadows' well-researched and well-written account traces the lives of Butch Cassidy (Robert LeRoy Parker) and the Sundance Kid (Harry Longabaugh) from their earliest days, although the book concentrates on what are thought to be their final two years, 1906-08, which were spent in Bolivia. The bones dug up in San Vicente, however, were not those of the outlaws. In this thoroughly enjoyable tale, readers join the author in pursuit of all the many leads she followed in the attempt to reconstruct the Bolivian finale. But Butch and Sundance have the last word; they remain elusive to the end.

Flora and Fauna

155 Plant hunters in the Andes.
Thomas Harper Goodspeed. New York; Toronto: Farrar &
Rinehart, 1941. 429p. maps. (Reprinted, London: Robert Hale, 1950.
2nd ed. rev. and enlarged, Berkeley: University of California Press,
1961).
This classic study discusses the collecting of plants and mapping of vegetation in Peru,
Chile, Bolivia, and Argentina over a twenty-five-year period. The volume is by no means
solely for botanists, however. Goodspeed also provides a highly readable narrative that
depicts the landscapes and the people in both the rural and urban environments,
particularly during the 1930s, and he illustrates his text with numerous photographs.

156 The species of birds of South America with their distribution.
Rodolphe Meyer de Schauensee. Philadelphia: Academy of
Natural Sciences of Philadelphia, 1966. 577p. bibliog.
An outstanding one-volume listing of the birds which can be found in South America. The
purpose of this work was to fill a gap in the ornithological literature and to provide an
authoritative source for both the professional and amateur ornithologist. It provides a
particularly useful study of distributional problems, and the numerous taxonomic notes
should be of value to students of anatomy and systematics. Also included is a country-by-
country bibliography.

157 A guide to the birds of South America.
Rodolphe Meyer de Schauensee. Wynnewood, Pennsylvania:
Academy of Natural Sciences of Philadelphia, 1970; Edinburgh:
Oliver & Boyd, 1971. 470p. maps. bibliog.
The bird fauna of South America is the richest in the world both in numbers and in variety
of species. This is an illustrated and systematic guide which updates the author's 1966
publication (see previous item), and also extends the geographical range of a number of

species included there. The work is clearly organized and easy to follow, an indispensable reference book.

158 Birds of South America: illustrations from the lithographs of John Gould.

John Gould, text by Abram Rutgers.   London: Eyre Methuen, 1972. 321p.

The plates contained in this impressive volume were selected from Gould's four monographs on the subject. John Gould (1804-81) was one of the 19th century's most outstanding ornithologists and natural history artists, whose magnificent collection comprised nearly 3,000 illustrations. Here, the beautiful colour plates are ably supported with the detailed descriptions by Rutgers, a leading Dutch ornithologist and author. Many of the birds recorded in this volume are found in Bolivia, while the whole study is as much a work of art as a work of science.

159 Bats of Bolivia: an annotated checklist.

Sydney Anderson, Karl F. Koopman, Ken G. Creighton.

New York: American Museum of Natural History, 1982. 24p. map.

This work, led by a noted scholar, lists species of bats found in Bolivia, and provides an early source of basic reference.

160 Notes on Bolivian mammals.

Sydney Anderson, William David Webster.   *American Museum Novitates*, no. 2766 (3 August 1983), p. 1-3.

Describes the first reporting of twenty-three bat species from the Department of Pando.

161 South American birds: a photographic aid to identification.

John S. Dunning.   Newtown Square, Pennsylvania: Harrowood Books, 1987. 351p. maps.

Over 2,700 species are included in this excellent illustrated field book which includes details for bird recognition as well as information on habitat and distribution. Dunning spent twenty-five years photographing the birds for this book in colour, a dedication that produced a unique volume to assist both the amateur and the professional ornithologist.

162 *Thyroptera discifera* (Chiroptera, Thyropteridae) in Bolivia.

Marcos P. Torres, Tomas Rosas, Sergio I. Tiranti.   *Journal of Mammalogy*, vol. 69, no. 2 (1988), p. 434-35. bibliog.

Reports the collection of bats (including *Thyroptera discifera*) and other mammals in the Itenez province, El Beni Department, as part of state-sponsored research into the origins and control of Bolivian haemorrhagic fever.

163 An annotated list of the birds of Bolivia.
James Vanderbeek Remsen, Jr, Melvin Alvah Traylor, Jr.
Vermilion, South Dakota: Buteo Books, 1989. 79p. map. bibliog.
Ornithologists will find this a helpful, easy-to-handle checklist of birds and their habitats in each of Bolivia's nine departments. The authors also provide a concise introduction to the richness of Bolivia's avifauna.

164 New records of bats from Bolivia.
Carlos Ibáñez, José Ochoa G. *Journal of Mammalogy*, vol. 70, no. 1 (1989), p. 216-19. map. bibliog.
Updates Sydney Anderson's 1982 checklist (see item no. 159) along with subsequent findings, by adding eight new species of bats not previously recorded in Bolivia, following a new inventory of fauna made in the Department of Santa Cruz.

165 Jaguar hunting in Mato Grosso and Bolivia: with notes on other game.
Tony de Almeida. Long Beach, California: Safari Press, 1991.
2nd ed. 275p. bibliog.
This is a profusely illustrated record of the author's expeditions in central South America, but for those with no appetite for big-game hunting, the book also includes a wealth of detail on the life of the jaguar and other animals in the Mato Grosso and eastern Bolivia (notably in the jungles along the Guaporé river), together with good observation on the region's general flora and fauna. Almeida provides a vivid description of the Pantanal, the huge expanse of floodwater and swamp around the river Paraguay, and one of the world's great wetlands.

166 In quest of the unicorn bird.
Oliver Greenfield. London: Michael Joseph, 1992. 211p. map.
A lighthearted account by an amateur ornithologist of a wildlife collecting trip to the Buena Vista region of Bolivia, northwest of Santa Cruz.

167 Ornithological gazetteer of Bolivia.
Raymond A. Paynter, Jr. Cambridge, Massachusetts: Harvard University; Bird Department, Museum of Comparative Zoology, 1992. 2nd ed. 185p. maps. bibliog.
Since the publication of the first edition in 1975, knowledge about Bolivian birds has increased so enormously that this new edition has been entirely rewritten and is more than twice the original size. Ornithologists and researchers will find Paynter's work particularly valuable since it not only maps all the observation localities, noting the physical features of each site, but also cites everyone who has worked at each field site, along with the dates and details of their publications. The work thus becomes a complete ornithological gazetteer and bibliography of Bolivia to the early 1990s, and an indispensable source of reference.

168 Rediscovery of the Bolivian recurvebill with notes on other little-known species of the Bolivian Andes.
T. A. Parker III, John M. Bates. *Wilson Bulletin*, vol. 104, no. 1 (March 1992), p. 173-78.

Reports on a survey of birds carried out in August 1989 in the upper Río Saguayo valley area of Amboró National Park, Department of Santa Cruz, in the eastern foothills of the Andes. The authors detail their field methods and findings in this exceptionally rich zone of Andean forest, and urge stronger legal protection for conservation of this region.

169 Where the wild things are.
Susan K. Reed. *People Weekly*, vol. 37, no. 2 (January 1992), p. 28-33.

Describes the work of Conservation International's Rapid Assessment Program in Bolivia's Gran Chaco region, Department of Santa Cruz. An experienced team of four biologists and ornithologists took a quick census of birds, plants and animals at locations chosen as representative of wider areas. In this case, they selected sites around the Parapetí river, and the article includes photographs of the field methods employed.

170 Avifauna of a Chaco locality in Bolivia.
Andrew W. Kratter (et al.). *Wilson Bulletin*, vol. 105, no. 1 (March 1993), p. 114-41. bibliog.

The study site, Estancia Perforación, lies in Cordillera province, Department of Santa Cruz, some eighty kilometres east of the Andean foothills. Vegetation varies dramatically in the Chaco from deciduous woodland to dry scrub, and this is reflected in the great diversity of bird life in the region. Expeditions in 1990 located six species found for the first time in Bolivia while, in all, well over 100 species were recorded. Detailed descriptions of bird calls, foraging behaviour and diet add to the value of this thorough investigation.

171 Benthic invertebrates of some saline lakes of the Sud Lipez region, Bolivia.
Claude Dejoux.   In: Proceedings of the Vth International Symposium on inland saline lakes, held in Bolivia, 22-29 March 1991, *Hydrobiologia*, vol. 267, nos. 1-3 (September 1993), p. 257-67. maps. bibliog.

Reports the findings of new research into the benthic (lake-floor) invertebrate fauna in the southern altiplano region of Bolivia, describing the sampling methods used, and illustrating the great diversity to be found in the fauna as a result of the differences in salinity and temperature that are produced by the various freshwater inflows to the lakes, and by the presence of hot and cold springs. The introduction to this comprehensive study of saline lakes worldwide, edited by Stuart H. Hurlbert, also reports a six-day excursion from Lake Titicaca by the symposium participants to all the major salt lakes and salt pans on the Bolivian altiplano.

172 Confessions of a plant inspector.
Douglas C. Daly. *Travel Holiday*, vol. 176 (November 1993),
p. 64-69, 110-11.

A sprightly account by a collector from the New York Botanical Garden of three of his
South American expeditions – to the Ucayali region of Peru, and in Bolivia, to the
northern forests of the Beni and the drier plateaux of the Serranía de Santiago in the
Department of Santa Cruz. The record is spiced with vivid, often humorous detail about
local characters and hair-raising travel, but the grandeur of much of the scenery is well
observed, and Daly also provides ample detail on his work as a professional botanist.

173 First observations of the blue-throated macaw in Bolivia.
Otto C. Jordan, Charles A. Munn. *Wilson Bulletin*, vol. 105, no. 4
(December 1993), p. 694-95.

Conservationists have long assumed that this species (*Ara glaucogularis*) is very rare and
possibly in immediate danger of extinction. But in August 1992, the authors found wild
blue-throated macaws in the Amazonian forest-and-savannah zone in the Department of
Beni. Although Bolivia outlawed the trapping and trading of macaws in 1984, smuggling
continues to satisfy the demands of international dealers. The authors therefore withhold
the exact locations of their study sites, while inviting personal queries from scholars.

174 Macaws: winged rainbows.
Charles A. Munn. *National Geographic Magazine*, vol. 185
(January 1994), p. 118-40. map.

Sixteen species of macaw inhabit the New World's tropical forests, from central Mexico
to northern Argentina. About half of them are endangered or under threat from hunters
and smugglers, as well as from the inroads made locally into the forests by loggers, gold
prospectors, and oil companies. Munn concentrates here on macaws in the Peruvian and
Bolivian rainforests, particularly those in Peru's Manu National Park, and presents
fascinating detail on their habitats, feeding practices, and flight. In turn, the photographs
by Frans Lanting offer dazzling pictures of the different species, capturing the brilliance
of their plumage in bursts of emerald green, ruby, blue, and gold.

**175 A new *Scytalopus* tapaculo (Rhinocryptidae) from Bolivia, with
notes on other Bolivian members of the genus and the
Magellanicus complex.**
Bret M. Whitney. *Wilson Bulletin*, vol. 106, no. 4 (December
1994), p. 585-614. map. bibliog.

A detailed report for specialists on work carried out in 1992 on tapaculo of the complex
genus *Scytalopus* in two areas of humid temperate forest in the Department of La Paz, and
a third area in Chapare province, Department of Cochabamba. The text is well supported
by illustrations (both in colour and in black and white), and by vocalizations, all reflecting
keen observation and recording by an experienced ornithologist working in Bolivia and
Peru.

176 Systematic relationships of the Bolivian tuco-tucos, genus
     ***Ctenomys* (Rodentia: Ctenomyidae).**
     Joseph A. Cook, Terry L. Yates.   *Journal of Mammalogy*, vol. 75,
     no. 3 (1994), p. 583-99. map. bibliog.

The tuco-tucos rodent, widespread in South America, has a long history in the region's literature; indeed it was noted on several occasions by Charles Darwin during his 19th-century voyage aboard HMS *Beagle*. In their scholarly investigation, the authors examine in detail the differences to be found in Bolivia between the tuco-tucos of the high Andes and the eastern plains, based on chromosomal, allozymic, and morphological variation, and argue that a simple highland–lowland dichotomy in the evolution of this group is no longer tenable.

177 The behaviour of mixed-species tamarin groups (*Saguinus*
     ***labiatus* and *Saguinus fuscicollis*).**
     S. M. Hardie.   PhD thesis, Stirling University, Scotland, 1995.

The tamarin is a small South American squirrel monkey (*Saguinus*). This field study in northern Bolivia confirmed that *Saguinus labiatus* and *Saguinus fuscicollis* form stable mixed-species groups in the wild, but that the species differed in the mean height used in the forest, in their method of locomotion, and in their preferred insect-foraging strategies. Subsequent studies of captive single-species and mixed-species groups made at Belfast Zoo found that these squirrel monkeys behaved in a similar way to their wild counterparts. The study turns on an analysis of the benefits that are derived from this mixed-species association.

178 Forest islands in an Amazonian savanna of northeastern Bolivia.
     Robert Peter Langstroth.   PhD thesis, University of Wisconsin,
     Madison, Wisconsin, 1996. 452p. bibliog.

At a study area east of Trinidad, the author investigates the various possible causes of the islands of forest that occur in the savannahs of the Beni. Having analysed the geomorphology, soils, vegetation, and archaeology in his area, Langstroth concludes that most of the forest islands are the result of the fragmentation and erosion of gallery forest along ancient natural levees above old river courses.

179 Conflict to conservation in Bolivia.
     Fiona McWilliam.   *The Geographical Magazine*, vol. 69 (June
     1997), p. 7.

The spectacled bear (*Tremarcos ornatus*) is the only species of bear to be found in South America, and in terms of evolution, is the most primitive of all bears. This note outlines the research project currently under way to record the extent of the damage done to crops and livestock by these bears in Bolivia, and examines the methods proposed to organize their future management and conservation.

Prehistory and Archaeology

180 Excavations at Tiahuanaco.
Wendell Clark Bennett. New York: American Museum of Natural History, 1934. 494p. bibliog.
This study by the leading United States scholar on the Central Andean region in the 1930s and 1940s remains a valuable starting-point for Tiahuanaco (Tiwanaku) archaeological investigation, since it allows the subsequent finds and interpretations, some of which overturn Bennett's assumptions, to be placed in the context of his pioneering work.

181 The domestication and exploitation of the South American camelids: methods of analysis and their application to circum-lacustrine archaeological sites in Bolivia and Peru.
Jonathan Dwight Kent. PhD dissertation, Washington University, St. Louis, Missouri, 1982. 645p. bibliog.
Focuses upon the development of techniques to analyse faunal assemblages from archaeological sites containing the remains of camelids, with emphasis on the domestication of animals and trade. These methods are then applied to two archaeological sites in Bolivia and Peru; the findings are instructive, and will interest archaeological research students in this field.

182 Marsh resource utilization and the ethnoarchaeology of the Uru-Muratos of highland Bolivia.
Darwin David Horn, Jr. PhD dissertation, Washington University, St. Louis, Missouri, 1984. 411p. bibliog.
The author discusses two aspects of man's use of marshes. He evaluates four characteristics of marsh vegetation: abundance (in terms of rates of primary productivity); nutritional composition; seasonal availability; and ease of harvest. In terms of these factors, marshes have the potential to support human populations. The second aspect of marsh utilization focuses on the Uru-Muratos, highland Bolivians who continue to exploit marshes in a traditional manner. Modern exploitation is also examined.

183 Raised fields without bureaucracy: an archaeological examination of intensive wetland cultivation in the Pampa Koani zone, Lake Titicaca, Bolivia.
Gray Clayton Graffam. PhD thesis, University of Toronto, Ontario, Canada, 1990. 398p. bibliog.

The author contends that raised-field agriculture in the southern Lake Titicaca Basin continued after the collapse of the Tiwanaku state, despite the high level of agricultural organization formerly exercised by the state's bureaucracy. Extensive stretches of raised fields were built well after Tiwanaku's decline, although the technology was simplified, and elaborate methods of artificial drainage were abandoned in favour of less sophisticated techniques.

184 The secrets of ancient Tiwanaku are benefiting today's Bolivia.
Baird Straughan. *Smithsonian*, vol. 21, no. 11 (February 1991), p. 38-49. map.

A popular account of the revival of raised-field agriculture on the Bolivian altiplano based on the ancient practices to increase food supplies developed during the Tiwanaku period between AD 500 and AD 1000. The raised platforms intersected by canals reduce the risk of frost damage and result in high yields of potatoes, grains, and vegetables. The article reviews earlier archaeological studies at Tiwanaku before concentrating on the fieldwork in progress, led by Alan Kolata and Oswaldo Rivera. Vivid colour photographs by Wolfgang Schüler enrich the text.

185 Pre-hispanic and early colonial settlement patterns in the lower Tiwanaku Valley, Bolivia.
Juan V. Albarracin-Jordan. PhD thesis, Southern Methodist University, Dallas, Texas, 1992. 419p. bibliog.

Examines the various types, and the continuity of settlement in the lower Tiwanaku Valley from the pre-Tiwanaku phase, through the Tiwanaku and Inca periods, to the early Spanish colonial years.

186 Prehispanic settlement and agriculture in the Middle Tiwanaku Valley.
James Edward Mathews. PhD thesis, University of Chicago, Chicago, Illinois, 1992. 306p. bibliog.

A useful discussion of the strengths and weaknesses of the three major archaeological/anthropological models that have been advanced to explain the emergence of the Tiwanaku state; in summary: (1) Murra's 'Vertical Archipelago' model which holds that ethnic groups from the Andean plateau gradually colonized a number of varied ecological zones which were able to provide vital resources unavailable on the altiplano; (2) Browman's 'Altiplano' model which, like Murra's, is based on the assumption that the Titicaca Basin was ecologically incapable of feeding large numbers and that state growth therefore depended on long-distance trade with other regions; and (3) the 'Agricultural Production' model put forward by Kolata and others from the early 1980s onwards, which holds that key areas of the altiplano should be regarded not only as agriculturally self-sufficient in pre-hispanic times, but also capable of producing large-scale agricultural surpluses. Land reclamation and major agricultural projects in the Titicaca Basin (including raised-field agriculture) were essential elements of state policy in the Tiwanaku IV and V periods, permitting unprecedented population growth and state expansion. Mathews sets out clearly his methods for testing the three models, and the relative importance of the evidence (or lack of it) on which he bases his conclusions.

187 **Sacred peaks of the Andes.**
Johan Reinhard. *National Geographic Magazine*, vol. 181 (March 1992), p. 84-111. maps.
Reinhard records his twelve years of climbing and research among the lands of the Inca empire. In that time he made over one hundred ascents above 17,000 feet (c. 5,200 metres), finding ritual platforms and other Inca ruins at more than 22,000 feet (6,700 metres), and pioneering as he did so the study of high-altitude archaeology. Reinhard concludes that these Inca and pre-Inca structures scattered among the Andean peaks were built for venerating the mountains themselves, for sun worship, and for important astronomical observations. The author's own photographs make a splendid addition to his text.

188 **Agricultural biodiversity and peasant rights to subsistence in the Central Andes during Inca rule.**
Karl S. Zimmerer. *Journal of Historical Geography*, vol. 19, no. 1 (1993), p. 15-32. maps. bibliog.
Identifies two distinct features of central Andean agriculture during the 15th and 16th centuries. The Incas' state-run economy concentrated on large-scale organization specializing in the cultivation of a few selected crops, and on the production of a regular surplus for distribution within the empire. At the same time, subsistence farming, involving a much greater variety of crops, was left to the small individual peasant households. The landscape contrasts between 'surplus fields' and 'subsistence fields' was discernible at least until the end of the 17th century.

189 **Climate and collapse: agro-ecological perspectives on the decline of the Tiwanaku state.**
Charles R. Ortloff, Alan K. Kolata. *Journal of Archaeological Science*, vol. 20 (1993), p. 195-221. maps. bibliog.
In this sharp, scholarly paper, the authors discuss the possible reasons for the disintegration of the Tiwanaku state as a major political force in the Central Andes. The cause, or causes, of Tiwanaku's collapse between c. AD 1000 and AD 1100 after centuries of growth and expansion has been vigorously debated, but Ortloff and Kolata argue that the failure of Tiwanaku's intensive agricultural economy, the foundation of empire, was triggered by increasing regional drought conditions after AD 1000. The correlation here between Tiwanaku's decline and a devastating climatic change is based on Quelccaya ice-core analyses undertaken over the years by L. G. Thompson *et al.* (see, for example, items 37, 39, 41), and on sediment cores from Lake Titicaca. The value of the paper is enhanced by the drawing together of recent research carried out by others, both in Tiwanaku's imperial outposts and in its altiplano heartland. Ortloff and Kolata do not claim that the 'great drought' is a complete explanation for Tiwanaku's collapse, but that the post-AD 1000 shift to chronic drought conditions was the proximate cause. The state's skilled agro-engineers were simply incapable of responding to a drought of such unprecedented

duration and severity; decline and dispersal of the population were to follow. This stimulating analysis should be read by all specialists in the field.

190 The Inka empire's expansion into the Coastal Sierra region west of Lake Titicaca.
Peter Thomas Bürgi. PhD thesis, University of Chicago, Chicago, Illinois, 1993. 315p. bibliog.

Bürgi's archaeological investigations lead him to conclude that the Incas' imperial expansion into the Coastal Sierra west of Lake Titicaca did not rely on the takeover of existing settlements, but on the creation of a new political infrastructure of their own. Selecting the Torata Valley as representative of the high western valleys, Bürgi examines the sites of Capanto and Sabaya, and argues that the Inca state annexed and integrated this Coastal Sierra region in a more direct fashion than had hitherto been suspected. In pointing to this direct rule, he rejects the proposition that Inca imperial administration was carried out vicariously by a surviving chain of Lupaqa communities in the Coastal Sierra.

191 The pre-hispanic occupation of Chayanta, Bolivia: an introduction to the archaeology of the region.
Anne Marie Hensley-Marchbanks. PhD thesis, University of Texas at Austin, 1993. 505p. bibliog.

Ceramic evidence forms the basis for this reconstruction and discussion of the Chayanta region's cultural history in pre-hispanic and early colonial times. The study provides a most useful introduction to the methodology of archaeological fieldwork in this northern section of the Department of Potosí, including excavation, collection, and site-dating.

192 The role of the camelid in the development of the Tiwanaku state.
Ann Demuth Webster. PhD thesis, University of Chicago, Chicago, Illinois, 1993. 421p. bibliog.

A well-organized and meticulously documented study which evaluates the contribution of llama and alpaca herding to the development and maintenance of the Tiwanaku state. Archaeological fieldwork was carried out at the urban centres of Tiwanaku and Lukurmata, and at eight smaller rural sites in the Tiwanaku Valley. Webster's analysis is based on large quantities of excavated animal bones and teeth, along with other items, representing a long time-span. There is clear evidence that the hunting of wild guanaco and vicuña continued throughout the period. Her findings also suggest that increasing division and specialization took place between Tiwanaku's pastoralists and farmers, and then between pastoralists managing llama or alpaca herds on controlled grazing grounds, as Tiwanaku's state organization expanded across the altiplano into contrasted Andean environments. Webster reviews the varying uses of the domesticated camelids for meat, wool, hides, tools, ornaments, and as pack animals, but gives particular attention to the butchering and distribution of meat, and to the composition and physical characteristics of herds in differing locations. Few individuals have looked directly at camelid remains from Tiwanaku sites in order to study pastoralism in the context of state emergence; here Webster makes a valuable contribution to this area of research.

193 The Tiwanaku: portrait of an Andean civilization.
Alan L. Kolata. Cambridge, Massachusetts; Oxford: Blackwell, 1993. 317p. maps. bibliog.

Analyses the development of the Tiwanakan culture around Lake Titicaca from c. 1000 BC by tracing the expansion of colonization, economic production, and long-distance trade in the Central Andes, an exchange that included the Pacific coast, altiplano and Yungas region. Tiwanaku's role both as a ceremonial centre and, between AD 500 and AD 1000, as the focus of a dynamic economic (not military) empire is clearly examined in the light of modern excavation and new interpretations. In addition to the maps, the volume is well illustrated with photographs, plans and diagrams, and provides a stimulating study for the specialist as well as for the general reader.

194 Climate and the collapse of civilization.
Tom Abate. *BioScience*, vol. 44, no. 8 (1994), p. 516-19.

Presents a concise summary of the archaeological debate on whether there is a direct link between climate change and the collapse of civilizations. Most agree that climate change alone (specifically increasingly aridity) is insufficient to cause a collapse, since well-organized élites have traditionally been capable of building irrigation systems when necessary. Research into the collapse of civilizations in both the Old World and the New World suggests that increasingly dry conditions have a contributory rather than a causal role.

195 Lukurmata: household archaeology in prehispanic Bolivia.
Marc Bermann. Princeton, New Jersey; Chichester, England: Princeton University Press, 1994. 307p. maps. bibliog.

Lukurmata, lying on the southern shore of Lake Titicaca and earlier thought to be no more than a provincial centre of the Tiwanakan state, is now known to be of much greater antiquity. Bermann's excavations of this settlement reveal a sequence of domestic occupation of which only the later stages mark its incorporation into the Tiwanakan system. This is an exemplary study in its clarity and presentation. Examining domestic remains and household units, the author records evidence of local flora and fauna, dwelling construction, burial sites, artefacts, pottery, food preparation, dietary changes, and raised-field agriculture in a text which is well supported by diagrams, tables, and photographs.

196 State and local power in a pre-hispanic Andean polity: changing patterns of urban residence in Tiwanaku and Lukurmata, Bolivia.
John Wayne Janusek. PhD thesis, University of Chicago, Chicago, Illinois, 1994. 497p. bibliog.

Basing his findings on extensive archaeological excavations in residential areas of two Tiwanaku urban centres in the southern Lake Titicaca Basin, the author identifies two contrasted periods in their social organization. From AD 400 to 800, urban social organization was segmentary, diversified, and grounded in local economic management. After AD 800, ruling groups attempted to assert greater control over the local networks prompting, it is suggested, tense and probably violent reaction. The thesis is presented in two volumes.

197 The origins of Andean irrigation.
Karl S. Zimmerer. *Nature*, vol. 378 (30 November 1995),
p. 481-83. map. bibliog.

Zimmerer places his fieldwork in the Department of Cochabamba in the context of the complex systems of irrigation (including canals, aqueducts and raised fields), which sustained intensive agriculture in the high Andes from about AD 530 and reached its climax during the Tiwanaku and Inca civilizations. Investigation of the great alluvial fan below the town of Tarata has revealed an extensive and integrated system of floodwater control and canal irrigation which was in use by about AD 719, but which Zimmerer estimates to have been functioning as early as 3500 years before the present (BP). The work is based on sediment and geomorphological analysis, including ^{14}C dating of charcoal buried in the massive silt layers deposited by irrigation in the Tarata fan. The author contends that these findings suggest a parallel with the early history of irrigation in the coastal and low Andean valleys of western South America, where farmers had adopted irrigated agriculture by 3500 BP. This is a valuable contribution to the literature for all those interested in the development of pre-hispanic irrigated agriculture within the Andes. Indeed, modern-day equivalent practices continued to be in use around Tarata until the early 1990s.

198 Heat and moisture dynamics in raised fields of the Lake Titicaca region, Bolivia.
Diego Sánchez de Lozada. PhD thesis, Cornell University, Ithaca, New York, 1996. 186p. bibliog.

Concentrating on the physical processes involved in frost reduction in raised-field agriculture as practised in the Lake Titicaca Basin, the author's research confirms that the circulation of humid air from the intervening canals to the crop on the raised platforms appears to be more significant in frost reduction than heat flow from the water to the soil.

199 Prehispanic settlement and land use in Cochabamba, Bolivia.
Alvaro Higueras-Hare. PhD thesis, University of Pittsburgh, Pittsburgh, Pennsylvania, 1996. 348p. bibliog.

A study of the evolution of pre-hispanic settlement and land use in the Cochabamba valleys. Despite the widespread use there of Tiwanaku-style pottery during the Intermediate Ceramic Sequence, the author rejects the belief that this represents evidence of Tiwanaku imperial expansion eastwards into agricultural regions more productive than those on the altiplano. The assumption is that expansion would have been on to the best agricultural land in the valleys, yet there was no correlation at the study sites between this and the distribution of Tiwanaku-style pottery.

200 Tiwanaku and its hinterland: archaeology and paleoecology of an Andean civilization.
Edited by Alan L. Kolata. Washington, DC: Smithsonian Institution Press, 1996. 323p. maps. bibliog. (Smithsonian Series in Archaeological Inquiry, No. 1, Agroecology).

This is the first of a two-volume set that will draw together data and interpretations from a combined, long-term University of Chicago–Bolivian National Institute of Archaeology project of interdisciplinary research at the Tiwanaku site and its sustaining hinterland.

This well-illustrated volume focuses on the nature, technology, and social organization of agricultural production, with twelve essays variously examining the soils, climates, and geomorphology of the Tiwanaku region, along with ancient and modern raised-field agriculture, engineering and nutrient systems, and studies of the local indigenous communities. Between them, the authors present a meticulously researched and finely presented piece of work on the Tiwanaku culture, and on its legacy in the farming practices of today.

201 **Valley of the spirits: a journey into the lost realm of the Aymara.**
Alan L. Kolata. New York; Chichester, England: John Wiley & Sons, 1996. 288p.

Chapters 3-5 are based on Kolata's 1993 publication on the Tiwanaku culture (item no. 193). Introductory material and the final two chapters, however, focus on the descendants of the Aymara people, and on the present-day lives of those living along the shores of Lake Titicaca in Bolivia and Peru. The author finds significant continuity with the past, especially in the traditional symbolism of mountain peaks, sacred shrines, and ceremonial pilgrimages. But the Aymara Indians of today are not living wholly in the past; they are eager to find new opportunities to improve their standards of living, notably through improved agricultural production, and in the revival of raised-field cultivation.

202 **Tiwanaku and the anatomy of time: a new ceramic chronology from the Iwawi site, Department of La Paz, Bolivia.**
Joellen Burkholder. PhD thesis, State University of New York at Binghamton, 1997. 263p. bibliog.

With the aid of a computer database, computer-based graphics and radiocarbon dating, the author records a range of newly defined ceramic styles for the Tiwanaku culture and its local antecedents, based on work at the Iwawi site. The styles described range in date from c. 1000 BC to AD 1000, although the conclusion drawn here is that the Tiwanaku cultural phenomenon was both late and brief, emerging after AD 600 and disappearing before AD 1000.

203 **'Above, below and far away': dualism, hierarchy and exchange in highland South America (Peru and Bolivia).**
David Jenkins. PhD thesis, Brandeis University, Waltham, Massachusetts, 1998. 519p. bibliog.

This study applies graph theory to selected aspects of the Andean societies of Peru and Bolivia in pre-hispanic times, including their social hierarchies, their early road systems and highland–coast trade networks, and the symbolic relationships between the people and their gods.

204 **The cities of the ancient Andes.**
Adriana von Hagen, Craig Morris. London; New York: Thames and Hudson, 1998. 240p. maps. bibliog.

A richly illustrated study which investigates the evolution of village settlements, religious centres, empires and city states (including Tiwanaku) in relation to their contrasted geographical settings along the coast, the high Andes, and the jungle fringes. The book also includes many colourful entries on textiles, pottery and gold artefacts, as well as up-to-date information on archaeological excavations currently under way.

205 The agricultural base of the pre-Incan Andean civilizations.
Arthur Morris. *The Geographical Journal*, vol. 165, no. 3 (1999), p. 286-95. maps. bibliog.

A disappointingly superficial, and in places misleading, review of the topic. Morris's claim that his paper offers a new challenge to, or a modification of, what is already known about the early high levels of agricultural production in the Lake Titicaca region is not substantiated. Apart from a short description of the current experimental project in the Puno-Juliaca area, Morris appears to be unaware of the extensive research work on Tiwanaku's agro-economy that has been published since the early 1990s – for example, items 189, 195, 197, 200 – as he makes no reference to any of them, either in the text or in the bibliography.

206 Interpreting the meaning of ritual spaces: the temple complex of Pumapunku, Tiwanaku, Bolivia.
Alexei N. Vranich. PhD thesis, University of Pennsylvania, Philadelphia, Pennsylvania, 1999. 457p. bibliog.

The Pumapunku temple complex is one of the largest and most important ritual precincts at Tiwanaku, comprising buildings, platforms, plazas, courtyards, and stairways. Vranich argues that, together, they were designed to present a sequence of images, 'to funnel groups of people across specially constructed architectural spaces, and to display a series of symbolically important and ritually charged experiences'. Moreover, the temple complex may also have afforded an architectural representation of the centre of the Andean world, its layout a model of *axis mundi*.

History

General

207 Nueva historia de Bolivia. (A new history of Bolivia.)
Enrique Finot. La Paz: Gisbert y Cía, 1980. 368p. bibliog.
An excellent interpretation of Bolivian history from the pre-Inca civilization of
Tiahuanaco to the 1930s. The topics discussed include Tiahuanaco and the Inca conquest,
the Spanish conquest of 1538 and the colonial era, the establishment of the Republic in
1825, *caudillo* politics of the 19th century, the War of the Pacific (1879-84), the rise of
the conservative élites, and the Chaco War (1932-35).

208 Historia de Bolivia. (History of Bolivia.)
Augusto Guzmán. La Paz: Editorial 'Los Amigos del Libro', 1981.
6th ed. 454p. bibliog.
A prize-winning survey of Bolivian history which discusses in a chronological framework
the following topics: pre-Columbian cultures, the colonial period, Independence, the
Republic, the age of dictators and miners, and the revolution of 1952.

209 The Andean past: land, societies, and conflicts.
Magnus Mörner. New York: Columbia University Press, 1985.
300p. bibliog.
Using John Murra's thesis of reciprocity, Mörner traces social development from the
earliest times through the colonial and national periods. There are three noteworthy
features of the work: the coverage of the prehistoric period; the development of a regional
study of Andean space rather than artificial nation-state divisions; and its readable, and
sympathetic treatment of the subject.

210   Bolivia: the evolution of a multi-ethnic society.
Herbert S. Klein.   New York; Oxford: Oxford University Press,
1992. 2nd ed. 343p. maps. bibliog.

Updates the first edition (1982) of this comprehensive and well-balanced study of Bolivia
with a revision of chapter nine ('The Military Interregnum, 1964-82'), a new final chapter
ten on events of the late 1980s, and an expanded bibliography.

The colonial period (16th-early 19th centuries)

211   Technical aid to Upper Peru: the Nordenflicht Expedition.
Rose Marie Buechler.   *Journal of Latin American Studies*, vol. 5
(1973), p. 37-77. map. bibliog.

A detailed study of the urgent technological improvements that were proposed by a
foreign team of advisers to the Spanish Crown during the 1790s in an attempt to raise
productivity in the silver mines, particularly at Potosí. See also A. Z. Helms, *Travels from
Buenos Ayres, by Potosí, to Lima*, item no. 126.

212   Tales of Potosí: Bartolomé Arzáns de Orsúa y Vela.
Edited with an introduction by R. C. Padden, translated by Frances
M. López-Morillas.   Providence, Rhode Island: Brown University
Press, 1975. 209p. bibliog.

These tales are drawn from Bartolomé Arzáns' monumental account of the history of
Potosí from its founding in 1545 until 1736, the year of his death. The stories include
private lives and public pageantry, and range from the dazzling splendour of the 'City of
Silver' to titbits of local gossip and scandal. Arzáns was born in Potosí, lived there his
entire life, and left future generations with a vivid record of the power and prestige of a
city which, during much of the 17th century, was the largest city in the New World.

**213   An abolitionism born of frustration: the Conde de Lemos and
the Potosí *mita*, 1667-1673.**
Jeffrey A. Cole.   *The Hispanic American Historical Review*,
vol. 63, no. 2 (1983), p. 307-33. bibliog.

This article examines the attempts made by Viceroy Conde de Lemos to abolish the Potosí
mita, or forced labour system. What is clear to the author is that the 'flexibility' attributed
to the Habsburg bureaucracy also existed in the American colonies. The transformation
of the *mita* to a part draft-labour system and a part-cash subsidy for the mine and mill-
owners demonstrated that fundamental decision-making could take place in the colonies.

214 The Cambridge History of Latin America, vol. 2, Colonial Latin America.
Edited by Leslie Bethell. Cambridge: Cambridge University Press, 1984. 912p. maps. bibliog.

Helpful background on conditions in colonial Upper Peru (now Bolivia), and on the general setting of the region in relation to other parts of colonial Spanish America, is included in the following chapters: 1. 'Population' (Nicolás Sánchez-Albornoz); 3. 'Urban development' (Richard M. Morse); 4. 'Mining' (Peter Bakewell); 6. 'Rural economy and society' (Magnus Mörner); 7. 'Aspects of the internal economy: labour, taxation, distribution and exchange' (Murdo J. MacLeod); 8. 'Social organization and social change' (James Lockhart); and 11. 'Indian societies under Spanish rule' (Charles Gibson). See also Asunción Lavrin, 'Women in Spanish American colonial society', item no. 646.

215 Miners of the Red Mountain: Indian labor in Potosí, 1545-1650.
Peter John Bakewell. Albuquerque: University of New Mexico Press, 1984. 213p. maps. bibliog.

Bakewell's perceptive study of Potosí's silver production during this turbulent century examines the sources and characteristics of the industry's huge Indian labour force, particularly the degree of coercion involved in securing it. Contrary to widespread belief that the *mita* (forced labour) dominated the system, by the start of the 17th century, hired wage-labourers formed half the workforce, a dual structure of forced and voluntary labour (*mitayo* and *minga*) which lasted throughout the colonial period and had its origins in Inca and pre-Inca times. Bakewell sifts and presents his evidence in fluent style to provide an illuminating monograph which is both concise and informative. This is an excellent contribution to the socio-economic history of colonial Spanish America.

216 The Potosí *mita*, 1573-1700: compulsory Indian labor in the Andes.
Jeffery A. Cole. Stanford, California: Stanford University Press, 1985. 206p. bibliog.

Examines the late 16th- and 17th-century *mita* after it was formalized by the Viceroy of Peru, Francisco de Toledo. When the Indians learned about working conditions at the Potosí mine, they attempted to escape obligatory service, some by moving away, but many more by attempting to purchase their freedom. This is a sound study of specific aspects of the forced labour system, particularly its institutional and administrative structures rather than its impact on Indian everyday existence.

217 Cochabamba, 1550-1900: colonialism and agrarian transformation in Bolivia.
Brooke Larson. Princeton, New Jersey: Princeton University Press, 1988. 376p., expanded edition 422p. maps. bibliog.; Durham, North Carolina: Duke University Press, 1998. rev. ed.

During the colonial period, the fortunes of the Cochabamba agricultural region were always closely associated with the silver-mining economy in the high Andes, and here the study of Cochabamba is linked to the economic cycles of the mines, especially at Potosí. In such a prosperous farming area, both agricultural and commercial activities were expanded by the indigenous population in order to avoid the *mita* (forced labour system) during the boom periods in silver production, while during periods of recession in

Potosí's mining industry, particularly between the 1680s and 1730s, local *hacendados* (owners of large estates) found the small peasant farmers not only encroaching on *hacienda* lands but also challenging the landowners in the marketplace through the sale of their produce. Ethnic, class, and political relationships are all examined in this scholarly analysis, which in fact begins with the 14th-century background and extends well beyond 1900 into the 20th century.

218 **Silver and entrepreneurship in seventeenth-century Potosí: the life and times of Antonio López de Quiroga.**
Peter John Bakewell. Albuquerque: University of New Mexico Press, 1988. 250p. maps. bibliog.; Dallas, Texas: Southern Methodist University Press, 1995. 2nd ed.

Bakewell examines the career of this extraordinary Spanish immigrant from Galicia, noting that 'he must rank as one of the most diverse and capable businessmen to appear in the whole span of the Spanish empire in America'. During his lifetime (c. 1620-1699), López was outstandingly successful as a mine-owner, silver refiner, trader, investor, landowner, and sponsor of a wide range of other enterprises. López had arrived in Potosí in 1648 where he was to combine great wealth with an eye for new opportunities and remarkable powers of organization. The author provides a vivid account of this astute individual, whose biography is skilfully used to trace the turbulent economic and social history of Potosí.

219 **Archbishops, canons, and priests: the interaction of religious and social values in the clergy of seventeenth-century Bolivia.**
Lincoln Arnold Draper. PhD thesis, University of New Mexico, Albuquerque, New Mexico, 1989. 289p. bibliog.

An investigation into the manner in which the formal religious values of Spanish Catholicism interacted with the values of secular creole society during the first half of the 17th century. Challenge to the authority of the Catholic Church in Upper Peru came from both provincial and local officials – an example of the clashes which occurred between the cultural values of metropolitan Spain and those of Spaniards born in the Americas. Nonetheless, the study reveals that clerical responses to local needs and demands were by no means uniform, with hearts and minds often torn in different directions.

220 **Migration in colonial Peru: an overview.**
Noble David Cook. In: *Migration in colonial Spanish America.* Edited by David J. Robinson. Cambridge: Cambridge University Press, 1990, p. 41-61. map. bibliog. (Cambridge Studies in Historical Geography, No. 16).

The size and importance of migration in the Andean region during the colonial period have received increasing attention from historians and historical geographers in recent years. In reviewing the literature, the author discusses what is now known about migration in colonial Peru, including Upper Peru (later Bolivia), its Inca antecedents, the origins and types of migrants involved, the main patterns of migration, and directions for future research. This is an authoritative contribution to the historical demography of Spanish America, and recommended reading for students and scholars working in this field.

221 **Migration processes in Upper Peru in the seventeenth century.**
Brian Evans. In: *Migration in colonial Spanish America.* Edited
by David J. Robinson. Cambridge: Cambridge University Press,
1990, p. 62-85. maps. bibliog. (Cambridge Studies in Historical
Geography, No. 16).

Focusing here on Upper Peru (later Bolivia), the author draws on two major statistical
sources: census material in the *Visita General* of Viceroy Toledo (1575), and that in the
Numeración General of Viceroy Palata (1683-86). The discussion concentrates on the
migration patterns and population redistribution that occurred between the dates of the
two surveys, a period when, as Evans notes, 'Alto Peru was a society in movement'. The
strengths and weaknesses of the census data are examined, and selected settlements
investigated in more detail. This is a clear, tautly argued essay whose value is further
enhanced by its accompanying population distribution maps, and other figures.

222 **Crisis in Upper Peru, 1800-1805.**
Enrique Tandeter. *The Hispanic American Historical Review*,
vol. 71, no. 1 (1991), p. 35-71. map. bibliog.

In a meticulous and illuminating study, the author analyses the baptismal, death, and
marriage registers for selected parishes within the city of Potosí and in the northern
province of Chayanta to reveal the effects on prices and production of the exceptionally
severe successive droughts experienced there at the start of the 19th century. Attention is
also paid to the impact of crises in the mining industry and the outbreak of smallpox. At
the local level, historians, with the help of parish registers, have been extending their
research into weather conditions, crop and livestock losses, famines and epidemics, and
Tandeter provides a well-written, exemplary contribution to the economic and
demographic literature.

223 **Trade, war and revolution: exports from Spain to Spanish
America, 1797-1820.**
John Fisher. Liverpool, England: Institute of Latin American
Studies, University of Liverpooi, 1992. 145p. (Monograph Series,
No. 16).

A quantitative study of commercial movements between Spain and Spanish America
during the final years of empire. The monograph is largely based on the analysis of ships
registers, registered exports, ports of departure and destination, and by regional
destination. The text is greatly extended by appendices and tables. Evaluation of the
quantitative data traces the various causes of trade fluctuation within this period, and the
changing fortunes of the major ports.

224 **Coercion and market: silver mining in colonial Potosí, 1692-
1826.**
Enrique Tandeter. Albuquerque, New Mexico: University of New
Mexico Press, 1993. 322p. maps. bibliog.

A detailed and scholarly analysis of the Potosí *mita*, the system of forced Indian labour
drawn from a huge area in the Central Andes on which the city's legendary silver
production depended. The study devotes particular attention to the administration and

organization of the workforce, and the difficulties encountered by Spain's colonial officials in maintaining order and safety in the mines.

225 *Haciendas* and *ayllus*: rural society in the Bolivian Andes in the eighteenth and nineteenth centuries.
Herbert S. Klein.   Stanford, California: Stanford University Press, 1993. 230p. bibliog.

Basing the greater part of his analysis on notarial records and Indian tribute censuses from the province/intendancy of La Paz, the author develops a detailed study of the *haciendas* (large estates) and the Indian communities (*ayllus*) in this region, emphasizing the complexity of the relationships between them. The central theme is that at least some of the great landowners were more active and more market-orientated than generalizations about them have suggested, while at the same time, the Indian communities were not the uniformly downtrodden masses that earlier stereotyping has proposed – reassessments that have been made increasingly by scholars in recent years. The Indians' determination to preserve their land led to a continuing struggle in some cases with the *haciendados*, during which the Indians developed considerable staying-power. The book is weakened by its complete lack of maps. These would not only have located the places mentioned in the text (an indispensable aid in this case), but would also have revealed significant distribution patterns in the landscape that here remain buried in the statistical tables.

226 Regional markets and agrarian transformation in Bolivia: Cochabamba, 1539-1960.
Robert Howard Jackson.   Albuquerque: University of New Mexico Press, 1994. 283p. maps. bibliog.

This thought-provoking and well-documented study examines the development and transformation of Cochabamba's agricultural economy over four centuries, with particular attention paid to the impact of market forces on the *hacienda* system. Jackson challenges Larson's conclusion (item no. 217) that the decline of the Potosí market in the 17th and 18th centuries triggered structural changes in the *haciendas*, and contributed to the subdivision of land and the growth in the number of peasant smallholders. Instead, he argues that alternative markets were still available for Cochabamba flour and grain at that time, and that fundamental changes in the *hacienda* economy did not occur until the late 19th and early 20th centuries, when the growth of railways from the Pacific ports captured the major markets on the altiplano and in Cochabamba and Potosí, and brought in cheaper foreign wheat. See also Jackson's article, 'The decline of the hacienda in Cochabamba, Bolivia: the case of the Sacaba Valley, 1870-1929' (*The Hispanic American Historical Review*, vol. 69, no. 2 [1989], p. 259-81. maps. bibliog.).

227 Power and violence in the colonial city: Oruro from the mining renaissance to the rebellion of Tupac Amaru (1740-1782).
Oscar Cornblit, translated by Elizabeth Ladd Glick.   Cambridge: Cambridge University Press, 1995. 227p. maps. bibliog.

Examines the origins of this important Andean silver-mining centre together with its social, economic, and political development during the 18th century. Unlike the *mita* of Potosí, Spain did not introduce a forced labour system in Oruro, where work was paid for largely on a free-market basis. The author provides much detail on Spain's administrative organization, the lives and attitudes of government officials, and the endless confrontations and lawsuits that characterized the 1740s. The analysis of Oruro's urban politics is perceptive and will interest scholars of the period. This is an uneven book, however. Despite its chosen span, the study moves from the 1740s to the uprisings in 1780-81 with relatively little attention given to the intervening decades.

228   **They eat from their labor: work and social change in colonial Bolivia.**
Ann Zulawski.   Pittsburgh, Pennsylvania: University of Pittsburgh Press, 1995. 283p. maps. bibliog. (Pitt Latin American Series).
Examines the development of the Indian workforce in Upper Peru (Bolivia) during the 17th and early 18th centuries by means of two contrasted case-studies: the silver-mining centre of Oruro, and the agricultural province of Pilaya y Paspaya which helped to supply the city markets, especially Potosí. Using census and other records, the author traces the varied origins and characteristics of the indigenous labour force, its migration patterns, marketing skills, and the extent to which ethnic networks were adapted and maintained through periods of both boom and recession. This is a discerning contribution to colonial economic history.

229   **Colonial crisis, community, and Andean self-rule: Aymara politics in the age of insurgency.**
Sinclair Stephen Thomson.   PhD thesis, University of Wisconsin, Madison, Wisconsin, 1996. 392p. bibliog.
Traces the causes of the conflicts against Spanish colonial rule which developed among the Aymara communities in the La Paz region during the 18th century, and which culminated in the rebellion of 1780-82. Special attention is given to the political power shift that followed the insurrection, down from the Indian leaders (*caciques*) to the base-level members of the community, an enduring legacy seen in the peasant political culture of highland Bolivia today.

230   **Disputed images of colonialism: Spanish rule and Indian subversion in northern Potosí, 1777-1780.**
Sergio Serulnikov.   *The Hispanic American Historical Review*, vol. 76, no. 2 (1996), p. 189-226. bibliog.
Examines the Indian protest movement and insurrection against the Spanish authorities which took place in the town of Macha in Chayanta province following the changes in tribute and service introduced by the Bourbon reforms, which brought in tighter bureaucratic controls. In a detailed study, the author provides a scholarly analysis of the distinctiveness of the Indian leader Tomás Katari and the communities of northern Potosí, placing it in the context of the wider Indian uprisings against Spanish rule that erupted during this late colonial period.

231 The 'port' of Potosí.

J. Valerie Fifer. In: *The Master Builders: structures of empire in the New World. Spanish initiatives and United States invention.*
J. Valerie Fifer. Bishop Auckland, Durham: Durham Academic Press, 1996. 320p. maps. bibliog.

A study in which the basic principles of structural engineering are applied to the historical development of the Spanish and United States empires in the Americas – a comparative analysis of the two most daring compression and tension structures ever built in the New World. Within this broader interpretive study of the contrasted development of the Hispanic and United States empires, Spain's perception of Upper Peru's location is revealing since, essentially, Upper Peru (later Bolivia) had a structural, not a geographical, location. It was the true end-fixture of the great oceanic tie-beam. Thus, Potosí was a port, a great inland port, a 'port of the mountains' in true medieval Castilian style. In terms of Upper Peru's structural ties with imperial Spain, it is argued that the concept of the 'port' of Potosí was also to influence Spain's perception of long-distance overland transport in the Americas, which, unlike the United States, was to remain *interoceánico*, not transcontinental.

232 The economic aspects of Spanish imperialism in America, 1492-1810.

John R. Fisher. Liverpool, England: Liverpool University Press, 1997. 238p. maps. bibliog.

A clear, comprehensive survey of the economic relations between Spain and Spanish America during the colonial period. Students seeking background on Bolivia will find useful discussion on the wealth of Potosí, and the mining and trade of Upper Peru in general. Although the book is written for the non-specialist in economic history, specialists also will appreciate this readable, informative overview.

233 *Encomienda*, family, and business in colonial Charcas (modern Bolivia): the *encomenderos* of La Plata, 1550-1600.

Ana Maria Presta. PhD thesis, Ohio State University, Columbus, Ohio, 1997. 363p. bibliog.

In Spanish America, *encomenderos* were colonists granted land by the Crown with the added responsibility for the welfare and protection of the Indians living on it. This study analyses the economic activities of a group of *encomenderos* living in the city of La Plata (Chuquisaca, later Sucre), and discusses the ways in which they developed family networks to expand their business enterprises through inheritance, investment, and access to labour. Four family hierarchies are examined: Almendras, Pamagua de Loaysa, Zarate, and Ondegardo.

234 The American finances of the Spanish empire: royal income and expenditures in colonial Mexico, Peru, and Bolivia, 1680-1809.

Herbert S. Klein. Albuquerque, New Mexico: University of New Mexico Press, 1998. 221p. maps. bibliog.

Uses tax revenues to analyse the economies of the three major silver-producing regions in the Spanish American empire, and to determine long-term trends in both the colonial economy and the royal finances from the late 17th to the early 19th centuries. The tax categories examined include mining, trade, monopoly taxes, and tribute taxes. The text is well supported by tables and graphs, and the most relevant section here on Bolivia (Audiencia of Charcas/Upper Peru) is recommended to economic historians specializing in the colonial period.

The struggle for Independence (1809-25)

235 Simón Bolívar and Spanish American Independence, 1783-1830.
John J. Johnson.   Princeton, New Jersey: Van Nostrand, 1968. (Reprinted, Malabar, Florida: Krieger Publishing, 1992, with the collaboration of Doris M. Ladd). 223p. map. bibliog. (Anvil Series).

Johnson provides a thoughtful, compact study of Bolívar as soldier, state-maker, political theorist, idealist, and pragmatist, noting that at the end of the 20th century, the Bolivarian Andean States are once again turning to the Liberator as a rallying symbol. The text also includes seventeen annotated selected readings by Bolívar and others, including the Jamaica Letter (1815), the Angostura Address (1819), and the Bolivian Constitution of 1826.

236 Simón Bolívar.
Gerhard Masur.   Albuquerque, New Mexico: University of New Mexico Press, 1969. 2nd ed. 572p. maps. bibliog.

An outstanding study which remains the best biography of Bolívar in English. Masur handles an immense amount of research material with great skill and assurance. His chapter on Bolivia includes discussion of Bolívar's new Constitution for the country, and also of the Liberator's ambivalent attitude to the Independence of Upper Peru – his reprimand to Sucre for having authorized the act when Independence should legally have awaited the approval of Argentina and Peru; his realization that Upper Peru's Independence was almost certainly inevitable, and that in any case it was probably for the best. It would be folly to allow the region's great wealth in silver to fall into the hands of either Buenos Aires or Lima. In its range and its assessments, this is a book that stands the test of time.

237 The emergence of the Republic of Bolivia.
Charles Wolfgang Arnade.   New York: Russell & Russell, 1970. rev. ed. 269p. maps. bibliog.

First published in 1957, this is an excellent analysis of the events which culminated in the Independence of Upper Peru in 1825. Arnade documents the complex internal rivalries and ambitions within both the Royalist forces and the separatist ranks, revealing the daunting problems inherited, and those still to be faced, by the newly independent state of Bolivia.

238 General Francis Burdett O'Connor.
Eric Lambert. *The Irish Sword*, vol. 13, no. 51 (1977), p. 128-33. bibliog.

A brief biography of Francis Burdett O'Connor (1791-1871) which is mainly anecdotal, but which provides interesting early family background in Ireland and draws on O'Connor's own recollections. The young Irishman originally planned to emigrate to the United States, but circumstances led him instead to South America in 1818 with the Irish Legion. He served as an officer under Bolívar, and later under Sucre in the liberation of Upper Peru. O'Connor was to remain in Bolivia for the rest of his life, becoming a leading citizen and landowner in Tarija.

239 Participación popular en la independencia de Bolivia. (Popular participation in Bolivian independence.)
René Arze Aguirre. La Paz: Editorial Don Bosco, 1979. 271p. maps. bibliog.

A prize-winning monograph and the first scholarly attempt to document popular participation in the campaigns for Bolivian independence. This study, which is based on extensive documentation, argues that lower-class participation was both extensive and important during the first phase of the Independence movement, but that this participation was limited to the early years.

240 The Spanish American revolutions, 1808-1826.
John Lynch. New York: W. W. Norton, 1986. 2nd ed. 448p. maps. bibliog.

A masterly analysis and synthesis of the complex events and widely scattered campaigns that eventually led to the collapse of Spain's American empire. Lynch's chapter on Bolivia discusses the roles of the three major figures – Bolívar; Sucre, Bolívar's most able commander; and General Pedro Antonio Olañeta, who commanded the Spanish army in Upper Peru: 'a Spaniard more royalist than the viceroy, more absolutist than the king'. The book as a whole combines sharp insights with supple prose, an excellent text for both the scholar and the general reader.

241 El Libertador: Simón Bolívar.
Brian Hodgson. *National Geographic Magazine*, vol. 185 (March 1994), p. 35-65. map.

A well-illustrated general account of Bolívar's life and, through it, the story of Spanish America's liberation from Spain in the early 19th century. There is a sad, haunting quality to the piece as Bolívar's dreams of unity fade into the reality of entrenched regionalism and political turbulence that plagued most of the newly independent states.

242 Simón Bolívar: South American liberator.
David Goodnough. Springfield, New Jersey: Enslow Publishers, 1998. 112p. maps. bibliog. (Hispanic Biographies Series).

Written for young readers in the 11-15 age range, this book provides them with a comprehensive biography of Bolívar, including his background, early life, campaigns in the Wars of Independence, and his final weary pessimism about what Latin America's future will be. The text and layout are clear, maps and photographs give good support, there is a useful glossary of unfamiliar terms, and several points for discussion emerge regarding events in Europe and conditions in Latin America at the time. This is an attractive book, easy to handle and thought-provoking for its intended readership.

243 **The third man: Francisco Burdett O'Connor and the emancipation of the Americas.**
James Dunkerley. London: University of London Institute of Latin American Studies, 1999. 23p. bibliog. (Occasional Paper, No. 20).

First presented as an inaugural lecture, the paper provides an engaging review of O'Connor's life, his service in the wars of liberation and in the early years of Bolivia's independence. In 1825, Sucre had put O'Connor in command of the operation to hunt down the remaining Royalist forces in Upper Peru under General Pedro Olañeta, and the Irishman is depicted here as the third man behind Bolívar and Sucre, and later behind Sucre and Andrés Santa Cruz. O'Connor settled in Tarija, where one of the Department's provinces keeps his name. The author draws on O'Connor's published recollections, and additional sources, in this short but eloquent biography of one of the many Irishmen who never went home. Instead, Francis Burdett O'Connor exemplified the distinctive Irish connection with Latin America during the emancipation period, a connection which was subsequently absorbed, where luck held, into the region's prosperous land-owning élite.

244 **Cochabamba's heroic mothers.**
Anne W. Tennant, photography by Mike Ceaser. *Américas*, vol. 52, no. 3 (2000), p. 26-31. map.

Recalls the day in May 1812 when a group of women on the outskirts of Cochabamba fought and died in their struggle to repel Royalist troops commanded by General José Manuel de Goyeneche. Tennant sets this event, which is still commemorated annually in the city, against the background of other scattered rebel movements in Upper Peru during the first stages of the War of Independence, reminding readers that Cochabamba was one of the main early centres of resistance against Spain.

245 **Liberators: Latin America's struggle for independence, 1810-1830.**
Robert Harvey. London: John Murray, 2000. 561p. maps. bibliog.

A lively, well-researched study of Latin America's independence from Spain and Portugal based on seven key liberators – Miranda, Bolívar, San Martín, O'Higgins, Cochrane, Iturbide, and Pedro I. Harvey's magnificent seven have clearly been selected both for their own exceptional qualities and for their regional significance, since between them their stories cover the continent, and emphasize the huge scale of the campaigns. Antonio José de Sucre, so vital in the endorsement of Bolivia's independence (and the country's first elected President), is not a major player in this collection but his main exploits are included in the text. Harvey captures the drama, ovation, and tragedy of the conflict; his characters are listed as *dramatis personae* and, inevitably, Bolívar occupies centre-stage. In the scenes set in Upper Peru, we follow his late, triumphant progress into Bolivia, his rapturous reception in La Paz, Potosí and Chuquisaca, and his new Constitution for the country, where Bolívar's earlier irritation at Upper Peru's breakaway movement was somewhat mollified on arrival by his discovery of the strength of local feeling for Independence, and by the delegates' shrewdly chosen name for their new creation. The volume conveys the heroism, follies, cruelties, and idealism that marked this bitter struggle, overshadowed before its end by disillusion and despair. The book is well illustrated, the campaigns clearly mapped – altogether a stimulating addition to the huge existing literature on the subject.

The new Republic after 1825 (19th century)

246 The promise and problem of reform: attempted social and economic change in the first years of Bolivian Independence.
William Lee Lofstrom. Ithaca, New York: Cornell University Press, 1972. 626p. bibliog.

A scholarly monograph which examines the administration of Antonio José de Sucre, the first elected president of Bolivia (1826-28). This lengthy work may well be the definitive study of the attempted social and economic reform of the Sucre presidency. It demonstrates why the reforms were largely unsuccessful, but that although they failed, the Bolivian example does provide a necessary case-study of the reform effort.

247 Report on Bolivia, 1827, by Joseph Barclay Pentland.
Edited, with an introduction, by J. Valerie Fifer. London: The Royal Historical Society, 1974. 98p. maps. bibliog. (Camden Miscellany, Vol. 25).

Pentland's report is significant as the first major description of Bolivia at a very early period in its history. Appointed by the Foreign Office in 1825 to assist the British Consul General in Lima, Pentland was instructed soon after his arrival to undertake a fact-finding tour of Bolivia, known before Independence as Upper Peru. He travelled extensively through Bolivia's Andean region, noting physical features, population, settlement patterns, and agriculture, all of which are summarized in the Introduction to this volume. Then follow, in full, the longest and most detailed sections of his report: 3. 'A review of the present state of the mines, and of their former produce'; 4. 'A review of the commercial relations, foreign and domestic'; 5. 'A short view of the present political state of Bolivia, embracing the history of the country since its independence, its government, laws, and institutions'. Together, they provide a unique and well-observed picture of Bolivia's prospects and problems at the start of Independence.

248 Sub-regional integration in nineteenth century South America: Andrés Santa Cruz and the Peru–Bolivian Confederation, 1835-1839.
Philip Parkerson. PhD dissertation, University of Florida, Gainesville, Florida, 1979. 384p. bibliog.

Examines the attempts of Andrés Santa Cruz in the 1830s to unite Bolivia and Peru into a confederation. The study will be of particular interest to students working on the early

19th-century history of these two states, and on the attitudes of their neighbours to such a perceived power bloc.

249 **Historia de Bolivia.** (History of Bolivia.)
Alcides Arguedas.   La Paz: Librería y Editorial 'Juventud', 1981.
5 vols. bibliog.
An outstanding history of Bolivia by a noted intellectual (1879-1946). It traces Bolivian history from Independence (1825), to the 1880s. Each volume is well written and enjoyable to read, and each is written so as to stand independently of the others. The volumes are entitled: 1. 'The foundation of the Republic'; 2. The 'Educated *caudillos*'; 3. 'Dictatorship and anarchy'; 4. 'People in action'; and 5. The 'Barbaric *caudillos*'. These volumes are based on Arguedas' seminal work *Historia general de Bolivia: el proceso de la nacionalidad, 1809-1921*, which was published in La Paz in 1922.

250 **The Brazilian monarchy and the South American republics, 1822-1831.**
Ronald L. Seckinger.   Baton Rouge, Louisiana: Louisiana State University Press, 1984. 187p. maps. bibliog.
An interesting monograph which includes the early conflict between Brazil and Bolivia over the former's attempt, soon after Bolivia's Independence, to annex the province of Chiquitos in eastern Bolivia. General/President Sucre stood firm, tempers cooled, and war was averted.

251 **Commerce and credit on the periphery: Tarija merchants, 1830-1914.**
Erick Detlef Langer, Gina L. Hames.   *The Hispanic American Historical Review*, vol. 74, no. 2 (1994), p. 285-316. maps. bibliog.
The authors analyse the accounts, diaries and correspondence of the major landowners and leading import–export merchants in Tarija after Independence, and discuss the nature and extent of cross-border trade with northern Argentina (at Salta and Jujuy) and with the Chiriguano Indians. The company histories, patterns of credit, and customer distribution provide a valuable addition to the literature on this frontier region. But despite the peripheral location noted in the title, Langer and Hames make some exaggerated claims for Tarija's importance; for example, the absurd statement concerning 'Tarija's preeminent position in the continent's commercial network' during much of this period. In addition, their map showing the extent of the railroad c. 1900 is inaccurate.

252 **Colombia's military and Brazil's monarchy: undermining the republican foundations of South American independence**
Thomas Millington.   Westport, Connecticut: Greenwood Press, 1996. 228p. map. bibliog.
The book examines the effects in the early years of Independence of the juxtaposition of the weak, fragmented Spanish American republics and the strength of monarchic rule in Brazil, arguing that the latter served to accelerate the decline of republican politics in South America. The author, a political scientist, builds his case around the conflict between Sucre and Bolívar over their differing political strategies for the region

immediately after Bolivian Independence, although Millington's interpretation of events remains controversial.

253 Incas sí, Indios no: notes on Peruvian creole nationalism and its contemporary crisis.
Cecilia Méndez G. *Journal of Latin American Studies*, vol. 28, no. 1 (1996), p. 197-225. bibliog..

Although developed in relation to Peru, the article is based on what is seen as the initial influence of the short-lived Peru–Bolivian Confederation (1836-39) in shaping early Peruvian creole national consciousness. In this context, Méndez considers the Bolivian President Andrés Santa Cruz's vision of his new post-Independence confederate state, contrasting the greater support for it in southern Peru with opposition to it (both to Santa Cruz personally, and to the Confederation) from the commercial élites in Lima and the northern coast. There, economic interests were more closely linked to trade with Chile, whose army went on to defeat and destroy the Confederation in 1839.

254 Quinine and *caudillos*: Manuel Isidoro Belzu and the *Cinchona* bark trade in Bolivia, 1848-1855.
Carlos Pérez. PhD thesis, University of California, Los Angeles, 1998. 342p. bibliog.

Traces the growth of the *Cinchona* bark trade in Bolivia during the mid-19th century. As the basis of quinine manufacture, *Cinchona* bark commanded high prices in Europe at this period, and Pérez argues that these revenues were crucial in funding Belzu's populist administration, and in marking an early phase of Bolivia's export economy.

The modern period (20th century)

General

255 Revolution and reaction: Bolivia, 1964-1985.
James M. Malloy, Eduardo A. Gamarra. New Brunswick, New Jersey; Oxford: Transaction Books, 1988. 244p. bibliog.

Reviews the twenty-year period of military or military-dominated national politics between the overthrow of civilian president Víctor Paz Estenssoro in November 1964 and his return to office in August 1985. Against the wider framework of military authoritarianism in South America in this period, the authors examine the varying nature of the military regimes in Bolivia over the two decades, and the major internal military, political, and economic pressures which led to the restoration of civilian administration. This is a discerning addition to the literature both for the specialist and the general reader.

256 Bolivia since 1930.
Laurence Whitehead. In: *The Cambridge History of Latin America.*
Edited by Leslie Bethell. Cambridge: Cambridge University Press,
vol. 8, 1991, p. 509-83. bibliog.
Examines the eventful period from the 1930s to the 1980s, concentrating on the major
political and economic upheavals that the country has experienced since the Chaco War.
The author presents a detailed, well-balanced discussion of the changing external
pressures and internal policies during this fifty-year period, including the continuing, if
somewhat reduced, role played by Bolivia's traditional élites – political, social, and
economic – in the country's recent development.

257 Bolivia.
Laurence Whitehead. In: *Latin America between the Second World
War and the Cold War, 1944-1948.* Edited by Leslie Bethell, Ian
Roxborough. Cambridge: Cambridge University Press, 1992,
p. 120-46. bibliog.
The years 1944-1948 represent a transitional period in Bolivia rather than a discrete unit
of study. Whitehead reviews the previous decades before examining the early 1940s more
closely, when Bolivia's importance as a source of strategic raw materials ensured its
significance in the Second World War, a time of conflicting internal alignments between
the Axis powers, the USSR, and the United States. The essay presents a detailed
chronology of events, the power play between the rival parties, and the political and social
forces that combined to bring about the successful revolution of 1952.

258 Oil, politics, and economic nationalism in Bolivia, 1899-1942: the case of the Standard Oil Company of Bolivia.
Jayne Spencer. PhD thesis, University of California, Los Angeles,
1996. 246p. bibliog.
A study of economic nationalism which focuses on the responses of successive Bolivian
governments during this period to the activities and attitudes of the Standard Oil
Company of Bolivia. The work includes an examination of the company's contracts, its
de facto nationalization in 1937, and the Bolivian military's negotiations with the United
States for enlarged markets during the Second World War.

The Chaco War (1932-35)

259 The conduct of the Chaco War.
David Zook. New Haven, Connecticut: Bookman Associates,
1960. 331p. maps. bibliog.
Discusses the political, economic and military aspects of the Chaco War fought between
Bolivia and Paraguay, 1932-35. One of the first, and still one of the best, books written
on this war in any language.

260 Politics of the Chaco Peace Conference 1935-1939.
Leslie B. Rout, Jr.   Austin, Texas; London: University of Texas
Press, 1970. 268p. maps. bibliog. (Latin American Monograph,
No. 19).

Examines the three major aspects of the Chaco dispute which led to war between Bolivia
and Paraguay and the inter-American Peace Conference which settled it. Agreements
were achieved in total secrecy. This text is based on extensive primary documentation
from Brazilian, Argentine, Uruguayan and Bolivian archives.

261 The Chaco War: Bolivia and Paraguay, 1932-1935.
Bruce W. Farcau.   Westport, Connecticut; London: Praeger, 1996.
254p. map. bibliog.

A readable and well-researched account of the war, with particular use made of published
material and personal reminiscence by those who were involved on the Bolivian side.

Che Guevara

**262 The defeat of Che Guevara: military response to guerrilla
challenge in Bolivia.**
Gary Prado Salmón, translated by John Deredita.   New York:
Praeger, 1990. 288p. maps. bibliog.

This is a detailed record and analysis of the campaign by the officer commanding the unit
which tracked, captured and killed Che Guevara in 1967. Che's failure to gain support
from the local population became a fundamental flaw in his grand design, but Prado's
study is particularly notable for its objective assessment of the weaknesses in preparation,
communication and field operation that characterized both the guerrillas and the army
from time to time during the campaign.

263 The Bolivian diary of Ernesto Che Guevara.
Edited by Mary-Alice Waters.   New York: Pathfinder Press, 1994.
467p. maps. bibliog.

This volume draws on additional documents released by the Bolivian authorities and
others to amplify Daniel James's edited translation of Che Guevara's Bolivian diaries and
other associated documents which was first published in 1968. Waters's skilful editing
preserves Che's style, corrects inaccuracies that have since come to light, and among the
many varied publications issued during the nineties to mark the 30th anniversary of Che's
death in 1967, provides one of the best original sources of reference on the diaries now
available for English-speakers.

264 Che: a memoir by Fidel Castro.
Edited by David Deutschmann.   Melbourne: Ocean Press, 1994.
168p. (US distributor, New York: Talman Co.).

The book consists of a collection of excerpts from speeches, interviews, and writings by
Fidel Castro about Che Guevara. The two men first met in Mexico in 1955, and the

extracts reveal details of how the relationship began and developed. The text is well illustrated, and includes biographies of the main figures of the period.

265 Che Guevara: a revolutionary life.
Jon Lee Anderson.   New York: Grove Press, 1997. 814p. maps. bibliog.
A long and highly sympathetic biography of Che Guevara, based on many interviews, and on family and other archive sources in Argentina, Paraguay, Bolivia, Mexico, Cuba, Britain, Sweden, Russia, and the United States.

266 Pombo: a man of Che's *guerrilla*: with Che Guevara in Bolivia, 1966-68.
Pombo (*nom de guerre* of Harry Villegas Tamayo).   New York: Pathfinder, 1997. 365p. maps.
A detailed field journal of Che Guevara's Bolivian campaign by Harry Villegas, a young Cuban fighter and a key member of the would-be revolutionary unit both before and after Che's death in October 1967. The isolation, dangers, and helplessness of the group are clearly revealed in the diary's text and illustrations, which serve to underline the combination of ignorance and ineptitude that characterized the guerrillas' entire venture.

267 The fall of Che Guevara: a story of soldiers, spies, and diplomats.
Henry Butterfield Ryan.   New York: Oxford University Press, 1998. 224p. maps. bibliog.
Basing his study on newly released US government documents, including those of the State Department and the Central Intelligence Agency, Ryan reviews the history of US counter-insurgency practices as they developed after the Second World War. He goes on to examine the US responses, often uncertain and contradictory, to the activities of Che Guevara in Bolivia in 1966-67. In presenting a detailed and objective analysis of the roles of America's diplomatic and intelligence agencies at the time, the author provides a valuable addition to the substantial literature on Guevara, with additional incisive comment on other major personalities and events of the period.

Politics

268 Parties and political change in Bolivia, 1880-1952.
Herbert S. Klein. Cambridge: Cambridge University Press, 1962.
451p. bibliog.

The best available study in English of the political culture and the political system which existed in Bolivia in the seventy years before the MNR revolution. It examines the nature of intra-class political rivalries, the party structure, and the ideological considerations and position of the national and regional élites of Bolivia.

269 The Latin American military as a socio-political force: case studies of Bolivia and Argentina.
Charles Corbett. Coral Gables, Florida: Center for Advanced International Studies, University of Miami, 1972. 143p. bibliog.

Compares and contrasts the political role of the military in Bolivia and Argentina. The analysis combines an evaluation of professionalism, a consideration of the formation of political élites, and an examination of security doctrines. Also included is an historical review of the military's participation in 20th-century coups.

270 From national populism to national corporatism: the case of Bolivia: 1952-1970.
Melvin Burke, James M. Malloy. *Studies in Comparative International Development*, vol. 9, no. 1 (1974), p. 49-73.

Traces the developments in Bolivia during this period which turned a populist revolutionary government into a military regime. Political factionalism so weakened the parties that they turned to the military for support and opened the door for a *golpe de estado* (*coup d'état*).

271 The legacy of populism in Bolivia: from the MNR to military rule.
Christopher Mitchell.   New York: Praeger, 1977. 167p. map. bibliog.

This was the first English-language book on Bolivian populism to be fundamentally critical of Bolivia's most important populist party, the MNR (Movimiento Nacionalista Revolucionario). Mitchell examines the nature of the MNR, a party made up of heterogeneous forces but dominated by the middle class, which became conservative once it attained power and its most basic objectives were achieved in 1952-53. Focusing on events between the 1930s and the late 1970s, the study analyses the relationship between the MNR and the military, and the conflicts among various cross-class interest groups that created tension and raised obstacles to continued political coalition and stable government. Mitchell's argument is extended to place new emphasis on what he sees as the political continuity between the MNR's civilian populism and the military regimes after 1964 – 'a transition to an even more vigorous and rigid middle-class domination than existed before'.

272 Miners as voters: the electoral process in Bolivia's mining camps.
Laurence Whitehead.   *Journal of Latin American Studies,* vol. 13, no. 2 (1981), p. 313-46. bibliog.

An examination of the politicization of Bolivian miners prior to the MNR revolution of 1952. The 1940 elections were the key to turning miners into political activists and Víctor Paz Estenssoro was significant in bringing them into the MNR fold.

273 Bolivia: past, present, and future of its politics.
Robert Jackson Alexander.   New York: Praeger, 1982. 157p. bibliog.

A well-drawn, analytical political history of Bolivia by a noted scholar, which provides a general survey of the country before focusing in greater detail on the post-Chaco War era. This remains an excellent introduction to contemporary Bolivia.

274 Bolivia, 1980-1981: the political system in crisis.
James Dunkerley.   London: University of London Institute of Latin American Studies, 1982. 48p. (Working Paper, No. 8).

Dunkerley examines the collapse that year of the election process in Bolivia. The crisis stemmed from the inability of any of the political parties to overcome sectarianism and put forward a coherent political solution. This sectarianism has its roots in Bolivia's parliamentary tradition and the ambiguous legacy of the populist MNR movement.

275 **The Ciza and Ucureña War: syndical violence and national revolution in Bolivia.**
James V. Kohl. *The Hispanic American Historical Review*, vol. 62, no. 4 (1982), p. 607-28. bibliog.
Concentrates on the patronage system as it developed in rural Cochabamba during the 1952 revolution, and the political infighting in the *sindicato* (union movement) of the national revolution. The paper explores the high point of union power in rural areas, the nature of the power élites, and the ties between rural peasant leadership and the national movement.

276 **Oil and politics in Latin America: nationalist movements and state companies.**
George D. E. Philip. Cambridge: Cambridge University Press, 1982. 577p. maps. bibliog.
A very useful introduction to the politics of oil in modern Latin America. It includes a section on Bolivian oil and trade relations with Argentina to the end of the 1970s.

277 **Transformation of a revolution from below: Bolivia and international capital.**
Susan Eckstein. Boston, Massachusetts: *Comparative Studies in Society and History*, vol. 25, no. 1 (1983), p. 105-35.
Argues that, in the 1960s, foreign capital became so important to development that it contributed to the breakdown of the populist coalition which brought the MNR to power. In particular, capital benefited large-scale farmers who became a political force of some consequence. See also Susan Eckstein's 'Revolutions and the restructuring of national economies: the Latin American experience' (*Comparative Politics*, vol. 17 [July 1985], p. 473-94).

278 **Rebellion in the veins: political struggle in Bolivia, 1952-82.**
James Dunkerley. London: Verso, 1984. 385p. maps.
Describes a rich period in Bolivian development and the four major actors in Bolivia's contemporary drama: the MNR, the tin miners, the military and the United States. The book is strongest in its explanation of the details of MNR politics and the role of the United States. This work is solid and offers keen insights into Bolivian political evolution. Photographs and tables are also included.

279 **How the last became first.**
The Economist, vol. 312 (12 August 1989), p. 33, 36.
Examines the power play in the 1989 presidential election between Hugo Banzer, Gonzalo Sánchez de Lozada, and Jaime Paz Zamora. The last-named finished third but became president with the support of Banzer, who remains an influential figure behind the scenes. See also 'Toughing it out' (*The Economist*, vol. 311 [13 May 1989], p. 48, 73); and 'When a winner cries foul' (*The Economist*, vol. 312 [1 July 1989], p. 36).

280 Political transition and economic stabilisation: Bolivia, 1982-1989.

James Dunkerley. London: University of London Institute of Latin American Studies, 1990. 81p. bibliog. (Research Paper, No. 22).

Reviews party politics, party coalitions, and government changes in the 1980s, and provides a concise commentary on the state of the Bolivian economy both before and after the austerity measures and structural reforms introduced in 1985. Tables and appendices support the text.

281 Social revolution: a Latin American perspective.

Alan Knight. *Bulletin of Latin American Research*, vol. 9, no. 2 (1990), p. 175-202. bibliog.

Discusses the place of the Mexican, Bolivian, and Cuban revolutions within the broader category of social revolution in Europe and Asia, and then analyses the similarities and contrasts between the three Latin American examples themselves. Here, the author finds changing urban and rural class relations, rather than the drive towards new state construction, to be the key to social revolution in Latin America.

282 Taxes and state power: political instability in Bolivia, 1900-1950.

Carmenza Gallo. Philadelphia: Temple University Press, 1991. 174p. bibliog.

Explains the central features of Bolivia's state formation and political instability in the first half of the twentieth century, tracing the various alliances that developed during this period between the government, and the élite land-owning and mine-owning classes. The frail bureaucracy, the weaknesses of the tax structure and the widespread tax evasion were aggravated by Bolivia's regional frictions, appalling poverty, and the growing divisions within the army in the 1930s. Together, they helped to pave the way for social revolution as shown in this well-researched study, which is recommended for specialists in the field.

283 Bolivia's transformist revolution.

Fernando García Argañarás. *Latin American Perspectives*, vol. 19, no. 2 (1992), p. 44-71. bibliog.

A study of the period between the 1952 revolution and the mid-1960s which traces the changing policies, political alliances, and shifting class support during these years between the middle class, the mining and urban proletariat, and the military.

284 The divided world of the Bolivian Andes: a structural view of domination and resistance.

Dwight R. Hahn. New York: Crane Russak, 1992. 143p. bibliog.

Traces the growing political awareness among the Bolivian peasantry over a fifty-year period from the Chaco War in the 1930s to the mid-1980s, and secondly, since the agrarian reform of 1952-53, the changing nature of the relationships between capitalist and non-capitalist modes of production.

285 Letter from Bolivia.
Alma Guillermoprieto.   *The New Yorker*, vol. 68 (March 1992),
p. 95-107. map.

An excellent account for the general reader of the political and economic scene in Bolivia in the early 1990s. The author travelled widely to interview, among others, government personalities in La Paz, miners in Potosí and Porco, and coca growers in the Chapare. The writing is lively, the comments perceptive. Recommended to all those seeking an informative overview of Bolivia's problems and prospects, and how these affect the day-to-day lives of the people.

286 Democracy in the making? Political parties and political institutions in Bolivia, 1985-1991.
Domingo Villegas.   DPhil thesis, University of Oxford, England,
1993.

Presents an institutional analysis of Bolivian politics in the late eighties to early nineties which considers the extent to which democratic government had been consolidated since 1985. The author concludes that although it was still early days to estimate how durable the democratic system and its institutional changes would be, the new structures put in place over the six-year period were on the whole operative, and showing evidence of resilience.

287 The Bolivarian presidents: conversations and correspondence with presidents of Bolivia, Peru, Ecuador, Colombia, and Venezuela.
Robert Jackson Alexander.   Westport, Connecticut; London:
Praeger, 1994. 283p. bibliog.

In his section on Bolivia (p. 1-93), Alexander records his personal conversations and correspondence with Víctor Paz Estenssoro, Hernán Siles, René Barrientos, Luís Adolfo Siles, Walter Guevara Arce, Lidia Gueiller, and Jaime Paz Zamora. While most of the contacts recorded with these Bolivian presidents are very brief, Alexander's longest acquaintance and most extensive report is on Víctor Paz Estenssoro, and this comprises four-fifths of the Bolivian entry. Although disconnected, the conversations and letters have a refreshing informality and are of interest for the light they shed on the politics, economics and international affairs of their period, as well as for the frank opinions expressed about some of the prominent figures of the time.

288 Bolivia: structural reforms, fiscal impacts and economic growth.
Vicente Fretes Cibils, Deborah Bateman.   Washington, DC: World
Bank, 1994. 197p. map. (Document of the World Bank, 13067-130).

This paper provides an early, useful assessment of the Popular Participation Law of 20 April 1994, emphasizing its role as the vehicle of Bolivia's new decentralization process. The law completely 'municipalizes' the country, by creating 198 new municipalities to bring the national total up to 314, with responsibilities to administer, maintain and improve education, health and sports facilities, local roads, and irrigation works.

289 A door to a new millennium.
Wilson T. Boots.   *The Christian Century*, vol. 111, no. 12 (April 1994), p. 374-75.
Welcomes the inauguration in 1993 of an Aymara, Víctor Hugo Cárdenas, as the elected vice-president of Bolivia. In his formal address to the people to mark the occasion, Cárdenas had underlined the historical significance of an indigenous leader achieving such high office for the first time. He urged all Bolivians to develop an inclusive society, multi-ethnic and multilingual, stressing the point by delivering his address in four languages – Aymara, Quechua, Guaraní, and Spanish.

290 From populism to the coca economy in Bolivia.
Washington Estellano, translated by Kathryn Nava-Ragazzi.
Latin American Perspectives, vol. 21, no. 4 (1994), p. 34-45. bibliog.
A brisk, business-like survey which examines how the powerful populist coalition of workers, miners and peasants of the 1952 revolution was weakened, and in part shattered politically, by the growth of a new military right wing, and by the force of the New Economic Policy led by Paz Estenssoro after 1985. Finally, the study considers the degree of success achieved by these austerity measures, and the crucial input of the coca/cocaine industry into the national economy by the 1990s.

291 Tradition and revolution: the struggle for community control at Bolivia's Chojlla mine, 1944-1964.
Andrew Patrick Boeger.   PhD thesis, University of Texas at Austin, 1994. 335p. bibliog.
Traces the growth of community spirit and revolutionary action at the Chojlla mine both before and after the social revolution of 1952. This is a useful case-study of Bolivian miners' grassroots politics, since the research is extended into the reactions of the Chojlla miners to falling mineral prices and to heavy lay-offs in the 1950s and early 1960s.

292 Bolivia: making the leap from local mobilization to national politics.
Xavier Albó.   *NACLA Report on the Americas* (North American Congress on Latin America), vol. 29, no. 5 (March/April 1996), p. 15-20.
The 1990s witnessed increasing protest from indigenous groups in lowland Bolivia over encroachment by logging companies on their traditional lands, but Albó observes that demonstrations and marches achieve little in the long run; protesters need to hone their political skills. New opportunities to do this may be at hand. The Educational Reform Law and the Popular Participation Law both aim to decentralize power to hundreds of new municipalities. The legislation has had a mixed reception, but time is needed to show how effective these new initiatives can become at local level.

293 Bolivia's silent revolution.
René Antonio Mayorga. *Journal of Democracy*, vol. 8, no. 1 (1997), p. 142-56. bibliog.

Here, the term 'silent revolution' is applied to Bolivian politics since the mid-1980s. While noting the economic reforms in this period, the author concentrates on the extent to which Bolivia is developing a moderate, as opposed to a polarized and fractured, party system. He examines internal party organization and finds that political parties in general have become much less ideological and class-based. Even so, old habits die hard; problems of patronage, bureaucratic inefficiency, and bloated state payrolls persist in some sectors. The administration of justice is still slow and often corrupt. The New Economic Policy since 1985 has not yet managed to achieve all that its architects hoped for, while the labour movement contains many disaffected and radicalized groups. Mayorga offers a comprehensive and well-balanced assessment suited to both the general and more specialized reader. More reforms are needed, but the article is largely optimistic in tone.

294 Hybrid presidentialism and democratization: the case of Bolivia.
Eduardo A. Gamarra. In: *Presidentialism and democracy in Latin America*. Edited by Scott Mainwaring, Matthew Sobert Shugart. Cambridge: Cambridge University Press, 1997, p. 363-93. bibliog.

Examines the complex nature of the Bolivian presidential system which combines features of both presidentialism and parliamentarism. Gamarra reviews the period from the late 1970s to the late 1990s, including the electoral laws and party system, the state bureaucracy, the economic crises, and the powerful patronage networks. With nearly thirty political parties in Bolivia and the fragility of many coalitions, the key role small parties can play in the election of the president becomes a crucial factor in the process. This is a clear and detailed survey for those specializing in the intricacies of Bolivian political institutions.

295 Latin American political yearbook, 1997.
Edited by Robert G. Breene, Jr. New Brunswick, New Jersey: Transaction Publishers, 1998. 290p.

This specialized yearbook, the first in a new series, covers the whole of 1996 and provides a chronological record of events for those requiring detailed information on the political parties, elections, trade, and economic developments that were of importance during that year. Yearbook 1998, covering 1997 and published in 1999, is much enlarged and includes more information on Latin America's regional organizations. The editor is head of the Latin American News Syndicate in San Antonio, Texas.

296 A new time and place for Bolivian popular politics: an introduction.
Robert Albro. *Ethnology*, vol. 37, no. 2 (1998), p. 99-115. bibliog.

Reviews the on-going, if locally uneven, development of national citizen awareness in Bolivia since the 1950s, including the role of the *Kataristas*, named after the 18th-century rebel Tupac Katari (the title adopted by the Aymara leader, Julián Apaza, to link the 1780-83 uprising with the earlier Aymara protest farther south led by the Katari family). Among the new wave of *Kataristas* were young Aymara students in the city of La Paz. Far from rejecting their past in the pursuit of a modern identity, they drew deeply during the 1970s and 1980s on the Aymaras' collective historical memory, forging a new urban–rural linkage in their search for a shared heritage and for new political inspiration.

297 The 1997 Bolivian election in historical perspective.
James Dunkerley. London: University of London Institute of Latin American Studies, 1998. 35p. bibliog. (Occasional Paper, No. 16).
Concentrating on the decade or so preceding the 1997 election, Dunkerley presents a crisp overview both of the political parties and personalities of the period, and of the sweeping economic and administrative changes which provided the context of events, including the Popular Participation Law and the Capitalization legislation of 1994. The final section on the death of Che Guevara and on Bolívar is misplaced, however; it is not convincingly related to the theme of the paper, and weakens the impact of an otherwise well-focused analysis.

298 Colonial legacies and plurinational imaginaries: indigenous movement politics in Ecuador and Bolivia.
Robert James Andolina. PhD thesis, University of Minnesota, Minneapolis, Minnesota, 1999. 385p. bibliog.
The author traces the formation and behaviour of contemporary indigenous people's movements in Ecuador and Bolivia, including the surviving influences from colonial times, and the manner in which indigenous movements today enlist the support of other agencies such as labour unions, non-governmental organizations, and selected political parties. The trend, he argues, is away from traditional protests, boycotts, and armed struggle, towards the forging of new, more sophisticated political alliances. Several good points are made, although Andolina dismisses too readily the results that can be achieved by peaceful mass protest when the issues touch the wider interests of Bolivia's population.

299 Hazarding popular spirits: metaforces of political culture and cultural politicking in Quillacollo, Bolivia.
Robert D. Albro. PhD thesis, University of Chicago, Chicago, Illinois, 1999. 664p. bibliog.
A case-study based on the provincial capital of Quillacollo, Department of Cochabamba, showing how successful local politicians juggle populism and ethnic interests. Albro contends that much depends on the leader's ability to move back and forth across cultural boundaries, and to remain sensitive to, and locally to exploit, rival *mestizo* and urban *cholo* factions.

300 Local misrule.
The Economist, vol. 352 (31 July 1999), p. 52, 54.
The Bolivian government's decentralization policy has involved a major shift of responsibility from central to local government, and this has exposed differing levels of inexperience, inefficiency and corruption in municipal administration, along with the urgent need to do something about them. Political, often short-term, appointments to the mayor's office are a major weakness, since they encourage showy projects at the expense of routine maintenance. The case of La Paz is considered here, with fourteen mayors in twelve years, and the growing risk of eclipse by Santa Cruz as foreign companies

increasingly choose to set up in the eastern city, not only because of its lower altitude but because it is seen as being better organized and more sympathetic to business. The report stresses the need for a career civil service at local government level if decentralization is to succeed, and notes that the Bolivian Congress is now considering a local government reform bill.

301 An overdue reform of justice.
The Economist, vol. 351 (10 April 1999), p. 32, 34.

Bolivia's political élite have long fought, and still fight, to maintain their influence on the country's judicial system. With the recent appointment of a people's ombudsman, a constitutional tribunal, and an independent judicial council, the Banzer administration hopes to achieve a much-needed reform of the judiciary, and also greater accountability of the police force, by the year 2001. While some international observers agree that Bolivia is now on the right road to reform of its justice system, all acknowledge that fundamental progress is likely to be slow.

302 The political analysis of legal pluralism in Bolivia and Colombia.
Donna Lee Van Cott. *Journal of Latin American Studies*, vol. 32, no. 1 (2000), p. 207-34. bibliog.

Takes up the issue of the difficulties faced by the state in its efforts to find the best way to incorporate different ethnic groups within the population into a single polity without threatening, or extinguishing, the groups' cherished identities. As this useful comparative study shows, the key difference is the size of the indigenous populations. Unlike those in Colombia, Bolivia's Indians form the majority of the population; they are also more rural and more widely dispersed. Legislation to modernize the Bolivian judicial system was prepared in 1994 during the Sánchez de Lozada administration, and subsequently introduced by President Banzer, but implementation has proved difficult, particularly the coordination of indigenous and national jurisdictions. When faced with deadlock, the author notes, 'the tradition in Bolivia is to negotiate rather than adjudicate'. Community solidarity, isolation, and the low priority among many judges given to acquiring expertise in legal pluralism or multiculturalism, all widen the gap between the theory and practice of the law.

303 Resistance and the arts of domination: miners and the Bolivian state.
Harry Sanabria. *Latin American Perspectives*, vol. 27, no. 1 (2000), p. 56-81. bibliog.

Sanabria's stated purpose at the outset 'is to suggest that we center more of our efforts on *ineffective* and *unsuccessful* resistance in order to understand better the contexts in which successful resistance can be achieved'. But his chosen example – the continuing weakness of the Bolivian miners' organized labour movement when confronting neoliberal government policies – is not an instructive case-study for finding a formula for successful resistance, given the national and international causes for the collapse of tin mining in the mid-1980s. In fact, the author does not pursue his intended line of enquiry to the end. Instead, in an article that is more descriptive than analytical, Sanabria reviews how neoliberal politics, economics, and ideology combined to frame and implement a policy of 'destroying state mining and smashing miners'.

304   The UDP government and the crisis of the Bolivian Left (1982-1985).
Enrique Ibáñez Rojo.   *Journal of Latin American Studies*, vol. 32, no. 1 (2000), p. 175-205. bibliog.

A perceptive account of the chaotic period in the early 1980s during which the powerful Central Obrera Boliviana (COB) moved to open confrontation with the Unión Democrática y Popular (UDP) – a new, weak, democratically elected coalition government whose attempts to arrest economic decline were vetoed by the COB with ritual demands for higher wages. Ibáñez Rojo contends that sharper political skills among the union's leadership could have stemmed the COB's dramatic loss of power. Its decline into a mainly spent force after 1985 is one of the remarkable features of recent Bolivian politics. In effect, the author argues that the COB dug its own grave.

Foreign Relations

General

305 Latin American diplomatic history: an introduction.
Harold Eugene Davis, John J. Finan, F. Taylor Peck.   Baton Rouge,
Louisiana: Louisiana State University Press, 1977. 301p. bibliog.

Emphasizes foreign relations among Latin American countries rather than their ties to
external states, although as the study moves on to the 20th century, the authors discuss
Latin America in wider perspective, notably the effects on the region of the Great
Depression, the Second World War, the Cold War, and the Alliance for Progress. For
Bolivia, the book concentrates on the War of the Santa Cruz Confederation (1836-39), the
War of the Pacific (1879-84), and the Chaco War (1932-35).

306 Hacia una nueva política exterior Boliviana. (Towards a new
foreign policy for Bolivia.)
Fernando Salazar Paredes.   La Paz: Ediciones CERID, 2000.
1249p. maps. bibliog.

A scholarly, comprehensive study by a noted Bolivian academic and diplomat which
examines Bolivia's relations with its immediate neighbours from the time of
Independence to the present day, as well as relations with the United States, the European
Union, and other international organizations. This is an objective analysis that assesses
past failures and identifies new priorities. Two-thirds of the volume comprises the texts
of Bolivia's major diplomatic treaties and other documents since 1825.

With the United States

307   In defense of neutral rights: the United States Navy and the wars of independence in Chile and Peru.
Edward Baxter Billingsley.   Chapel Hill, North Carolina: University of North Carolina Press, 1967. 266p. map. bibliog.

Examines the nature of US naval operations off the coasts of Chile and Peru during the Independence period, where the main concern was to minimize the interruption to United States commerce. Meetings between US Naval officers and major figures engaged in the fighting, both Royalist and Revolutionary, are recorded in this well-researched study, which also analyses the events' short-term and long-term impact on inter-American relations.

308   My missions for revolutionary Bolivia, 1944-1962.
Víctor Andrade.   Pittsburgh, Pennsylvania: University of Pittsburgh Press, 1976. 200p. (Pitt Latin American Series).

Víctor Andrade, Bolivian ambassador to the United States at intervals between 1944 and 1962, offers a unique perspective on United States–Bolivian relations during this period. The book contains candid, and often awkward, views of United States foreign policies and actions. It also includes records of meetings with Franklin D. Roosevelt, Truman, and Eisenhower, as well as accounts of how Andrade negotiated massive economic and military aid for Bolivia after the MNR revolution of 1952.

309   The United States and the Andean republics: Peru, Bolivia, and Ecuador.
Fredrick B. Pike.   Cambridge, Massachusetts: Harvard University Press, 1977. 493p. maps. bibliog.

This book presents the reader with much more than the title suggests. Pike provides an excellent comparative study of the political and cultural development of the three republics from Independence to the mid-1970s, and shows how Andean cultural patterns contrast sharply with those of the United States. From these contrasts in culture ensues a great deal of incompatibility between the two regions and prospects for reducing this incompatibility are seen as slight.

310   The dismantling of the Good Neighbor Policy.
Bryce Wood.   Austin, Texas: University of Texas Press, 1985. 290p. bibliog.

This volume is based on documents from the US National Archives and State Department, and the Public Record Office in London, enabling Wood to provide the conclusion to his classic study, *The making of the Good Neighbor Policy*. The policy remained in effect during the Second World War (with the notable exception of Argentina), was codified in the Charter of the OAS in 1948, and reasserted by President Truman in 1948-50. Wood includes an interesting section on events in 1954 when the Good Neighbor Policy began to be dismantled in Guatemala but was continued in Bolivia, a decision influenced by the non-Communist nature of the MNR's Social Revolution, a favourable report by the President's brother, Milton Eisenhower, and the positive role played by Bolivia's Ambassador in Washington, Víctor Andrade. After 1954, however, the term 'Good Neighbor Policy' was dropped.

311 Decisions on intervention: United States response to Third World nationalist governments, 1950-1957.
John Stephen Zunes.   PhD thesis, Cornell University, Ithaca, New York, 1990. 472p. bibliog.

This is a carefully researched and well-reasoned commentary on contrasted aspects of United States foreign policy during the 1950s. Two sets of examples are examined, one of non-intervention, the other of intervention by the United States – Bolivia and Guatemala, and Iran and Egypt – with discussion of the dominant arguments in Washington in each case.

312 Dependent revolution: the United States and radical change in Bolivia and Cuba.
Jennifer Leigh Bailey.   PhD thesis, University of Denver, Denver, Colorado, 1990. 410p. bibliog.

Selecting two major revolutionary movements in Latin America during the 1950s, Bailey contrasts the United States reaction to the Bolivian National and Social Revolution of 1952-53, with its reaction to the Cuban revolution of 1959. She considers geographical location, and the differing pre-revolutionary relationships of the two states with the USA, against the backdrop of global politics in this eventful decade.

313 A hemisphere to itself: a history of US–Latin American relations.
Frank Niess, translated by Harry Drost.   London; Atlantic Highlands, New Jersey: Zed Books, 1986, 1990, 229p. maps. bibliog.

Translated from a text first published in Germany, this study provides a concise overview of the history of United States–Latin American relations since the Monroe Doctrine of 1823. As Niess observes, what contemporary historians and political analysts formally and euphemistically call the 'asymmetry of power' between the two regions has led to a turbulent relationship between two unequal neighbours, to say nothing of the secondary ranking by the United States caused by the huge internal inequalities within Latin America itself. Here, Niess bases his analysis on the conflict between the industrialized North and the developing South in a clearly written, informative volume of value both to students and to the general reader.

314 The United States and the Bolivian revolutionaries, 1943-1954: from hostility to accommodation to assistance.
Naoki Kamimura.   PhD thesis, University of California, Los Angeles, 1991. 640p. bibliog.

A study of the dramatically changing attitudes towards Bolivia shown by the United States during this ten-year period. The author traces at length the influences and decision-making in Washington, DC under the Eisenhower administration which eventually led to

American political support and economic assistance for the Bolivian National and Social Revolution of 1952-53.

315 The United States and Latin America: myths and stereotypes of civilization and nature.
Fredrick B. Pike. Austin, Texas: University of Texas Press, 1992. 442p. bibliog.

The author brings a lifetime of scholarship to this polished, stimulating study of United States–Latin American relationships, which combines a masterly grasp of events with shrewd insights into the contrasted cultural heritage, and the rocky sequence of economic and diplomatic exchanges that have marked the last 200 years. Pike is even-handed in his praise and his criticisms. Overt and more subtle images of the frontier over time underpin some of the most powerful myths and stereotypes associated with the value systems of the two regions, and these, along with other influences, are analysed in Pike's rich brew of history, politics, literature, music and art. Changing perceptions chase each other down the years but often provide only new variations on old themes. Indeed, Pike finally admits that, in the early 1990s, he cannot perceive a clearly happy ending for the story of American hemispheric relations. The book closes on a reflective note, particularly over the unprecedented surge of Hispanic immigration into the United States. Undoubtedly, a depression or even a stiff recession would sharpen US prejudice against this influx, but 'even if depression is avoided, Americans will continue to disagree, sometimes passionately, over whether [Hispanic] immigration constitutes an economic boon or the lamentable transfer of Third World conditions to the United States'. This thought-provoking assessment of 19th- and 20th-century attitudes and imagery is recommended to all who are interested in the development of the United States' relationships with the countries of Latin America.

316 United States trade and investment in Latin America: opportunities for business in the 1990s.
Chris C. Carvounis, Brinda Z. Carvounis. Westport, Connecticut: Quorum Books, 1992. 200p. bibliog.

A brisk, systematic analysis and ranking of those states of Latin America which are identified by the authors as justifying US investment under the Enterprise for the Americas Initiative (EAI). The placing of Bolivia among the 'first-tier' candidates for such investment is not based on the size or vibrancy of its economy, nor even on the country's potential to develop one. Instead, it is based on the degree of success achieved by Paz Estenssoro's economic reform package of 1985 – 'pioneering, bold, and (initially at least) a solo flight'. This is not a rose-tinted assessment, nor are the problems of restoring growth in the Bolivian economy played down, but fundamental groundwork is judged to be firmly in place. The book's wide coverage of the Latin American states allows valid comparisons of their different economies to be made, while there is also a useful introductory chapter on the significance to the United States of increasing global economic regionalism, and its likely impact on future US–Latin American trade relations.

317 Bolivia and the United States: a limited partnership.
Kenneth D. Lehman. Athens, Georgia: University of Georgia
Press, 1999. 296p. map. bibliog.

A thoughtful and well-written analysis of the uneven relationship between the United States and Bolivia, which surveys the diplomatic history of the 19th and 20th centuries before concentrating on events in the last twenty-five years. Lehman's stated intention is to examine in more detail the period since the publication of Pike's important work in 1977 (item no. 309), while concentrating exclusively on the US–Bolivia relationship. This is an articulate commentary on the new challenges that have emerged in the late 20th century. 'Different and distant' has long summed up the opinion of both states about each other. Now, Lehman finds a degree of change and fresh optimism in the relationship: 'Never has there been a time so opportune or so appropriate for Bolivia and the United States to transcend the patron–client features that have consistently limited true partnership to this point.'

318 The second century: US–Latin American relations since 1889.
Mark T. Gilderhus. Wilmington, Delaware: Scholarly Resources,
2000. 282p. bibliog.

A deft analysis of 20th-century relations between the United States and Latin America which captures the self-interest, good intentions, false assumptions, and stark realities which characterized the period. The author examines the core issues of commerce, politics, and security from the 1889 Pan American Conference and Spanish-American War, to the Good Neighbor Policy, the Second World War, the Cold War and Cuban crisis, the post-Cold War period and the 1990s NAFTA agreements. Gilderhus pegs his analysis to the historical sequence of US Presidents and their advisers, as he discusses the building, demolition, or tinkering with the country's policies towards Latin America throughout the 20th century. Given the United States' continuing dominance in the political, commercial, and technological fields, among others, little change is expected in the future, although Gilderhus raises the question of what effect the huge influx into the United States of illegal Latin American immigrants, mainly Mexican, may soon have on US attitudes, and on US society itself. The author brings a sure touch and a fluent style to this study, which should attract a wide readership.

See also items 545-54 on US–Bolivia relations on the drugs issue.

The Andean Community and MERCOSUR

319 The Andean Pact: a selected bibliography.
Compiled by Elizabeth G. Ferris. *Latin American Research
Review*, vol. 13, no. 3 (1978), p. 108-24.

The creation of the Andean Pact in 1969 attracted renewed interest in Latin American integration, with scholars approaching the study of the Pact from different academic disciplines, ideological positions, and methodological backgrounds. Initially descriptive in nature, the commentaries gradually became more analytical as crises and dilemmas plagued the group. Ferris's bibliography, after a 10-year period, draws on a wide range of publications in English and Spanish which she groups into general studies, studies of specific Andean Pact programmes, and studies of individual member states' experiences within the Pact. This is an indispensable source of reference (by no means exclusively bibliographical) for those examining the early evolution of the Andean Pact.

320 The Andean Group at the ten year mark.
Gordon Mace. *International Perspectives* (Ottawa), September-December 1979, p. 30-34.

The Cartagena Agreement of 1969 initiated the process of economic integration among Andean Pact members. The encouraging progress of the first four years ended in 1974, primarily because of changes in the economic development models of member nations and also because of the loss of Chile as a Pact member. At the end of the 1970s, the Pact has been unable to avoid the difficulties that have affected similar efforts in the Third World.

321 National support for the Andean Pact.
Elizabeth G. Ferris. *Journal of Developing Areas*, vol. 16, no. 2 (1982), p. 249-70.

An update specifically on Bolivian participation in the Andean Pact.

322 The politics of crisis and cooperation in the Andean Group.
William P. Avery. *Journal of Developing Areas*, vol. 17, no. 2 (1983), p. 155-84.

Progress towards regional co-operation has halted because of profound political and economic problems in the area. The instability of member governments, and the fact that systems of government range from military dictatorships to democracies, make co-operation very difficult.

323 Whither the Andean Pact?
Thomas G. Sanders. Indianapolis, Indiana: *UFSI Reports* (1985). 10p.

The post-1980 recession has posed the greatest challenge yet to the Pact's survival, though new initiatives, such as those presented by the Andean Business Consultation Council, hold some promise for the future.

324 The potential of biotechnology for mining in developing countries: the case of the Andean Pact Copper Project.
A. C. Warhurst. PhD thesis, University of Sussex, England, 1986.

Advances in biotechnology present opportunities for developing countries to exploit the emerging potential of bacterial leaching, in this case, of copper. Bacterial leaching is a low-cost technology which extracts residue metals from ancient mine dumps, a process that can be increased by using specially designed heaps or confined systems. The Andean Pact Copper Project was a unique collaborative programme of technology development in bacterial leaching undertaken by Bolivia and Peru in the 1970s; its added purpose was to foster Andean Pact integration.

325 An empirical evaluation of the trade effects of the Andean Trade Preference Act.
Kefu Wu.   PhD thesis, University of Arkansas, Fayetteville, Arkansas, 1993. 87p. bibliog.

Under the provisions of the United States' Andean Trade Preference Act (effective 4 December 1991), the US government introduced some duty-free imports from Bolivia, Colombia, Ecuador and Peru in order to encourage an increase in legal exports through diversification into non-traditional sectors, e.g. the fish and vegetable industries, cut flowers, clothing, and iron and steel. The author's early analysis suggests that the duty-free list was too narrowly based; the impact on trade is likely to be disappointing, with Colombian cut-flower export destined to become the main beneficiary.

326 Evaluating Bolivia's choices for trade integration.
Sarath Rajapatirana.   Washington, DC: World Bank; Operations Policy Department, Operations Policy Group, 1996. 36p. bibliog. (Policy Research Working Papers, No. 1632).

Debates Bolivia's trading options with reference to the Andean Group and to MERCOSUR (the Southern Common Market), noting that MERCOSUR, whose full members are Argentina, Brazil, Paraguay and Uruguay, dominates both Bolivia's import and export trade. Internally, however, Bolivia's commercial and political interests are divided, and links to the Andean Group are unlikely to be severed. Negotiation which maintains membership of the Andean Group while seeking preferential access to MERCOSUR is advised here.

327 Business guide to MERCOSUR: research report.
New York: Economist Intelligence Unit, 1998. 99p.

A comprehensive analysis of the membership, functioning, market opportunities, infrastructure, future potential, and obstacles to integration in this Southern Common Market, created in 1991. Chile has joined Argentina, Brazil, Paraguay, and Uruguay (though as an associate member of MERCOSUR), while Bolivia also became an associate member in 1996, and aspires to full membership. The report concludes that Bolivia, the poorest member of the group, has much to gain as a partner in MERCOSUR. This is a sound, balanced piece of research, a valuable source of information and comment both for the specialist and the general reader.

328 The Alfonsín administration and the promotion of democratic values in the Southern Cone and the Andes.
Dominique Fournier.   *Journal of Latin American Studies*, vol. 31, no. 1 (1999), p. 39-74. bibliog.

A well-focused review of Argentina's bilateral foreign policies with its immediate neighbours during President Raúl Alfonsín's administration (1983-89), which followed the defeat of Argentina's military dictatorship. Relations with Brazil, Uruguay, Paraguay, Bolivia, and Chile are discussed in turn, the author arguing that Argentina's strategy to defend and promote democratic values was framed both on principle, and on the need to strengthen its own fragile democracy at a time in the early 1980s when most of Argentina's neighbours were still ruled by the military. Alfonsín's efforts met with varying degrees of success but helped to pave the way, Fournier suggests, for the creation of MERCOSUR's regional common market agreement in 1991. Although the undoubted added force of international pressure upon the region as a whole to adopt democratic institutions is not considered here, the author provides a helpful analysis for the student of Latin American politics, of Argentina's own bilateral diplomatic initiatives during this critical transitional period to democracy.

329 How to do business in the Andean Community: trade and investment guide.
Lima: Andean Community General Secretariat, 1999. 187p.
The Andean Pact (Andean Group), created by the Cartagena Agreement in May 1969 between Bolivia, Chile (which later withdrew), Colombia, Ecuador, Peru and Venezuela, was reformed as the Andean Nations Community in June 1997. This is a detailed prospectus of the Community – its membership, objectives (both economic and political), institutions, economy, tariffs, and foreign policy. Prepared specifically for trading partners and foreign investors, the guide is a good, informative source of reference in English for those seeking background on the Andean Community.

Non-governmental organizations

330 To stem the tide of world suffering.
James M. Wall. *The Christian Century*, vol. 109, no. 25 (1992), p. 763-65.
By the early 1990s, a growing number of non-governmental organizations (NGOs) from the United States were working in Bolivia. The author studied the activities of two of them, the Christian Children's Fund and the Andean Rural Health Care programme, finding that such organizations are often closer and more sensitive to the needs and hopes of local people than the official US government aid networks. Wall therefore urges government officials to consult more frequently with the NGOs working in Bolivia, even when no financial support is available to help these non-governmental agencies, in order to make the best use of official US funding.

331 Non-governmental organizations and the state in Latin America: rethinking roles in sustainable agricultural development.
Anthony Bebbington, Graham Thiele, Penelope Davies, Martin Prager, Hernando Riveros. London; New York: Routledge, 1993. 290p. map. bibliog. (Overseas Development Institute Non-Governmental Organizations Series).
This excellent study focuses on three major issues: the extreme poverty of many rural areas in Latin America; the help that collaboration between the state and non-governmental organizations (NGOs) can provide; and the pitfalls that such collaboration

can create. The proliferation of NGOs in Latin America has been spectacular, leading in some places to duplication of activities and a total lack of co-ordination. More interaction between NGOs, and between NGOs and government institutions, is called for here. The authors' presentation of their material is exceptionally clear, with the main text interspersed with boxed insertions which present case-studies drawn from the whole region, together with notes on the points such case-studies reveal. In Bolivia, projects in the Alto Beni, Chapare, Santa Cruz and the eastern lowlands are examined in relation to the methods adopted to improve rural technology and the modernization of agriculture. The book is effective on both the theoretical and practical levels. It pulls no punches, but remains fair and even-handed, offering sound analysis, judicious comment, and concrete recommendations.

332 Non-governmental organizations and poverty in Bolivia.
Sonia Arellano-López, James F. Petras. *Development and Change*, vol. 25, no. 3 (1994), p. 555-68. bibliog.

Despite the central role played by non-governmental organizations (NGOs) established to alleviate poverty in Bolivia during the 1980s and early 1990s, the authors question whether NGOs are now any more successful than state agencies in maintaining direct contact with the country's many poor local communities. As massive international aid was increasingly awarded to Bolivia after the mid-1980s, NGOs strengthened their links with the international donors and with central government rather than with grassroots organizations, which, it is claimed, became politically marginalized by the relative weakening of their direct contact with the state agencies. The authors present a sweeping judgement, without examples or exceptions. In fact, notable differences are to be found among the hundreds of non-governmental organizations working in Bolivia, including those working in cooperation with state agencies at local level. Despite some valid points, the argument is weakened by its blanket generalization.

333 Falling from grace? The political economy of non-governmental organizations: a study of competition and dysfunction in Bolivia.
Guillermo Francisco Monje. PhD thesis, Ohio State University, Columbus, Ohio, 1995. 191p. bibliog.

Two sites in Bolivia were chosen at which various non-governmental organizations (NGOs) and government programmes were all serving the same poor, rural population. This discussion concentrates on the role of the NGOs, and examines the difficulties that can arise locally where their individual policies are incompatible, and where NGOs are forced to compete with each other for scarce international funding.

334 The debt-for-nature swap experience: structuring a transnational domain.
Tamara A. Hennings. PhD thesis, University of Pennsylvania, Philadelphia, Pennsylvania, 1996. 290p. bibliog.

Focuses on some of the ways in which debt-for-nature agreements (in Bolivia and Costa Rica) promote new and improved working relationships between non-governmental organizations (NGOs), international funding bodies, and national governments.

335 Linking livelihood strategies to development: experiences from the Bolivian Andes.
Annelies Zoomers.   Amsterdam: Royal Tropical Institute/Centre for Latin American Research and Documentation (CEDLA), 1999. 107p. map. bibliog.

A gritty piece of self-analysis by an experienced rural agricultural adviser in Bolivia who acknowledges that project designers, though well-intentioned, often adopt an incomplete or biased view of the local situation and the local priorities. She reports the findings of a joint Bolivian-Dutch research team working between 1983 and 1997 in the Departments of Chuquisaca and Potosí, and asks how meaningful many agency projects are to the farmers themselves. Are the suggested strategies what they want and need? This is a well-balanced, objective study which stresses that the *campesinos'* rejection of a particular project does not mean that they are resistant to change.

Population and Other Statistics

336 Anuario estadístico. (Statistical yearbook for Bolivia.)
La Paz: Instituto Nacional de Estadística, 630p. maps.
This is the primary source of the official national statistics on Bolivia. These detailed figures are prefaced by a series of coloured maps of the country and of each of its nine departments, which also show the provincial subdivisions and the municipal regions. The social statistics record population, standards of living, health and nutrition, education, employment, and social security provision. The economic statistics include agriculture, mining, industry, construction, transport, tourism, trade, government accounts, and banking.

337 Estadísticas socio-económicas. (Socio-economic statistics.)
La Paz: Muller & Asociados/Banco Santa Cruz. 428p. Published annually.
A useful abstract of the official Bolivian national socio-economic statistics presented in a handy compact form, and well supported with graphs and diagrams.

338 International financial statistics.
Washington, DC: International Monetary Fund. Published monthly, and as an annual volume (c. 830p.).
This is the IMF's principal statistical publication, and has been published since 1948 in English, French and Spanish. As a standard source of statistics on all aspects of international and domestic finance, the volumes and reports include data on a state's exchange rates, financial position, international liquidity, money and banking accounts, interest rates, prices, production, labour, international transactions, government finance, and national accounting. Bolivia is covered both in the World Tables, and at length in the Country Tables.

339 Statistical abstract of Latin America.
Edited by James W. Wilkie. Los Angeles: UCLA Latin American Center Publications. Published annually.

An excellent standard source of statistical information on Latin America. The individual countries are listed in the tabulated entries on a comprehensive range of topics: (1) Geography, land, and environment; (2) Transportation and communication; (3) Population, health, and education; (4) Politics, religion, and the military; (5) Working conditions and migration; (6) Illegal and legal industry; (7) Mining, energy, sea, and land production; (8) Foreign trade; (9) Financial flows; (10) National accounts, government policy and finance, and prices. The volume concludes with a number of individual essays on themes of current interest.

340 Statistical yearbook for Latin America and the Caribbean.
New York: United Nations Economic Commission for Latin America and the Caribbean.

Published annually in English and Spanish, this standard reference presents a compilation of demographic and social statistics for each state in the region, along with detailed information on its economy, resources, trade and transport. A list of the indicators applied for making a periodic appraisal of the development process in the region as a whole is also included.

341 A guide to Latin American and Caribbean census material.
Edited by Carole Travis. London: The British Library, Standing Conference of National and University Libraries/University of London Institute of Latin American Studies; Boston: G. K. Hall, 1990. bibliog.

The entry for Bolivia (p. 118-27) records the history of census-taking in the country from the general census of the Provinces in Upper Peru in 1796. This is followed by a list of Bolivia's subsequent census publications, including national, regional, departmental, urban, and special surveys.

342 Bolivia: situación de la población de la tercera edad.
(The condition of Bolivia's third-age population.)
La Paz: Instituto Nacional de Estadística, Ministerio de Hacienda, in association with the United Nations Population Fund, 1998. 63p.

Presents data on the demographic, social, and economic characteristics of Bolivia's population aged 60 and over, together with population projections and social security. The report is based on 1976 and 1992 census data.

343 Primer censo de gobiernos municipales. (First census of municipal governments.)
La Paz: Ministerio de Hacienda, Ministerio de Desarrollo Sostenible y Planificación, 1998. 297p.

Provides the first comprehensive data on Bolivia's new municipal governments – their services, business establishments, infrastructure, existing development, government information systems, government employees, tax payers, budget, and development projects. See also *Bolivia: un mundo de potencialidades. Atlas estadístico de municipios* (item no. 67).

Ethnic Groups and Minorities

Indigenous Indian population

344 The aboriginal cultural geography of the Llanos de Mojos of Bolivia.
William M. Denevan. Berkeley, Los Angeles: University of California Press, 1966. 160p. maps. bibliog. (Ibero-Americana Series, No. 48).

This monograph provides an excellent example of cultural geography, demonstrating as it does how well geography, anthropology, and archaeology can serve each other. Based on extensive field research, Denevan reviews the physical characteristics of the Llanos (plains) de Mojos, and the early settlement and organization of these Indian communities in a region that would later approximate to the Department of Beni. He then examines in detail the indigenous population's early economy, and the village patterns, mounds, causeways, canals, and field systems that were constructed in these huge, seasonally flooded savannahs. This is a scholarly study, well supported by striking air and ground photographs.

345 The Bolivian Aymara.
Hans C. Buechler, Judith-Maria Buechler. New York: Holt, Rinehart & Winston, 1971. 114p. map. bibliog. (Case Studies in Cultural Anthropology).

This study by two noted anthropologists remains an engaging introduction for the general reader to the Aymara peasant society of highland Bolivia. It can also be read as a more detailed community analysis of Compi, on the shores of Lake Titicaca, particularly of its kinship, ritual and agricultural networks. The authors trace the settlement's evolution from the colonial *hacienda* era to the major changes that occurred in Compi's land-holding system and market economy after the Agrarian Reform of 1953.

346 Andean kinship and marriage.
Ralph Bolton, Enrique Mayer. Washington, DC: American
Anthropological Association, 1977. 298p. maps. bibliog.
A book of essays by noted Andean anthropologists, which had previously been circulated
privately among scholars. Essays include: Lambert's 'Bilaterality in the Andes' (p. 1-27);
William E. Carter's 'Trial marriage in the Andes'; Ralph Bolton's 'The Qolla marriage
process' (p. 217-35); William T. Stuart's and John M. Hickman's 'Descent, alliance and
moiety in Chucuito, Peru – an explanatory sketch of Aymara social organization' (p. 43-
59); and Norman Long's 'Commerce and kinship in the Peruvian highland' (p. 153-76).
A section entitled 'References cited' represents an important bibliographical tool.

**347 At the crossroads of the earth and the sky: an Andean
cosmology.**
Gary Dwayne Urton. Austin, Texas: University of Texas Press,
1981. 248p. maps. bibliog.
A study of indigenous religious beliefs that presents considerable detail of interest to the
specialist on Inca and Quechua cosmology. Among his other themes, the author discusses
the significance of the constellations representing the serpent, toad, llama and fox, and the
cross which, to the Quechua, represents an axis along which a state of equilibrium is
established and maintained. The text demonstrates clearly the continuing importance of
astronomical observation to Quechua communities, particularly in the ordering of their
agricultural calendar and seasonal ritual. Urton provides a valuable source of reference
for anthropologists specializing in the regulatory role of astronomy in Andean life.

348 Andean ethnology in the 1970s: a retrospective.
Frank Salomon. *Latin American Research Review*, vol. 7, no. 2
(1982), p. 75-128. bibliog.
The 1970s witnessed an outpouring of research on Andean cultural themes which was
sufficient to place Andean studies among the more well-established regional sub-
specialities of anthropology. Among the historic factors which helped to produce this
abundance was the emergence of generation of field-workers trained by John Murra, John
Rowe, Herman Trimborn and R. T. Zuidema. This essay points out the areas of progress
in Andean ethnology since the 1970s and provides an excellent listing of materials. Serves
both the specialist and the *aficionado*.

349 Andean societies.
John V. Murra. *Annual Review of Anthropology*, vol. 13 (1984),
p. 119-41. bibliog.
Remains recommended background reading for anyone interested in the evolutionary
development of the Andean region. It includes a scholarly review of ethnographic,
ethnohistorical and historical trends in the region. Murra presents the state of research
reached by the early 1980s in a readable, non-technical manner which is useful to both
specialists and students.

350 Oprimados pero no vencidos: luchas del campesinado aymara y qhechwa de Bolivia, 1900-1930. (Oppressed but not defeated: the struggles of the Aymara and Quechua peasants of Bolivia, 1900-1930.)
Silvia Rivera Cusicanqui.   La Paz: Historia Boliviana, 1984. 201p. bibliog.

A social and political history of Bolivian peasants' attempts to gain political, social and economic integration in the years before the Chaco War. An English version is available, entitled *Oppressed but not defeated. Peasant struggles among the Aymara and Qhechwa in Bolivia, 1900-1930* (Geneva: United Nations Research Institute for Social Development, 1987. 222p.).

351 Pueblos indígenas de Bolivia. (Indigenous people of Bolivia.)
Dick Edgar Ibarra Grasso.   La Paz: Librería y Editorial 'Juventud', 1985. 506p. maps. bibliog.

A comprehensive overview of Bolivia's complex indigenous culture which includes a discussion of : Quechua-speaking and Aymara-speaking Indians in the colonial era; the Urus and Chipayas of today; the Tacanas and Panos; the Lecos, Mosetenes and Yuracares; the Arawak nations of Bolivia; the Tupi-Guaraní in Bolivia; the Chiquitos, Bororos, Zamucos and Guatos; and the Tobas and Matacos of the far Chaco.

352 The fiscal role of the Andean *ayllu*.
Ricardo A. Godoy.   *Man*, vol. 21, no. 4 (1986), p. 723-41. bibliog.

The traditional indigenous mechanism for collecting rural taxes in the northern region of the Department of Potosí ensures that households meet their tax liability to the state irrespective of their ability to pay. From this study of the Jukumani *allyu* (Indian community), Godoy suggests that by taking on the fiscal responsibility where necessary, the *ayllu* protects families from the danger of eviction, and that such protection may explain why these social groups have survived.

353 Class conflict or ethnic oppression? The cost of being Indian in rural Bolivia.
Jonathan Kelley.   *Rural Sociology*, vol. 53, no. 4 (1988), p. 399-420. bibliog.

From a detailed analysis of data drawn from a large representative sample of male heads-of-household, Kelley concludes that inequality in rural Bolivia is basically a matter of class, not ethnic discrimination. The determining factor is the level of education. In those few cases where the Indian's education and family position were comparable with the Spanish/*mestizo* experience, the author finds that, regardless of ethnicity, the type of occupation, standard of living, and social class were also the same.

354 Domination and cultural resistance: authority and power among an Andean people.
Roger Neil Rasnake.   Durham, North Carolina; London: Duke University Press, 1988. 321p. maps. bibliog.

In this book on the Yura peasant farmers near Potosí, Rasnake describes their settlement patterns, agricultural practices, and hierarchical *ayllu* (Indian community) organization. His main discussion is focused on the *kuraqkuna* (indigenous authorities) whose role in tax collection, law and order, service obligations, and fiesta rituals, for example, is a major factor in maintaining the cohesion of this Quechua-speaking society and defining its cultural identity – a challenge that becomes increasingly important as many young adults seek seasonal wage-labour in lowland Bolivia and in Argentina. This is an informative study, well supported with diagrams, tables, and photographs.

355 Economic change and rural resistance in southern Bolivia, 1880-1930.
Erick Detlef Langer.   Stanford, California: Stanford University Press, 1989. 269p. maps. bibliog.

Argues that resistance to change by Bolivia's Indian communities in the late 19th and early 20th centuries was more widespread than previously thought. The focus here is on the Department of Chuquisaca, where four contrasted regions are selected to illustrate the varying responses by rural communities to the changing economic and political conditions around them in this period. Adaptation, resistance, and rebellion were to be found in different areas, all set against the wider background of the recession in silver mining, and Chuquisaca's growing isolation and decline.

356 Folk literature of the Ayoreo Indians.
Edited by Johannes Wilbert, Karin Simoneau.   Los Angeles: UCLA Latin American Center Publications, University of California, 1989. 802p. map. bibliog.

This is an outstanding piece of compilation and skilled editing which contains 566 narratives of the Ayoreo Indians, and represents one of the richest indigenous collections from anywhere in South America. The narratives are grouped under: (1) Cosmogony and cosmology; (2) Creation and the ordering of human life; (3) Animals; (4) Plants; and (5) Unclassified. They are accompanied by interpretive essays by several contributing authors. The Ayoreo are traditionally hunters and gatherers, numbering about 1,800 in all. Some remain nomadic, but most are now clustered in scattered groups along the Santa Cruz-Corumbá railway. The volume contains a distribution map of the Ayoreo and other tribes in the Chaco, and records interesting observations on the impact of the outside world, including Bolivia's colonization zones, on the Ayoreos' old way of life.

357 Yuquí foragers in the Bolivian Amazon: subsistence strategies, prestige, and leadership in an acculturating society.
Allyn MacLean Stearman.   *Journal of Anthropological Research*, vol. 45, no. 2 (1989), p. 219-44. bibliog.

Among the Yuquí, prestige is both earned and expressed by success as a hunter, and this in turn allows the distribution of fish and game after the hunt to other members of the group to confirm the relative standing and leadership role of the donor. Quantitative data are presented here to analyse the ranking of the hunters within their small community.

358 **Liberal democracy and *ayllu* democracy in Bolivia: the case of northern Potosí.**
Silvia Rivera Cusicanqui, translated by Charles Roberts.
The Journal of Development Studies, vol. 26, no. 4 (1990), p. 97-121. bibliog.

Argues that the economic and political reforms imposed on the *ayllus*, Bolivia's indigenous rural communities, in the name of modernization and democracy have actually reinforced long-standing colonial forms of oppression. *Ayllus*, which have formed the basic unit of social organization and communal land-holding since pre-hispanic times, conflict with the more broadly based, modern concepts of national citizenship, political parties, agrarian reform, and peasant unions, all of them more closely associated with the *mestizo*/creole urban minority than with the rural majority, particularly in northern Potosí. Perhaps the differences between them are irreconcilable. The writer is strong on the factors which have weakened the *ayllu* system, but offers no solutions as to how a viable, harmonious co-existence might be achieved.

359 **Faces of Latin America.**
Duncan Green.   London: Latin America Bureau, 1991. 211p. map. bibliog.

These faces of Latin America are the faces of the poor. The author's commentary includes some historical background, but concentrates on modern conditions in such areas as land ownership, migration, indigenous populations, politics, the Church, and the military. Green's themes throughout are those of hardship, exploitation, and discrimination. There are no success stories here; even the note on Bolivia's ambitious colonization programme for hitherto landless farmers is entirely pessimistic. The book is built upon a negative appraisal, unrelieved by any positive note of optimism or genuine hope for the future.

360 **Political organization among the Izoceno Indians of Bolivia.**
Silvia Maria Hirsch.   PhD thesis, University of California, Los Angeles, 1991. 311p. bibliog.

A study of skilful political management. The author discusses the successful political organization of Bolivia's Izoceno Indians, whose leaders have adapted well to the demands of establishing a Bolivian national image without surrendering their ethnic identity. Relationships with government and non-government organizations have been carefully nurtured in order to acquire resources for the community, while at the same time, group solidarity and decision-making have remained intact.

361 **Chimane resource use and market involvement in the Beni Biosphere Reserve, Bolivia.**
Avecita del Carmen Chicchon.   PhD thesis, University of Florida, Gainesville, Florida, 1992. 285p. bibliog.

The Beni Biosphere Reserve lies in the northeastern portion of the Chimane Indians' traditional territory. This study examines the various ways in which the Chimane adapt the rhythms of hunting, fishing, and farming to their own food requirements and, in hard times, to the opportunities to sell or barter their produce in nearby markets.

362 Indian communities, political cultures, and the state in Latin America, 1780-1990.
Florencia E. Mallon. *Journal of Latin American Studies*, vol. 24 (Quincentenary Supplement), 1992, p. 35-53.
Seeks to define and explain the factors which differentiate the modern histories of Peru, Bolivia and Mexico in terms of past and future potential contributions of the indigenous political cultures to the ongoing formation of these three Latin American states. Clearly written and jargon-free, the comparison is well managed, with shrewd observation on the differing paths taken and the results so far achieved.

363 The politics of pacha: the conflict of values in a Bolivian Aymara community.
A. L. E. Canessa. PhD thesis, London School of Economics, England, 1993.
A study of ethnic identity under threat in the modern world. The author discusses the various ways, many of them successful, in which the people of the small Aymara village of Pocobaya seek to prevent their language, values and customs from being absorbed into the surrounding 'national' metropolitan culture.

364 Agricultural changes and drinking among the Bolivian Camba: a longitudinal view of the aftermath of a revolution.
Dwight B. Heath. *Human Organization*, vol. 53, no. 4 (1994), p. 357-61. bibliog.
Basing his analysis on the changing drinking patterns of the Camba (lowland dwellers) in the Santa Cruz colonization region over four decades, Heath provides a flowing yet detailed account of changing land-ownership among the Camba since the 1952 revolution. He notes that a return to the old ritualistic pattern of formalized drinking has occurred among some of the older generation who, by the 1990s, had sold their land. By reviving an important earlier method of social bonding, these landless Camba appear to be expressing their heritage and group identity once more.

365 Autonomy and power: the dynamics of class and culture in rural Bolivia.
Maria L. Lagos. Philadelphia: University of Pennsylvania Press, 1994. 206p. maps. bibliog.
Tiraque, a province in the highlands of Cochabamba, provides the case-study for this analysis of a distinctive rural merchant class and a maturing land-owning peasantry which have both emerged since the land reform of 1952-53. Complex, sometimes conflicting, relationships produce new alliances and new social groupings, but always within what remains a strongly interdependent community.

366 Ethnicity and peasant struggle in Bolivia.
Aimee Sullivan. Amherst, Massachusetts: Latin American Studies
Consortium of New England, 1994. 78p. bibliog. (Occasional Paper,
No. 2).

A brief survey of indigenous peasant politics in Bolivia, including a historical review of
Andean peasant resistance and rebellion both before and after the social revolution of
1952. The most useful section investigates the rise of the Aymara *Katarista* movement,
and its influence within the peasant unions during the 1970s and 1980s.

**367 From *indio* to mestizo ... to *indio*: new indianist movements in
Bolivia.**
Juliana Ströbele-Gregor, translated by Bert Hoffman and Andrew
Holmes. *Latin American Perspectives*, vol. 21, no. 2 (1994),
p. 106-23. bibliog.

Focuses on the growing protest among the lowland Indian communities of eastern Bolivia
concerning the destruction of their traditional rights and living space as the harsh realities
of the economic reforms introduced in the mid-1980s have taken hold. One result has
been the growing self-awareness of these indigenous groups, and their demand to be
heard. But as the author points out in an informative and well-balanced survey, the Indian
communities in Bolivia do not speak with one voice; there are conflicts of interest not
only between the Andean and the lowland Indians, but also between the lowland
indigenous groups themselves. Besides which, the prospects for any fundamental policy
changes on any government's part are not encouraging.

368 Gods and vampires: return to Chipaya.
Nathan Wachtel, translated by Carol Volk. Chicago: University of
Chicago Press, 1994. 153p. maps. bibliog.

This study becomes something of a sentimental journey as Wachtel returns to his earlier
research area in an altiplano village populated by Chipaya and Uru Indians, to meet old
friends and to monitor changes that have taken place in this enclave set within a region
dominated by Aymara Indian settlement. The result is a distinctive and engaging account
that will interest both the specialist and the general reader.

**369 Losing game: coaxed out of Bolivia's vanishing wilderness, the
last Yuquí are reluctant to give up the hunt.**
Allyn MacLean Stearman. *Natural History*, vol. 103 (January
1994), p. 6-10.

An account of the changing world of the Yuquí Indians, an isolated group of some 130
hunters and gatherers in the forests fifty miles northwest of the city of Santa Cruz.
Increasing colonization of this region since the 1950s has brought rapid forest clearance,
and with it, a sharp reduction in the Yuquí's sources of game, fruit and fish. But although
by the 1990s they had become completely surrounded by colonists, the Yuquí cling to
tradition, and are reluctant to turn to farming. See also the same author's article, 'The
effects of settler incursion on fish and game resources of the Yuquí' (*Human
Organization*, vol. 49, no. 4 [1990], p. 373-85).

370 'The coming of the white people'. Reflections on the mythologisation of history in Latin America.
Olivia Harris. *Bulletin of Latin American Research*, vol. 14, no. 1 (1995), p. 9-24. bibliog.
Indigenous peoples in Latin America frequently do not divide the past into the historical periods familiar to Europeans. A review of the literature on the subject suggests that, in particular, the arrival of the Spanish and Portuguese is not necessarily regarded as a universal epoch-making event among the indigenous populations of Latin America who give meaning to the past in other ways.

371 Living on the edge: Sirionó hunting and fishing in lowland Bolivia.
Wendy R. Townsend. PhD thesis, University of Florida, Gainesville, Florida, 1995. 169p. bibliog.
Describes the hunting and fishing practices of the Sirionó Indians who inhabit the Llanos de Mojos of eastern Bolivia. Townsend discusses the increase in the territory required to maintain the Sirionós' sources of game animals as their own population grows, and their ancestral lands are encroached upon by colonists, loggers, and cattle ranchers. Help from the Bolivian government, as well as adjustment to their own hunting practices by the Sirionó themselves, are advocated here.

372 The Chayanta rebellion of 1927, Potosí, Bolivia.
A. Grunberg. DPhil thesis, University of Oxford, England, 1996.
The Chayanta peasant rebellion swept through large parts of northern Potosí and northwestern Chuquisaca in the winter of 1927. The author investigates the years preceding the revolt, years of growing demand for protection of the Indians' civil and land rights, and for access to political appointments on the same terms as other citizens. This study rejects the argument that the Indians in 19th- and early 20th-century Potosí sought only to maintain their traditional tribute-paying and other identifying practices; in addition, it is suggested that they also sought entry to mainstream politics.

373 Culture and political practice of the Aymara and Quechua in Bolivia: autonomous forms of modernity in the Andes.
Juliana Ströbele-Gregor. *Latin American Perspectives*, vol. 23, no. 2 (1996), p. 72-90. bibliog.
This is a study of cultural survival. In tracing the ways in which many Aymara and Quechua peasants have adapted their basic principles of community, reciprocity, and collective action to the demands of the modern state, the author argues that they often show considerable skill and flexibility in coping with new ideas and procedures, without in any way abandoning their own modes of thinking and their traditional organization.

374 **Ethnobotany of the Chácobo Indians, Beni, Bolivia.**
Brian Morey Boom. Bronx, New York: Scientific Publications
Department, New York Botanical Garden, 1996. 2nd ed. 74p.
bibliog.

The Chácobo community, numbering about 260 Indians, inhabits the Amazonian
rainforest some seventy miles south of Riberalta. The major value of this monograph is
the first-hand information it provides on the Chácobos' intensive and varied use of the
forest, since the author's inventory of a one-hectare site revealed that 82 per cent of the
species and 95 per cent of the individual trees are utilized – for food, fuel, shelter,
transport, utensils, textiles, dyes, poisons, medicines, and other useful products. Boom
demonstrates clearly the Chácobos' profound knowledge of the rainforest, and discusses
the impact of deforestation programmes on indigenous forest people such as these.

375 **Land reform compromise deflates Bolivian protest.**
InterPress Service, NotiSur. *NACLA Report on the Americas*
(North American Congress on Latin America), vol. 30, no. 3
(November-December 1996), p. 46-47.

Notes that the new Agrarian Reform Law of October 1996 is already proving highly
controversial. Representatives of several indigenous organizations in lowland Bolivia,
together with coca growers in the Chapare, had assembled in Santa Cruz and marched to
La Paz, where their demands had included secure individual titles to their land, and the
creation of a community social and economic development fund which they would help
to administer. They had left La Paz dissatisfied, having made no headway with the
government on shared involvement in development funding or on land rights where these
conflicted with business interests or with productive large-scale land-holdings. Moreover,
they had been angered to discover that indigenous groups in Bolivia's northern
Amazonian forests had negotiated separately with the government and had been granted
title deeds for collective ownership of their lands.

376 **The use and abuse of ethnicity: the case of the Bolivian CSUTCB.**
Dwight R. Hahn. *Latin American Perspectives*, vol. 23, no. 2
(1996), p. 91-106. bibliog.

Considers the weaknesses of the indigenous-based *Confederación Sindical Unica de
Trabajadores Campesinos de Bolivia* (CSUTCB) as a inclusive organization for all
Bolivian peasants. While many Aymara and Quechua farmers in the Chapare have
adapted readily to land reform and the capitalist system, others, especially in lowland
Bolivia, have resisted the state's 'western-style' intrusion and in recent years have begun
to defend themselves against capitalist enterprise and the demands of an external market.
One focus of resistance has been the founding of the Centre for Indigenous Peoples of
Eastern Bolivia, based in Santa Cruz.

377 **Creating citizens, making men: the military and masculinity in
Bolivia.**
Lesley Gill. *Cultural Anthropology*, vol. 12, no. 4 (1997), p. 527-
50. bibliog.

In Bolivia, young male military conscripts come from the most powerless sections of
society – from Quechua, Aymara, and Guaraní peasant communities, and poor urban

neighbourhoods. Despite rough conditions, these men are generally eager to serve in the military; completed service is a prerequisite for many forms of urban employment, it provides escape from parental control, and builds self-esteem, masculinity, and citizen-awareness. Based mainly on interviews in the city of El Alto, the article considers the making of these citizen-soldiers, and contrasts the role of men's army training with that of women's domestic service, which remains marginalized, and without empowerment or the prospect of new opportunities.

378 The reproduction of community through communal practices in Kila Kila, Bolivia.
A. Klemola.   PhD thesis, University of Liverpool, England, 1997.
Investigates the cut and thrust of communal meetings and communal discourses in the *ayllu* of Kila Kila, demonstrating the crucial role that these meetings play in upholding the authority of the leaders, in displaying the rise or fall in status of individual family heads, and in performing the rituals which maintain the *ayllu*'s group identity. Thus, the heads of households debate, voice their grievances, and seek to lift their status among their fellows, while the successful leader of the *ayllu* exercises his ultimate decision-making role in the community.

379 Pathways of memory and power: ethnography and history among an Andean people.
Thomas Alan Abercrombie.   Madison, Wisconsin: University of Wisconsin Press, 1998. 603p. maps. bibliog.
Based on the Aymara community of Santa Bárbara (*ayllu* K'ulta), the study examines the relationships between the European sense of history and the indigenous ways of understanding the past. Complex Andean rituals hybridize the Spanish and indigenous traditions to shape the community's social memory. The author's historical approach to ethnography has involved his inclusion of extended general accounts of Spain's colonization of the Andes and of Spanish records of Indian contacts. These, combined with Abercrombie's own narrative-style account of his fieldwork, have unfortunately led to a protracted and often unwieldy book in which several of the crucial points he wishes to make are obscured. Even so, students of indigenous Aymara culture, and of the border zone between written and unwritten history, should be able to find interesting ideas and comparisons for their own work on this theme.

380 Political institutions and the evanescence of power: making history in highland Bolivia.
Stuart Alexander Rockefeller.   *Ethnology*, vol. 37, no. 2 (1998), p. 187-207. bibliog.
Examines the declining effectiveness of their political institutions in Bolivia's small rural Quechua community of Quirpini. The main thrust of the argument is that self-government by the Quirpini *campesinos*, such as it is, is possible in real terms only with the consent and co-operation of the Spanish-speaking *mestizo* élite in the nearby regional capital of San Lucas. Quirpini organization, it is argued, has been manipulated by the town to dominate the village, particularly in the demand for the *campesinos'* services by the urban authorities. The author notes that growing Bolivian national influence may be beginning to weaken the power of the local San Lucas élite, but that if this occurs, it is likely to be a slow process.

381 Strategies of rain-forest dwellers against misfortunes: the Tsimane' Indians of Bolivia.

Ricardo Godoy, Marc Jacobson, David Wilkie. *Ethnology*, vol. 37, no. 1 (1998), p. 55-69. bibliog.

Sets out to test the traditional view that the rainforest provides security, and that during misfortunes such as illness, death, or crop failure, the Indians increase foraging and other forms of dependence on the forest even when they have become exposed to the outside influences of market and wage labour. Investigation of some 200 Tsimane' households in nineteen villages reveals that death or crop loss still triggers greater clearance of old and secondary growth forest in the isolated villages, while proximity to town triggers requests for wage advance. Reciprocal obligations within the village in time of misfortune play a much smaller role than expected.

382 Ethnobotany of the Ese Eja: plants, health, and change in an Amazonian society.

Miguel N. Alexiades.   PhD thesis, City University of New York, 1999. 467p. bibliog.

The Ese Eja are a small indigenous group living in the tropical forests along the Beni and Madre de Dios rivers. Alexiades' research concentrates on the rich variety of flora and fauna in these forests, where over 190 plant species and 50 animal species were identified in his study area. These are used by the Ese Eja in a wide range of medical treatments, and in many social activities and rituals. The author describes present-day practices, and shows how these have changed and developed over time.

383 Nature and culture in the Andes.

Daniel W. Gade.   Madison, Wisconsin: University of Wisconsin Press, 1999. 287p. maps. bibliog.

Gade describes his book as 'the cultural history of nature and the ecological history of culture' at selected sites in the Andes in Ecuador, Peru and Bolivia. Well-chosen case-studies analyse the relationships between landscape, people, plants and animals over time, as the author adopts a holistic approach to his interpretation of the region. This is a carefully researched supplementary text, of value to students working in different disciplines but whose collective interests are focused on the Andes.

384 'Now my daughter is alone': performing kinship and embodying effect in marriage practices among native Andeans in Bolivia.

Krista Eileen Van Vleet.   PhD thesis, University of Michigan, Ann Arbor, Michigan, 1999. 418p. bibliog.

In her study of the Sullk'ata *ayllu* in Chayanta province, Department of Potosí, the author focuses on the relationships between mothers- and daughters-in-law and marriage partners, and the ways in which these are influenced by the internal kinship system and by external economic demands. In spite of the ideals of complementarity and caring between marriage partners, and of reciprocity and respect between mothers- and daughters-in-law, marriage creates contradictions and conflicts that are recognized in songs, stories, gossip, emotional displays, and physical violence.

385 The dynamics of Aymara duality: change and continuity in socio-political structures in the Bolivian Andes.
Astvaldur Astvaldsson. *Journal of Latin American Studies*, vol. 32, no. 1 (2000), p. 145-74. maps. bibliog.

In the altiplano community of Jesús de Machaqa, the author examines key aspects of the traditional Aymara socio-political structures which appear to have survived largely intact from colonial, and even pre-Columbian, times into the 20th century. Based on fieldwork, the study considers the changes that have occurred since the revolution of 1952, and includes a discussion of the methodological problems faced by those who seek to reconstruct the past of indigenous communities, particularly the difficulties that emerge when trying to match evidence from colonial documents with that from oral tradition.

386 The sound of the Pututos: politicisation and indigenous rebellions in Bolivia, 1826-1921.
Marta Irurozqui. *Journal of Latin American Studies*, vol. 32, no. 1 (2000), p. 85-114. bibliog.

A scholarly examination of the way in which politics among Bolivia's indigenous population became increasingly nationalized during the century after Independence, with landownership as the focus of rebellion, legal battles, and patronage agreements. The author argues that the Indians' aspiration was to participate as citizens in the shaping of one Bolivian nation, not to construct an alternative national identity. In doing so, she seeks to refute the image of the indigenous people collectively 'as pre-political, passive, incomprehensible, and alien to all that was Western'.

Immigrants and minorities

387 Alemanes en Bolivia. (Germans in Bolivia.)
Albert Crespo. La Paz: Editorial 'Los Amigos del Libro', 1978. 246p. bibliog.

A general introduction, complete with photographs, to Bolivia's German community, with an emphasis on the most prominent citizens.

388 Latin American Jewish studies.
Judith Laiken Elkin. Cincinnati, Ohio: American Jewish Archives, 1980. 53p.

An inventory of the status of studies at the end of the 1970s pertaining to Latin American Jewry.

389   Japanese settlement in eastern Bolivia and Brazil.

James L. Tigner. *Journal of Interamerican Studies and World Affairs*, vol. 24, no. 4 (1982), p. 496-517. bibliog.

Reviews major studies on Japanese immigration. Bolivia does not on the whole incorporate the Japanese into its social system, whilst Brazil does. The study is based on government documents from the three nations.

390   The economic and social condition of Jewish and Arab immigrants in Bolivia, 1890-1980.

Marc J. Osteweil. *Immigrants and Minorities*, vol. 16, nos. 1 and 2 (March/July 1997), p. 146-66. bibliog.

This well-balanced study notes that Arab immigration to Bolivia has been a long, orderly process, producing a stable minority with clear evidence of assimilation and acculturation. In contrast, Jewish immigration is characterized by large numbers arriving over a relatively short period; they have formed a less stable minority since many came as Second World War refugees and subsequently moved elsewhere. Those Jews who remained, like the Arab immigrants and their descendants, are found in the upper levels of society, mainly in La Paz and Cochabamba, where both groups are successfully involved in international trade, manufacturing and commerce, and are frequently associated with innovative business organization.

391   Hotel Bolivia: the culture of memory in a refuge from Nazism.

Leo Spitzer.   New York: Hill and Wang, 1998. 234p. bibliog.

An informative history of the experience of Jewish refugees who escaped to Bolivia in the 1930s. The author was born in La Paz of Austrian-Jewish immigrants, and incorporates his own memories with later extensive research in documentary archives, family memoirs, and videotaped accounts made with survivors in Bolivia and their children. This is a well-rounded study which also includes a record of earlier German immigration to Bolivia and the activities of Nazi sympathizers there at this time. The first-hand observations of life in La Paz during the 1940s are particularly valuable, while the illustrated text also provides a scholarly contribution to the wider study of Jewish history in the first half of the 20th century.

392   A high altitude congregation.

Larry Luxner. *Américas*, vol. 51, no. 4 (1999), p. 4-5.

Describes 'the highest synagogue on earth' in La Paz, whose members belong to the country's Circulo Israelita. The author also outlines the history of the Jews in Bolivia – in La Paz, Cochabamba, and Santa Cruz.

The Economy and Economic Reform

General

393 The Bolivian hyperinflation and stabilization.
Jeffrey Sachs. *American Economic Review*, vol. 77 (May 1987),
p. 279-83.

Bolivia's notorious surge into hyperinflation in 1984-85 was the most rapid in Latin American history and one of the highest-ever in world history. In that year, Bolivian prices rose by an average of 20,000 per cent, while between May and August 1985, prices had climbed by a dizzying 60,000 per cent. Sachs provides a clear, concise summary of the causes of this hyperinflation, and the main components of President Paz Estenssoro's New Economic Policy introduced as an emergency measure in August 1985. The policy went well beyond macroeconomic stabilization, however, into a radical reform of fiscal, trade, and public-sector organization.

394 Bolivia: 1952-1986.
Jeffrey Sachs, Juan Antonio Morales.   San Francisco: International
Center for Economic Growth/ICS Press, 1988. 48p. bibliog.
(Country Studies, No. 6).

A lucid, authoritative analysis of the background to, and main components of, Bolivia's mid-1980s stabilization programme which can be recommended to both the general and the specialist reader. Sachs, a professor of economics at Harvard University, was involved in preparing the strategy for Bolivia's stabilization policies adopted by the newly elected Paz Estenssoro administration in 1985, and he became an adviser on its implementation over a two-year period. The study also includes shrewd consideration of the major problems to be faced in Bolivia's economy and society after stabilization has been achieved. These are forecast to be severe; with possible solutions outlined, the study makes illuminating reading in its anticipation of some of the events in the 1990s.

395 Doing it by the book.

The Economist, vol. 307 (28 May 1988), p. 74-75.

A useful summary for the general reader of the major economic reforms introduced by President Víctor Paz Estenssoro following his election in 1985, when the annual rate of inflation in Bolivia was running at 20,000 per cent. Reforms included cuts in government spending, more efficient tax collection, lower import tariffs, and new credit arrangements, together with general debt buy-back terms with the International Monetary Fund and the World Bank. The article notes that foreign investors were being made to feel more welcome in Bolivia, and that by the late 1980s inflation had dropped rapidly to 11 per cent.

396 Inflation stabilization in Bolivia.

Juan Antonio Morales.   In: *Inflation stabilization. The experience of Argentina, Brazil, Bolivia, Israel, and Mexico.*   Edited by Michael Bruno, Guido Di Tella, Rudiger Dornbusch, Stanley Fischer. Cambridge, Massachusetts: MIT Press, 1988, p. 307-46. bibliog.

Morales examines the years between 1982 and mid-1987, outlining the causes of Bolivia's inflation and hyperinflation, and the components of the New Economic Policy introduced in 1985. Analysing the policy's intended and unintended results so far, the author finds the preliminary results on stabilization impressive, but goes on to consider what might have been achieved by an alternative, less drastic programme. No obvious alternative emerges, however, especially in the context of the tin market's collapse in 1985, and the need for foreign loans.

397 Orthodox and heterodox stabilization policies in Bolivia and Peru: 1985-1988.

Arthur J. Mann, Manuel Pastor, Jr.   *Journal of Interamerican Studies and World Affairs*, vol. 31, no. 4 (1989), p. 163-92. bibliog.

An article stressing the need for policy-makers to be ready to adjust their programmes quickly once stabilization is achieved. Bolivia's orthodox approach to stabilization through tight fiscal policy, reduced state subsidies, public-sector wage freeze and other measures should be followed by reactivation and growth of the economy through more investment spending. At this critical point, after years of deprivation, the challenge becomes one of maintaining popular support for the discipline still needed for the next stage of economic development.

398 Out of the basket (Chile and Bolivia).

The Economist, vol. 311 (10 June 1989), p. 67.

After examining the successes of Chile's earlier economic reconstruction, the article reviews the prospect for economic stability in Bolivia since the reforms of 1985. The writer is cautiously optimistic about the country's ability to achieve durable, export-led, non-inflationary growth. Bolivia remains heavily dependent on cash-flow from Argentina, which (in the late 1980s) was taking forty per cent of Bolivia's official exports in the form of natural gas. But sound economic growth in the future will depend on attracting a wide range of foreign investment.

399 A platform for growth.
The Economist, vol. 312 (23 September 1989), Third World Survey,
p. 16, 21-22, 25.
This is a thoughtful analysis of Víctor Paz Estenssoro's economic reforms introduced in
August 1985, the New Economic Policy, which was designed to be comprehensive,
simple, and to take immediate effect. The writer debates whether the catastrophic events
of 1985, which stifled party-political bickering and forced the acceptance of major
economic reform, will have a lasting effect. The widespread recognition throughout
Bolivia, however, that drastic reform must be endured as a necessary evil may be an
encouraging sign for the future, if the stabilization programme produces results.

400 Workers' benefits from Bolivia's Emergency Social Fund.
John L. Newman, Steen Jorgensen, Menno Pradhan. Washington,
DC: World Bank, 1991. 42p. bibliog. (Living Standards
Measurement Study Working Paper, No. 77).
The Emergency Social Fund (ESF) for Bolivia was one of the first World Bank-funded
efforts to address the huge social costs of the country's economic structural adjustment
during the 1980s by including a separate compensatory relief programme as part of the
deal. Concentrating on different sections of the workforce, the authors suggest that male
workers aged between 18 and 55 years, particularly those in the construction industry,
derived the greatest benefit from their participation in the ESF initiative.

**401 Bolivia's answer to poverty, economic crisis, and adjustment: the
Emergency Social Fund.**
Edited by Steen Jorgensen, Margaret Grosh, Mark Schacter.
Washington, DC: World Bank, 1992. 124p. bibliog. (World Bank
Regional and Sectoral Studies).
A comprehensive and authoritative study of Bolivia's Emergency Social Fund (ESF),
which was created in December 1986 for a three-year term and subsequently extended
until March 1991. The authors review the objectives of the scheme, analyse contrasted
case-studies, and identify reasons for the project's success, not least its low overheads, the
efficiency of the administrators, and the reduced discontent among rival government
ministries once the temporary nature of the ESF organization was confirmed. Although
the programme did not always reach the poorest of the poor or solve Bolivia's widespread
unemployment problems, it funded over 3,000 small projects in a fast, flexible manner,
and stimulated cooperation between hitherto isolated agencies. The study is well balanced
and exceptionally jargon-free, combining a wealth of information with a direct,
economical style.

**402 Inflation, stabilization, and debt: macroeconomic experiments in
Peru and Bolivia.**
Manuel Pastor, Jr. Boulder, Colorado: Westview Press, 1992. 176p.
bibliog. (Westview Special Studies on Latin America and the
Caribbean).
Examines the severe economic swings in Peru and Bolivia during the 1980s, and analyses
the macroeconomic experiments adopted by these two states in their attempts to achieve
stabilization. Pastor reviews Bolivia's stringent orthodox New Economic Policy of 1985,

acknowledging that there was probably no alternative to it at the time. Growth up to 1992, however, had been slow, with future progress dependent on foreign and domestic capital. The comparison between Bolivia and Peru is well sustained, and widened briefly to include the experiences of Chile, Brazil, and Argentina.

403 Interpreting social movements: Bolivian resistance to economic conditions imposed by the International Monetary Fund.
June Nash. *American Ethnologist*, vol. 19, no. 2 (1992), p. 275-93. bibliog.

Describes the great march to La Paz by members of the mining communities in 1986 to protest against the harsh measures imposed by the International Monetary Fund for the payment of Bolivia's national debt. Nash offers a sympathetic, first-hand account of the march and the desperation of the marchers, but fails to mention any other options open to President Paz Estenssoro in this period of national economic collapse.

404 The politics of protecting the poor during adjustment: Bolivia's Emergency Social Fund.
Carol Graham. *World Development*, vol. 20, no. 9 (1992), p. 1233-51. bibliog.

Established in 1986 to complement Paz Estenssoro's stringent New Economic Policy, the Emergency Social Fund (ESF) was designed as a short-term mechanism to protect the most needy until the economy revived and a more permanent solution could be sought. On the whole, the ESF proved to be well managed, remarkably free of political interference, and successful in reaching both the urban and many of the rural poor. It helped small businesses, farmers, and municipalities to select and organize their own local projects; indeed, the Fund reached large numbers of the poor who had previously been neglected by the state. This is a clear and detailed study based on a wide range of well-chosen examples.

405 Spreading the rewards of virtue.
The Economist, vol. 328 (11 September 1993), p. 46.

Reviews President Gonzalo Sánchez de Lozada's economic policies for Bolivia, including that of capitalization which differs from full-scale privatization of the state-owned companies by inviting foreign concerns to invest in them and manage them in return for half the equity, the remainder to be distributed in some form still to be decided among the Bolivian people.

406 Temporary external shocks and stabilization policies for Bolivia.
Juan Antonio Morales, Justo Espejo, Gonzalo Chávez. In: *External shocks and stabilization mechanisms*. Edited by Eduardo Engel, Patricio Meller. Washington, DC: Inter-American Development Bank; distributed by Johns Hopkins University Press, 1993, p. 173-217. bibliog.

Considers the financial measures necessary to reduce the adverse effects on countries whose major exports are subject to large fluctuations in world market prices. The examples of natural gas, tin, and zinc are examined, since together these provided 64 per cent of the annual value of Bolivia's legal exports between 1950 and 1990. The authors suggest actions that should be adopted to implement risk management, including tax reform, pricing, and marketing methods. This is a good, systematic study for specialists, well supported by tables and graphs. It also serves as a comparative exercise for the reader, as other chapters in this volume examine the case of Chile (copper), and of Venezuela (oil).

407 **Democracy, markets, and structural reform in Latin America: Argentina, Bolivia, Brazil, Chile, and Mexico.**
Edited by William C. Smith, Carlos H. Acuña, Eduardo A. Gamarra. New Brunswick, New Jersey; London: Transaction Publishers, in association with University of Miami, North-South Center, 1994. 331p.

Two chapters are devoted to Bolivia in this wider study of economic restructuring in Latin America. Eduardo Gamarra examines how support for stabilization and structural adjustment was secured for the New Economic Policy (NEP) in the 1980s through a series of pacts and alliances between key political parties in Congress. Juan Antonio Morales, assessing the achievements of the NEP by the early 1990s, concludes that Bolivia's poor economic performance in terms of growth, employment, wages, and access to public services may well be challenged in the future by an increasingly dissatisfied and restless electorate. Although it was too early to judge the effects of capitalization, there had been inadequate preparation so far for long-term growth.

408 **Market-oriented reforms and democratization in Bolivia.**
Eduardo A. Gamarra. In: *A precarious balance: democracy and economic reforms in Latin America.* Edited by Joan M. Nelson. San Francisco: Institute for Contemporary Studies; International Center for Economic Growth, 1994, vol. 2, p. 21-94. bibliog.

In a long, thoughtful review of the political and economic changes in Bolivia in recent decades, the author considers the events leading to the introduction of the reforms, and analyses the aims and side-effects of the austerity measures introduced in 1985 by the New Economic Policy. Arguing that these did not solve the country's deep structural problems, Gamarra discusses the difficulties still facing successive administrations in the post-stabilization phase and displays an ambivalent attitude to privatization, maintaining that the state will have to continue to play a key role in investment. Moreover, he contends that the future of democratization in Bolivia is by no means straightforward nor its outcome clear, since potential conflicts of interest remain between organized labour, the armed forces, the political parties, and the private sector.

409 **Share-out.**
The Economist, vol. 330 (26 March 1994), p. 51-52.

Expands upon Bolivia's new capitalization programme, for which the first six state-owned enterprises are now ready for private investment – oil and gas, telephones, electricity, smelting, railways, and the national airline. Foreign investors will receive half-stakes in the companies and full management control, bringing with them improved management techniques and advanced technology. The remaining half-shares will be issued to all 3.2 million Bolivians over twenty-one as contributions to their own pension funds, thus shifting pensions into the private sector.

410 State-owned enterprise reform through performance contracts: the Bolivian experiment.
Richard D. Mallon. *World Development*, vol. 22, no. 6 (1994), p. 925-34. bibliog.

Since the 1980s, increasing attention has been given worldwide to the problems of state-owned enterprises – their inefficiency, costliness, and waste. Combined with, or as a preparation for, privatization, performance contracts drawn up between the Bolivian government and individual state-owned enterprises have had mixed success; in general they appear to have stimulated improved performance, although in some cases they are shown to have been vulnerable to political interference. In an investigation that combines detail with clarity, Mallon analyses a number of Bolivian examples to provide an informative and well-balanced critique.

411 Unsettling statecraft: democracy and neoliberalism in the central Andes.
Catherine M. Conaghan, James M. Malloy. Pittsburgh: University of Pittsburgh Press, 1994. 303p. bibliog. (Pitt Latin American Series).

A first-rate study of the changing economic and political events during the 1980s in Bolivia, Peru, and Ecuador, as each introduced stabilization policies and neoliberal market reforms. The authors' approach is genuinely comparative, moving easily from one country to another in a cohesive analysis of contemporary events, including reports of discussions with local politicians, economic ministers and business leaders. While Bolivia's neoliberal policies under Paz Estenssoro were the most severe, they were also the most successful of the three in terms of a fundamental restructuring of the state's role in the economy. Policy-making is regarded as a historically conditioned process, and here, the gains and losses of Bolivia's uniquely styled neoliberal experiment are closely scrutinized in a book that can be highly recommended to both the specialist and the general reader.

412 Crisis and reform in Latin America: from despair to hope.
Sebastian Edwards. New York: Oxford University Press, for the World Bank, 1995. 364p. bibliog.

A detailed and dispassionate investigation of Latin America's major economic reforms, which started as an isolated process in Chile in the 1970s and became a sweeping movement affecting virtually every country in the region. Edwards concentrates on developments since the 1982 debt crisis, and analyses the different strategies, stabilization programmes, trade liberation, privatization, and social security reforms up to the 1994 Mexican currency crisis. These topics, and others, are included in the broader discussion on Bolivia. This is an authoritative study, of value both to policy-makers and students. The author notes that few analysts would have predicted in 1984 the depth and scope of Latin America's economic transformation a mere ten years later. Although Latin America's modernization processes are still largely unfinished, 'after decades of timid performance and spiralling inequalities, there are rays of hope'.

413   His way.
The Economist, vol. 336 (30 September 1995), p. 47, 50.

After reviewing progress to date on President Gonzalo Sánchez de Lozada's capitalization programme, the writer considers some of the pros and cons of the policy so far in more detail. Under this system, the government receives no one-off boost to state revenues as occurs in conventional privatization. This reduces the opportunities for corruption, but with the loss of the most profitable enterprises, it may make the implementation of other state commitments more difficult. The complaint is also made that some companies have been sold too cheaply; and finally, that many Bolivians have no hope of reaching the pensionable age of sixty-five.

414   Will Bolivians read *Forbes*?
Christopher Palmeri.   *Forbes*, vol. 155, no. 6 (March 1995), p. 47.

Palmeri hails the policies of Bolivia's president Gonzalo Sánchez de Lozada to encourage free enterprise and sell six state-owned companies. The sales are linked to the setting up of privately run pension funds for Bolivia, so that the process is known as capitalization, not privatization. The article's jaunty title emphasizes Bolivia's new era of capitalist economic reforms.

415   Economic policy in Bolivia after the transition to democracy.
Juan Antonio Morales.   In: *Economic policy and the transition to democracy: the Latin American experience*.   Edited by Juan Antonio Morales, Gary McMahon.   Basingstoke, England; London: Macmillan; New York: St Martin's Press, 1996, p. 30-48. bibliog. (Macmillan International Political Economy Series).

Extending his earlier analyses, the author provides a progress report on Bolivia's New Economic Policy introduced in 1985. The tone is cautious, even pessimistic, as Morales argues that by the mid-1990s some of the reforms, after initial success, have failed to produce sustained economic growth or social improvement. Bolivia must therefore seek to avoid populist movements growing in power and reversing what has clearly been achieved in terms of modernization.

416   Bolivia: the social consequences of debt.
Marie Dennis.   *NACLA Report on the Americas* (North American Congress on Latin America), vol. 31, no. 3 (November/December 1997), p. 37-41.

An objective and informative survey of the economic conditions during the 1980s and 1990s, illustrating how Bolivia's heavy debt burden narrowed the country's opportunities to choose policy options that would improve the quality of life of its poorest and most vulnerable communities. The New Economic Policy reforms of 1985-86 are analysed in detail, for and against, together with the economic and political effects of the expanding coca/cocaine industry on the country as a whole. The writing is clear and concise, providing a helpful summary for both the specialist and the general reader.

417 The Bolivian formula: from state capitalism to capitalisation.
Richard Bauer, Sally Bowen. Santiago: McGraw-Hill/
Interamericana de Chile Ltda, 1997. 114p.

A vigorous and informative study of Bolivia's capitalization programme. Neither a manual nor a consultant's report, the book is based on a very wide range of personal interviews with those close in one way or another to the capitalization process. The authors provide a stimulating analysis of the policies and personalities involved, together with details of the bidders, purchasers, costs and subsequent progress made on each of the six capitalized concerns. This is an excellent introduction to the topic for the general reader and a clear source of reference for the specialist.

418 Capitalization: a Bolivian model of social and economic reform.
Edited by Margaret Hollis Peirce. Washington, DC: Woodrow
Wilson Center; University of Miami, North-South Center, 1997.
467p.

Capitalization has been defined as the Bolivian version of privatization but with a social and an economic twist. Based on the legislation of 1994 and 1996, details of the six key sectors of the economy involved in capitalization are presented, along with the associated Pension Reform plan, and the Popular Participation and Administrative Decentralization programmes. These are discussed in a series of scholarly papers which emphasize the breadth and originality of this ambitious reform policy and its long-term goals. The contributors for the most part are cautiously optimistic about the future of the reforms, given time. The book is distinguished by its extensive coverage and its incisive comment, and provides the most detailed analysis of the capitalization programme yet available in English.

419 Capitalization: an example in the Andes.
The Economist, vol. 344 (9 August 1997), p. 29-30.

Discusses the future of Sánchez de Lozada's major economic reforms as he leaves office in favour of President Hugo Banzer and the new administration. The reforms, still in their early stages, are so far generally popular among the Bolivians, while they have also won initial approval from world bankers. The outlook appears favourable, since Banzer supports the stabilization programme and the free market, and has already declared that with regard to the broad thrust of the reforms, there will be no turning back. Some worries persist, however. Maintaining the role of independent regulators in the privatized/capitalized industries is crucial, while corruption in areas such as customs, police, and judiciary has scarcely been touched by the reforms so far.

**420 The Bolivian experiment: structural adjustment and poverty
alleviation.**
Edited by Pitou van Dijck. Amsterdam: Centre for Latin American
Research and Documentation (CEDLA), 1998. 270p. map. bibliog.

This collection of twelve essays on the benefits and shortcomings of Bolivia's New Economic Policy (NEP) of August 1985 strikes a good balance between empirical studies and theoretical assessment. In the short term, the policy proved remarkably successful in achieving stabilization and radical new thinking, but much less so over the next decade in securing overall economic growth and in alleviating poverty. Several key sectors are examined in their urban and rural setting. Some contributors, for example, maintain that the agricultural sector was given no particular role nor a well-defined policy under the NEP, and that major state investment will still be required to support growth and reduce rural poverty. Other authors analyse the difficulties faced by non-governmental organizations (NGOs) in implementing national policy in Bolivia (where more than 600 NGOs were working by the mid-1990s), although they reject the claim that NGOs have lost contact with local people and local needs. This is a well-integrated, scholarly compilation, recommended for its range and substance.

Economic reports

421   Bolivia: fact sheet and country profile.
US Department of State Dispatch, vol. 3 (March 1992), p. 170-71.
Summarizes Bolivia's political conditions since the 1970s, the major economic and trade issues (including relations with the United States and the counter-narcotics strategy), together with basic information on geography, population, and government. The material is regularly updated.

422   Bolivia: recent economic developments.
Compiled by Patricia Brenner, Benedict Clements, Paulo Drummond, Toma Gudec, Gerardo Peraza.   Washington, DC: International Monetary Fund, 1996. 119p. (IMF Staff Country Report, No. 96/42).
Focusing on the period 1990-95, this detailed report offers a close analysis of the significant trends in all the major sectors of Bolivia's economy, including production, employment, banking, investment, trade, capitalization, government expenditure, and prices. In addition to the statistical record, appendices also set out clearly, and comment on, the government's policies to attempt to reduce poverty, and to improve health and education. This is a well-arranged and informative source of reference.

423   Bolivia: country profile, 1999-2000.
London: Economist Intelligence Unit, 1995- . 54p. map. annual.
An annual publication which sets out briefly Bolivia's historical and political background before analysing in more detail the country's major resources, infrastructure, economic trends and economic potential. This is a concise, objective survey, well supported by tables.

424   Bolivia: country report.
London: Economist Intelligence Unit, 1995- . c. 20-30p. quarterly.
A quarterly publication designed to provide clear, up-to-date briefing for businesses, governments, and international organizations on economic and political developments, resources, output, trade, wages and employment, foreign loans, and significant long-term trends. It provides an excellent accessible source of regular information on Bolivia.

425 Bolivia: country risk service.
London: Economic Intelligence Unit, 1995- . quarterly.

A succinct report that provides lenders and investors with quarterly ratings of the riskiness of business and financial exposure in each of 100 highly indebted and developing countries. The report on Bolivia assesses political and economic policy, economic structure, banking, and liquidity, as well as offering insights into other risk factors where they occur, and into debt constraints.

426 Economic survey of Latin America and the Caribbean.
New York: United Nations, 1947- . annual.

This major source of economic information on the region reports first on macroeconomic policy, reforms, investment and employment, followed by sets of detailed statistics and text on the individual states. The volume published in 1997-98 was the 50th edition in the series. To mark this milestone, a special section was added: 'Fifty Years of the Economic Survey' (p. 343-68), which analyses the most significant features of the period, and provides an excellent critique, both for the specialist and the general reader, on the region's crises and achievements during the second half of the 20th century.

Economic history

427 The bankers in Bolivia, a study in American foreign investment.
Margaret Alexander Marsh.   New York: Vanguard Press, 1928.
233p. bibliog.

A now classic study of the penetration of foreign economic influence into an underdeveloped economy. Marsh focuses on the early years of the 20th century, particularly on the 1920s, when United States investment in Bolivia was greater than that by any other country – c. US$100,000,000 in tin mining, oil, railways, and financial loans. The analysis is crisp and objective, revealing the hostility and the nervousness that investment on this scale aroused both in Bolivia and the United States.

428 La economía de Bolivia. (The economy of Bolivia.)
Eduardo Arze Cuadros.   La Paz: Editorial 'Los Amigos del Libro',
1979. 578p. maps.

A survey of Bolivian economic history from 1492 to 1979, translated from French (originally a dissertation from the University of Paris). Included are theoretical chapters dealing with: dependency theory; regionalism; the historical context of regional development; the development of regional economic inequality; and the organization of regional development. The conclusions address the issue of regionalism and national integration. This represents a very competent work and an excellent starting place for students, scholars and interested general readers alike.

429 Debt, taxes, and war: the political economy of Bolivia, c. 1920-1935.
Manuel Eduardo Contreras. *Journal of Latin American Studies*,
vol. 22, no. 2 (1990), p. 265-87. bibliog.
Provides a useful panoramic view of the Bolivian economy in the 1920s, and of the
subsequent effects of the Chaco War. The author discusses the dominant role of tin, and
of the International Tin Cartel, but emphasizes that despite the boost provided by the
development of railways, banking institutions, and public utilities, the 1920s also
witnessed a series of lost opportunities. Contreras argues that the real barriers to economic
growth in the 1920s were the squandering of public funds through corruption and
unproductive prestige projects, while the early 1930s were marked, aside from the
debilitating effects of war, by the lack of investment opportunities for private capital.

Finance and Banking

430 Voluntary debt-reduction operations: Bolivia, Mexico, and beyond.
Ruben Lamdany. Washington, DC: World Bank, 1988. 28p.
bibliog. (World Bank Discussion Papers, No. 42).

The first half of this study sets out the main components of Bolivia's debt buy-back scheme in the mid-1980s, together with the issues faced by the 131 creditor banks involved, and the criteria used by these different banks to decide whether or not to participate in the buy-back programme. A brief but constructive comment on the future prospects of such operations concludes the paper.

431 Exchange rate rules, black market premia and fiscal deficits: the Bolivian hyperinflation.
Homi Kharas, Brian Pinto. *Review of Economic Studies*, vol. 56 (1989), p. 435-47. bibliog.

This paper offers an explanation for the dynamics of high inflation based on policy rules governing depreciation of the official nominal exchange rate when in the presence of high black market premia on foreign exchange. The authors develop a model that can assist the interpretation of countries like Bolivia, which jumped between plateaux of ever-higher inflation to the hyperinflation of 1984-85, rather than following a discernible upward trend.

432 Bolivia: hyperinflation, stabilisation, and beyond.
Manuel Pastor, Jr. *The Journal of Development Studies*, vol. 27, no. 2 (1991), p. 211-37. bibliog.

A detailed study of Bolivia's slide into inflation and hyperinflation in the early 1980s, followed by a discussion of the ways in which the New Economic Policy introduced in 1985 confronted the problem through exchange rate stability, slashing the budget, shifting the power away from labour, and attracting the support of the international lending institutions.

433 Debt reduction for Bolivia.
White House Fact Sheet, 22 August 1991. In: *US Department of State Dispatch*, vol. 2 (September 1991), p. 653.

Reports United States Presidential endorsement of an agreement between the US and Bolivian governments to reduce Bolivia's official bilateral debt owed to the US government on food assistance loans by eighty per cent, i.e. from approximately US$38 million to US$7.7 million. An Environmental Framework Agreement is also proposed whereby all interest payments on the reduced debt would be paid in local currency and channelled into an environmental fund established by Bolivia. A second agreement provides full cancellation of Bolivia's USAID debt to the United States, which is approximately US$341 million. The concessions are based on Bolivia's status as a least-developed country implementing strong macroeconomic and structural reforms.

434 Currency substitution: the recent experience of Bolivia.
Benedict Clements, Gerd Schwartz. *World Development*, vol. 21, no. 11 (1993), p. 1883-93. bibliog.

Bolivia has a long history of currency substitution, mostly in the form of US dollars substituting for domestic currency. Between 1986 and 1991, there had been a rapid increase in the share of foreign currency deposits in the Bolivian banking system, and the authors suggest that this trend is likely to continue whatever fiscal measures are adopted by Bolivia in an attempt to reverse the process. See also the same authors' working paper, WP/92/65, under the same title (Washington, DC: International Monetary Fund, 1992. 16p. bibliog.).

435 Decentralization and regional economic development: an econometric analysis of public expenditure, regional growth, and structural change in Bolivia.
Katherine Olga Baer. PhD thesis, Cornell University, Ithaca, New York, 1994. 232p. bibliog.

Analyses Bolivia's regional development patterns during the 1980s, the role of public investment in this development, and, in particular, the effects of decentralizing investment from the central to the regional and local government levels.

436 Exchange-rate depreciation, dollarization and uncertainty: a comparison of Bolivia and Peru.
Paul D. McNelis, Liliana Rojas-Suárez. Washington, DC: Inter-American Development Bank; Office of the Chief Economist, 1996. 23p. bibliog. (Inter-American Development Bank Working Paper, No. 325).

This paper discusses the persistence of dollarization in many Latin American countries despite improved macroeconomic conditions. Focusing here on Bolivia and Peru, the authors argue that dollarization, devaluation, and continued exchange-rate uncertainty are inter-related, and suggest that a reduction in uncertainty may require not only a credible and sustainable macroeconomic policy, but also effective supervision, accountability, and transparency of public and private institutions. In many dollarized countries, such requirements are still only at an early stage.

437 Financial innovation and the speed of adjustment of money demand: evidence from Bolivia, Israel, and Venezuela.
Martina Copelman. Washington, DC: Board of Governors of the Federal Reserve System, 1996. 29p. bibliog. (International Finance Discussion Paper, No. 567).

Examines the importance of money demand in the shaping of monetary policy, noting specifically the effects of Bolivia's innovative stabilization programme which, in 1985, included the introduction of extensive liberalization of all markets, and financial markets in particular.

438 Pension reform in Bolivia: innovative solutions to common problems.
Hermann von Gersdorff. Washington, DC: World Bank; Finance, Private Sector and Infrastructure Department, Private Sector Development Cluster, 1997. 26p. bibliog. (Policy Research Working Papers, No. 1832).

A sound analysis of Bolivia's Pension Reform Law (29 November 1996), which in some respects goes well beyond the Chilean prototype. The study combines detail with a wider perspective, examining the old, limited, and unsustainable state pension scheme alongside the new private pension fund administration. It considers the safeguards currently built into the system, and the challenges to its operation that may arise in the future.

439 Caught.
The Economist, vol. 347 (6 June 1998), p. 34, 36.

Reviews the uphill struggle facing President Banzer's government in its efforts to stamp out high-level corruption in Bolivia. The article reports the latest scandal – charges of theft of up to US$150 million from FOCSSAP, one of the old-style state pension funds for public-sector workers. The charges involve the fund's director, but the alleged misuse of pension-fund accounts is also likely to embroil some of Bolivia's banks, politicians, trade unionists, and civil servants when the case comes to trial, following the director's extradition from Argentina.

440 Financing small-scale enterprises in Bolivia.
Hans Buechler, Judith-Maria Buechler, Simone Buechler, Stephanie Buechler. In: *The third wave of modernization in Latin America*. Edited by Lynne Phillips. Wilmington, Delaware: Scholarly Resources, 1998, p. 83-108. bibliog. (Jaguar Books on Latin America, No. 16).

Life gets harder for small-scale traders in Bolivia as they struggle to compete with the effects of modernization policies and cheaper foreign imports, as well as with each other. The Buechlers examine the traders' access to credit using case-studies in La Paz and El Alto, outlining in particular the role of BancoSol, established in 1992 and the first commercial bank to specialize in helping microentrepreneurs. Small, low-interest loans without collateral are the key. The method is to lend only to 'solidarity groups' (not kinship groups), with each of the five to seven members responsible for ensuring the repayment of the entire loan, although loans are still made on an individual basis. It is an imaginative scheme, with low overheads, and acknowledges the fact that small enterprises can generate vital employment in the informal sector. Some failures have occurred, usually the result of inexperience. Here, the Buechlers provide a balanced debate on the strengths and weaknesses of a credit system which offers a lifeline to the poor, but which is still in its early stages.

441 Bolivia: the financial sector.
Martin Bell. London: British Trade International, September 1999. 19p.

A clear, judicious examination of the main characteristics of modern Bolivia's financial system, including banking, pensions, insurance and securities. Bell reviews changes in the banking sector since the mid-1990s, provides details on the major banks, and considers the potential for transparency and social benefit of the new pensions scheme, which is well explained here. Without ignoring the risks, the author identifies the strides forward that Bolivia has made in recent years, noting areas in which UK companies might well be interested in investing.

442 Credit for the poor: microlending technologies and contract design in Bolivia.
Sergio Navajas. PhD thesis, Ohio State University, Columbus, Ohio, 1999. 135p. bibliog.

Access to credit for the poor in Bolivia has improved dramatically in recent years. Here, the different lending policies of the two largest Bolivian microfinance organizations, BancoSol and Caja Los Andes, are analysed, particularly the difference in the degree of standardization of their loan contracts. BancoSol offers standardized contracts to all takers without collateral, with the relevant screening and monitoring delegated to joint-liability credit groups. Caja Los Andes, on the other hand, offers personal contracts after intensive screening and continued monitoring, and this approach is preferred by higher-productivity borrowers who wish to avoid cross-subsidizing others. Lower-productivity and poorer borrowers are thus more likely to borrow from BancoSol. This is a well-balanced contribution to an important aspect of Bolivia's growing microeconomy.

443 Facing up to inequality in Latin America.
Ricardo Hausmann, Eduardo Lora, Michael Gavin, Carmen Pagés, William Savedoff, Miguel Székely, Glenn Westley. Washington, DC: Inter-American Development Bank; Economic and Social Progress in Latin America, 1998-1999 Report. 282p. bibliog.

The world's largest *per capita* income inequalities are found in Latin America. This far-reaching report avoids superficial judgements while examining the causes of such extreme inequalities in detail, and identifying social policies which would make a real difference to the situation. Measures to increase women's participation in the workforce are seen as essential, particularly those which improve women's ability to seek and gain employment in good jobs. Access to credit by the poor, both men and women, is also discussed, and here, Bolivia's creation of several microenterprise financial institutions (MFIs), including BancoSol and Caja Los Andes, are cited as an important means of funding new microentrepreneurs: 'even better than just serving poor customers, the institutions seem to be helping to lift their borrowers out of poverty'. Income distribution in Latin American countries in the 21st century will depend heavily on government initiatives and government action. While more is often promised than the state can possibly deliver, there is great scope for new and effective legislation. This is a pungent analysis; the investigation is rigorous, forthright, and recommended reading for all politicians and other policy-makers involved in reducing income inequality in Latin America.

Employment and Trade Unions

444 Historia de los sindicatos campesinos: un proceso de integración nacional en Bolivia. (A history of peasant unions: a process of national integration in Bolivia.)
Luis Antezana E. La Paz: Consejo Nacional de Reforma Agraria, 1973. 436p.

This interesting and sympathetic study traces the history of peasant unions from the creation of the first syndicates in Cliza and Vacas in 1936, and considers their struggle against the socio-economic and political power structures. The second part deals with the era of passive resistance, from 1940 to 1946, and the post-1947 era. This was a period of reinvigorated struggle which led to the MNR triumph in April 1952 and the passage, and implementation, of the Agrarian Reform Bill in 1953. The account finishes in 1956.

445 A history of the Bolivian labour movement, 1848-1971.
Guillermo Lora. Edited by Laurence Whitehead, translated by Christine Whitehead. Cambridge: Cambridge University Press, 1977. 408p. bibliog.

An abridged edition of Lora's illuminating history of the Bolivian labour movement. Trade unionism in Bolivia played a fundamental role in bringing about the MNR revolution of 1952. Lora offers an excellent analysis of the major political events and ideological issues which gave the Bolivian labour movement a splendid and complex history, and it remains the best single volume on this subject.

446 Unemployment and underemployment in Bolivian agriculture: a critical survey of the literature.
Washington, DC: US Department of Agriculture, International Division; Bureau for Latin America, Rural Development Division, 1977. 70p. bibliog.

This critical review of rural unemployment, internal and external migration, wage rates and governmental involvement in rural Bolivian life retains its value to researchers.

447 Measuring rural underemployment in Bolivia: a critical review.
Clarence Zuvekas, Jr. *Inter-American Economic Affairs*, vol. 32
(spring 1979), p. 65-83.
Outlines the problems which confront researchers when attempting to calculate the levels
of underemployment and unemployment in a country such as Bolivia.

448 Workers' participation in the nationalized mines of Bolivia.
June Nash. In: *Peasants, primitives and proletariats.* Edited by
David Browman, Ronald Schwartz. New York: Mouton, 1979,
p. 311-27.
Traces the struggles concerning worker participation in the Bolivian mining industry
through a discussion of the organizational problems related to worker mobilization. The
author contends that worker participation in Bolivia has failed to introduce substantial
changes in working conditions; nor has it led to the miners playing a greater role in mine
management at the end of the 1970s.

**449 Workers from the north: plantations, Bolivian labor and the city
in northwest Argentina.**
Scott Whiteford. Austin, Texas: University of Texas Press, 1981.
189p. maps. bibliog. (Latin American Monographs, No. 54).
Studies the relationships between land, labour and the city in the frontier area of
northwest Argentina. Bolivian agricultural workers leave Bolivia seasonally to seek
employment in neighbouring Argentina, mainly for the 5-7-month sugar harvest, although
many of the poorest families hope to settle permanently in a town. Whiteford reviews the
historical and modern background to this migration and then concentrates on the
migrants' employment opportunities in Salta. This is a sound, well-focused piece of
research.

450 Ethnicity, education, and earnings in Bolivia and Guatemala.
George Psacharopoulos. Washington, DC: World Bank; Technical
Department, Latin America and the Caribbean, 1992. 23p. bibliog.
(Policy Research Working Papers; WPS 1014).
In this survey of Bolivian urban centres with over 10,000 people, the ethnic or indigenous
population is defined as those who usually speak one or more of Bolivia's vernacular
languages, even if they can also speak Spanish. Extensive sampling again demonstrated
that indigenous workers had much lower levels of education and earning power in the
labour market relative to the non-indigenous groups. At the same time, the better
educated, whether indigenous or not, earn more than the less educated.

451 Socioeconomic pacts during transitions to democracy.
Davide Grassi. PhD thesis, University of Chicago, Chicago,
Illinois, 1993. 224p. bibliog.
Examines the changing nature of government–trade union relations through three major
case-studies: Spain, Argentina, and Bolivia. In Bolivia, Grassi concentrates on the
changing fortunes of the once-powerful Central Obrera Boliviana (COB), which was
founded in April 1952 and quickly became the most important labour institution of the

128

Bolivian Left. Indeed, the COB performed many functions more typical of a political party than a workers' union. After the political and economic reforms of 1985, however, government funding was cut, and the relationship between the COB and the government became progressively more confrontational, as the power of both the radical Left (the COB) and the radical Right (the military) was curbed. The Bolivian and other case-studies are well handled in what is a clearly written, objective analysis.

452 Sector participation decisions in labor supply models.
Menno Pradhan.   Washington, DC: World Bank, 1995. 312p.
bibliog. (Living Standards Measurement Study Working Paper,
No. 113).

A report on the contrasted restrictions to mobility between the formal and informal sectors of Bolivia's urban labour market. Jobs in the formal sector have normally involved more rigid contractual agreements and wage-setting procedures which have determined entry and reduced subsequent mobility. Jobs in the informal sector, mainly small businesses with low capital investment, have had the advantages of free entry and virtually unrestricted mobility within the sector. Econometric models are used to analyse the varying patterns of job search, entry and movement within the two sectors, including the effects of age, ethnicity and gender.

**453 Challenging boundaries, redefining limits: the experience of
Bolivian handknitters in the global market.**
Janet Marie Page.   PhD thesis, City University of New York, 1999.
455p. bibliog.

A clear, well-focused study of the knitting industry in Bolivia, where several thousand women produce sweaters for export. These handknitters are to be found in some of the country's poorest rural areas where the work is put out and production controlled by middlemen. Page investigates the history and structure of Bolivia's knitwear industry, and the problems the women have encountered in attempting, unsuccessfully, to organize their own production and marketing cooperatives. This is a detailed and illuminating study of the interaction of local producers and global agencies in the handknit trade; it will also interest those concerned with women's involvement in grassroots politics.

**454 Labor market segmentation and migrant labor: a case study of
indigenous and *mestizo* migrants in Bolivia.**
Elizabeth Jimenez-Zamora.   PhD thesis, University of Notre Dame,
Notre Dame, Indiana, 1999. 267p. bibliog.

Indigenous migrant workers often fail to make a successful transition into wage employment in their new surroundings and instead remain straddled between subsistence agriculture and precarious jobs. The author's research among more than 200 indigenous and *mestizo* migrant workers in Bolivia leads her to conclude that indigenous migrants in particular are trapped in low-paid, unstable, and unprotected employment, not only by the lack of necessary skills and various forms of discrimination, but also because they are obliged to maintain their existing responsibilities in their distant home communities on which, in many cases, they depend for survival.

455 Bolivia: foreign labor trends.

La Paz: United States Embassy, for the US Department of Labor, Bureau of International Labor Affairs, Washington, DC. Published annually.

Summarizes key labour indicators for Bolivia, including data on population, literacy, employment, productivity, earnings, percentage of the population below the poverty level, health and safety, and child labour. Information is also provided on union organization, current labour legislation, and the main areas in need of legislative reform.

Agriculture

General

456 The potatoes of Bolivia: their breeding value and evolutionary relationships.
John Gregory Hawkes, J. Peter Hjerting.   Oxford: Clarendon Press, 1989. 472p. maps. bibliog.

The potato is one of the world's four major food crops, and this excellent monograph on the taxonomy (classification) of the wild and cultivated potato species in Bolivia is based on a series of expeditions which were designed to produce a broad genetic base for breeding new disease-resistant, high-yield varieties. Bolivia contains a huge diversity of indigenous potato (*Solanum*) species; already more than 1,600 have been recorded. The text is well supported by distribution maps, plant drawings, photographs, and tables, as well as by an interesting account of the history of potato sample collection and research in Bolivia since the 1920s. The result is a monograph that provides an indispensable work of reference for specialists in this field.

457 Petty producers, potatoes and land: a case study of agrarian change in the Cochabamba Serrania, Bolivia.
C. L. Sage.   PhD thesis, University of Durham, England, 1990.

Follows the changes that have occurred in a former *hacienda* estate in the Department of Cochabamba since Bolivia's 1953 Agrarian Reform, most notably the intensification of agriculture, and the emergence of small farmers as major potato producers in the region. The author assesses the role that truck operators and commercial intermediaries have played in this process, and analyses the new patterns of landownership, farm organization, and wage labour that have transformed the area.

458 **The potatoes of South America: Bolivia.**
Carlos M. Ochoa, translated by Donald Ugent.   Cambridge,
England: Cambridge University Press, 1990. 512p. maps. bibliog.
This substantial and scholarly study on the taxonomy of wild and cultivated potato
species in Bolivia also includes a historical review of collecting, and geographical detail
on the wild species habitats. Six distribution maps of Bolivia's wild potato species are
presented, along with many drawings and black-and-white photographs. In addition,
twenty-five coloured plates distinguish the volume, a fine series of watercolours by Franz
Frey. This is an important contribution to the literature on *Solanum*.

459 **Managing agricultural research for fragile environments:
Amazon and Himalayan case studies.**
John Farrington, Sudarshan B. Mathema.   London: Overseas
Development Institute, 1991. 99p. maps. bibliog. (Agricultural
Administration Unit, Occasional Paper, No. 11).
A study of environmental issues in Bolivia and Nepal which examines how limited
resources can be best applied to agricultural research and extension work in risk-prone
areas, whether these result from low and unreliable rainfall, poor soils, or hilly
topography. Farrington's case-study concentrates on the Santa Cruz region of Bolivia,
describing in particular the successful long-term collaboration between the British
Tropical Agriculture Mission and the Centro de Investigación en Agricultura Tropical
over research programmes and technical training. He also illustrates how practical, low-
cost techniques have been developed to improve cereals, livestock, pastures, and soil
fertility in order to limit damage by mechanized farming and to replace shifting
cultivation.

460 **Peanuts and peanut farmers of the Río Beni: traditional crop
genetic resource management in the Bolivian Amazon.**
David Edison Williams.   PhD thesis, City University of New York,
1991. 190p. bibliog.
Basing his fieldwork on peanut cultivation by a community of Tacana Indian farmers
living on the River Beni, the author sets out to discover the origin of the peanut's erect
subspecies *Arachis hypogaea fastigiata* Waldron. Six varieties of the erect subspecies are
planted extensively by the Tacana on riverine sandbars exposed during the low-water
season, and Williams's investigation leads him to suggest that this particular peanut
subspecies had its centre of origin in the vicinity of his study area. See also A. K. Singh,
'Groundnut. *Arachis hypogaea*' (item no. 471).

461 **High inflation and Bolivian agriculture.**
Ricardo Godoy, Mario de Franco.   *Journal of Latin American
Studies*, vol. 24, no. 3 (1992), p. 617-37.
Considers the view that stabilization programmes, inadvertently perhaps, have restricted
Bolivia's prospects for long-term economic growth, particularly, the authors contend, by
failing to offer clear direction on the strategies to be implemented after stabilization has
been achieved. The early argument is based on the period 1982-85, when increased
demand brought high food prices and rising rural wages. The subsequent downturn after
1985 (except for food exports) is blamed on the lack of a recipe for new growth.

462 **Genetics of reproductive development and reproductive strategies in the Andean grain crop quinoa (*Chenopodium quinoa*).**
J. E. Fleming.   PhD thesis, University of Cambridge, England, 1993.
Quinoa is a grain crop of Andean origin which is receiving increasing attention outside South America owing to its good nutritional qualities and potential industrial value. This study was designed to gain a fuller understanding of quinoa's genetic and environmental controls, and thus assist in the task of developing crossed strains for adaptation to British growing conditions. See also N. W. Galwey, 'Quinoa and relatives. *Chenopodium* spp.' (item no. 475).

463 **Potato-led growth: the macroeconomic effect of technological innovations in Bolivian agriculture.**
Mario de Franco, Ricardo Godoy.   *The Journal of Development Studies*, vol. 29, no. 3 (1993), p. 561-87. bibliog.
Using a Computable General Equilibrium model, the authors measure the wider economic improvements that could be achieved in Bolivia through improved agricultural technology (e.g. high-yielding crop varieties, and the greater use of fertilizers and pesticides). Four examples were selected: the relatively non-traded staples of potatoes and maize; an import crop, wheat; and an export crop, soybeans. The results showed that technological innovations in the production of potatoes would bring the greatest benefit to the Bolivian economy.

464 **Soil erosion and labor shortages in the Andes with special reference to Bolivia, 1953-91; implications for "conservation-with-development".**
Karl S. Zimmerer.   *World Development*, vol. 21, no. 10 (1993), p. 1659-75. map. bibliog.
Basing his findings on a case-study south of Cochabamba, Zimmerer reports that soil erosion in the Bolivian Andes increased in the period between 1953 and 1991 as growing numbers of peasant farmers shifted from labour-intensive conservation techniques such as maintaining drainage ditches, terraces, and retaining walls, and moved into non-farm employment, either permanent or seasonal. The paper assesses the environmental impact of these changes and considers possible future action by the remaining peasant farmers to reduce soil erosion.

465 **Soil erosion and social discourses in Cochabamba, Bolivia: perceiving the nature of environmental degradation.**
Karl S. Zimmerer.   *Economic Geography*, vol. 69 (July 1993), p. 312-27. bibliog.
This study examines the diverse perceptions of the causes of soil erosion among the peasant farmers living around Cochabamba. The older generation acknowledges that in some cases their ignorance of conservation practices has contributed to the problem in the past. The majority of young adult *campesinos* on the other hand blame government policies for the increasing erosion, and voice their complaints through the rural trade unions. The author's personal interviews and conversations with local farmers of all ages

add much to the value of the piece, revealing the interlocking economic, social, and religious attitudes held by the *campesinos* towards the land.

466 Local soil knowledge: answering basic questions in highland Bolivia.
Karl S. Zimmerer. *Journal of Soil and Water Conservation*, vol. 49, no. 1 (1994), p. 29-34. map. bibliog.

The severe soil erosion affecting parts of highland Bolivia is frequently attributed by government and external organizations to ignorance among the peasant land users. While this is not discounted, Zimmerer examines the ways in which many *campesinos* in the Department of Cochabamba have their own relatively accurate, inexpensive methods of monitoring soil erosion. Farmers classify soils by colour and texture, and then match their soil and terrain categories to the most appropriate land use necessary to conserve fertility. This well-observed paper also provides more detail on the farmers' use of retaining walls, terraces, run-off check dams, and wind-breaks as part of their management practice.

467 Report of expedition to collect wild species of potato: February 1–April 15, 1993 and January 1–February 26, 1994.
David M. Spooner, Ronald G. van den Berg, Willman García Fernández, María Luisa Ugarte. Washington, DC: US Department of Agriculture, Agricultural Research Service, 1994. 133p. maps. bibliog.

This is a detailed record of seed and tuber collections made in Bolivia during the expeditions of 1993 and 1994, and includes information on the routes taken, the methodology adopted, and a discussion of the results. Although prepared for a particular branch of agricultural research, the report provides a useful source of reference for collectors in general as well as for those specializing in potato species.

468 Rural credit markets and informal contracts in the Cochabamba valleys, Bolivia.
Jorge Antonio Muñoz. PhD thesis, Stanford University, Stanford, California, 1994. 172p. bibliog.

Discusses reasons for the frequent failure to provide subsidized credit to small farmers, and to minimize the role of moneylenders, in many developing countries. Rural borrowing behaviour and internal credit contracts in Cochabamba form the basis of this research which reveals the numerous formal and informal credit sources available (informal lenders provide more than half the loans), and the rich diversity in the uses of credit among peasant farmers in the Cochabamba region.

469 Andean fields and fallow pastures: communal land use management under pressure for intensification.
Karen Elaine Kraft. PhD thesis, University of Florida, Gainesville, Florida, 1995. 334p. bibliog.

Investigates communal management in the *ayllu* Chayantaka in the Department of Potosí with particular reference to crop–fallow rotation in open fields. The communities involved have faced the combined impact of declining land productivity, El Niño drought, population increase, and out-migration. Kraft considers ways in which these farmers could profitably modify their crop–fallow system, although successive droughts may reduce, or even exclude, future crop production in this highly marginal area of the Andes.

470 **Grain amaranths.** *Amaranthus* **spp. (Amaranthaceae).**
J. D. Sauer. In: *Evolution of crop plants.* Edited by J. Smartt, N. W. Simmonds. Harlow, England: Longman Group; New York: Wiley, 1995. 2nd ed., p. 8-10. bibliog.

Three main amaranth species were domesticated in the tropical and subtropical Americas well before the Spanish conquest, ranging in distribution from southwestern USA, through Mexico, to the high Andes. Like quinoa, amaranths are pseudo-cereals, i.e. they are not a grass but nevertheless produce large quantities of cereal-like grain. The cultivation of the Andean *Amaranthus caudatus* declined under Spanish rule, but it remains well adapted to dry soils and bright sunlight, and is, in addition, an excellent source of lysine, essential for balanced protein nutrition. *Campesinos* still grow grain amaranths on a small scale, but any plans to expand cultivation in South America are still in the experimental stage.

471 **Groundnut.** *Arachis hypogaea* **(Leguminosae-Papilionoideae).**
A. K. Singh. In: *Evolution of crop plants.* Edited by J. Smartt, N. W. Simmonds. Harlow, England: Longman Group; New York: Wiley, 1995. 2nd ed., p. 246-50. map. bibliog.

The groundnut (or peanut) is native to South America. The author discusses the evolution of this oil-rich, protein-rich plant, noting that the cultivated groundnut is believed to have originated in southern Bolivia/northwest Argentina, whence it spread into northern Bolivia, Peru, Brazil and beyond in the pre-Columbian period. Archaeological evidence from Peru indicates the existence of groundnut cultivation as early as 1500-1200 BC. Singh provides an interesting map of South America showing the distribution of wild *Arachis* species, the primary centre of origin of the cultivated groundnut, and the secondary and tertiary centres of diversity.

472 **Lupins.** *Lupinus.* **(Leguminosae-Papilionoideae).**
G. D. Hill. In: *Evolution of crop plants.* Edited by J. Smartt, N. W. Simmonds. Harlow, England: Longman Group; New York: Wiley, 1995. 2nd ed., p. 277-82. bibliog.

Native lupins are widely distributed in the Americas; in South America alone there are said to be between 1,200 and 1,500 wild lupin species. The earliest cultivation of lupins also occurred in South America – in the Peruvian Andes, probably as early as 2000-1000 BC, while in both Bolivia and Peru, *Lupinus mutabilis*, or *tarwi* was later cultivated as part of Tiwanaku's well-organized agricultural economy, and subsequently by that of the Incas. The lupin's advantages in crop rotation were not only the high protein and oil content of its seeds; it was also the only legume to grow at such high altitudes, and its natural capacity to improve soil fertility made it uniquely valuable in food production. Hill's informative study is recommended as a further reminder of the importance of the Lake Titicaca, the altiplano and surrounding regions of the high Andes as an agricultural core area, and of the pre-hispanic civilizations they sustained.

473 Management of tropical legume cover crops in the Bolivian Amazon to sustain crop yields and soil productivity.
Pedro Luna-Orea. PhD thesis, North Carolina State University, Raleigh, North Carolina, 1995. 94p. bibliog.

Loss of soil nutrients and heavy weed growth are two results of practising natural fallow methods as part of a system of shifting cultivation. Here, the author reports on a variety of experiments designed to improve productivity, particularly by replacing natural fallows with leguminous cover crops in the Chapare region of Bolivia, in order to reclaim lands that shifting agriculturalists have recently abandoned.

474 Potatoes. *Solanum tuberosum* (Solanaceae).
N. W. Simmonds. In: *Evolution of crop plants*. Edited by J. Smartt, N. W. Simmonds. Harlow, England: Longman Group; New York: Wiley, 1995. 2nd ed., p. 466-71. map. bibliog.

Archaeological and historical evidence suggests that in the 5000-2000 BC period, several wild potato tubers in South America were progressively selected to produce palatable, low-alkaloid varieties for everyday consumption, an important development for this future world staple food crop which was concurrent with the domestication of the llama. The first cultivation of the potato is assumed to have begun where the wild plants were most numerous and most variable, namely, on the Bolivian and Peruvian altiplano in the Lake Titicaca region. With the aid of diagrams and a diffusion map, Simmonds traces the evolution of the potato, its spread in the Americas from the Titicaca core area, its introduction into Europe by the Spanish c. 1570, and the subsequent development in the late 19th century of new, disease-resistant varieties, all founded genetically on the original *andigena* introductions. The author also records current research taking place on the altiplano, in a concise, scholarly survey designed primarily for the specialist.

475 Quinoa and relatives. *Chenopodium* spp. (Chenopodiaceae).
N. W. Galwey. In: *Evolution of crop plants*. Edited by J. Smartt, N. W. Simmonds. Harlow, England: Longman Group; New York: Wiley, 1995. 2nd ed., p. 41-46. map. bibliog.

The pseudo-cereal quinoa has a unique ability to produce high-protein grain under ecologically extreme conditions. Before the Spanish conquest, it was a staple crop among the Andean population, growing at altitudes of up to 4,000 metres (over 13,000 feet). Indeed, quinoa's tolerance of dry, poor soils made it second only to the potato in importance. This scholarly paper by an expert in the field traces the history of quinoa from its ancient centre of domestication in Bolivia and southern Peru, to its decline under Spanish rule in competition with barley, oats, and faba beans. Galwey then documents quinoa's remarkable revival in recent decades, as cultivation in the Andes has spread once more, and consumption in Europe and North America is increasing through promotion in the health-food sector.

476 **Rural–urban interactions in North Chuquisaca, Bolivia: flows of goods, relational exchange and power relations.**
A. M. Darbellay.   DPhil thesis, University of Oxford, England, 1995. [not paginated].

A discussion of the process of market integration in North Chuquisaca, using potatoes, wheat, and barley as examples. It explores the links between production, exchange and consumption, and the relative importance of social institutions in shaping and controlling market forces.

477 **Discourses on soil loss in Bolivia: sustainability and the search for socioenvironmental "middle ground".**
Karl S. Zimmerer.   In: *Liberation ecologies: environment, development, social movements.*   Edited by Richard Peet, Michael Watts.   London; New York: Routledge, 1996, p. 110-24. bibliog.

By the early 1990s, local press reports in Bolivia estimated that between 35 and 41 per cent of the country was experiencing moderate to extreme soil erosion. Here, the author draws together information on the growing concern about the problem since the 1970s, particularly among the local peasants and the international agencies, and expands his earlier study of the differing explanations for soil erosion, and the varying approaches to conservation, between the older peasants, and the young farmers and union leaders in the Cochabamba region. Zimmerer stresses the complexity of the economic, social and political setting, and the continuing gap between awareness of the problem and the search for an effective, sustainable remedy.

478 **Economic–environmental linkages in a small developing country: the case of Bolivia.**
Leslie Maria Fergerstrom.   PhD thesis, University of Notre Dame, Notre Dame, Indiana, 1997. 253p. bibliog.

The study examines the relationship between population growth and the expansion of agriculture, forestry, cattle-ranching, road-building and manufacturing in parts of lowland Bolivia since the mid-1950s. Particular attention is given to the wider effects of accelerated deforestation and soil degradation on agricultural productivity.

479 **Fewer people, less erosion: the twentieth century in southern Bolivia.**
David Preston, Mark Macklin, Jeff Warburton.   *The Geographical Journal*, vol. 163, part 2 (1997), p. 198-205. map. bibliog.

As well as providing a labour supply for other centres in Bolivia, the country's southernmost Department of Tarija has long been noted for its seasonal or longer-term out-migration to northern Argentina in order to provide wage-labour for sugar harvesting and production. This article concentrates on a small southwest section of the Department of Tarija, noting that where farming has declined in favour of the greater security of wage-labour elsewhere, decreasing pressure on the land has resulted in a denser vegetation cover on formerly cultivated areas and less soil erosion.

480 Policy variables and program choices: soil and water conservation results from the Cochabamba high valleys.
Michael S. Hanrahan, William McDowell. *Journal of Soil and Water Conservation*, vol. 52, no. 4 (1997), p. 252-59. map. bibliog.

A report on one of the projects funded by the United States Agency for International Development (USAID) designed to improve and diversify agriculture in the high, semi-arid valleys of Cochabamba Department, and thus offer a viable alternative to illegal coca/cocaine production in the neighbouring Chapare province. The key strategy is to secure regular water supply and reduce soil erosion by simple methods, including wells, pumps, small dams, canals, catchment-ponds, and contour ploughing. The authors examine ten case-study sites and find increased rural employment and higher rural income at all of them. Readers in turn glimpse a series of small miracles achieved at low cost and enthusiastically adopted during the 1990s by the region's highly practical farmers.

481 Social capital and rural intensification: local organizations and islands of sustainability in the rural Andes.
Anthony Bebbington. *The Geographical Journal*, vol. 163, part 2 (1997), p. 189-97. map. bibliog.

Throughout much of the rural Andes, economically successful communities (here called 'islands of sustainability') flourish amid regions of poverty, environmental degradation, and out-migration. Six localities in Ecuador and Bolivia at varying levels of prosperity or poverty are investigated here. One Bolivian example is drawn from the south of the Department of Potosí where, in a region of mine closures and general decline, the community of Quiwi Quiwi has developed a successful system of rural land use, including water management and intensive horticulture. In the Department of La Paz, certain villages in the Alto Beni have specialized in high-value agricultural products, for niche markets among Bolivia's urban middle class or overseas. Success depends on close co-operation with local organizations, access to modern technology, transport, and often personal contacts with resourceful individuals. Growing self-confidence and initiative within the most vibrant communities then play their part in stimulating further development. See also the same author's 'Organizations and intensifications: *campesino* federations, rural livelihoods, and agricultural technology in the Andes and Amazonia' (*World Development*, vol. 24, no. 7 [1996], p. 1161-77).

482 Tree-crop interactions and nutrient dynamics in agroforestry systems in Bolivia.
Angel Alejandro Salazar. PhD thesis, North Carolina State University, Raleigh, North Carolina, 1997. 123p. bibliog.

Investigates the various methods of simultaneous, interacting tree-and-crop cultivation in the Chapare region of Bolivia, including the effects of mulching, pruning, and root competition. Salazar's conclusions are that on acid, infertile soils, crop yields (particularly of cereals) and soil nutrients are reduced by simultaneous intercropping because of root competition. Sequential planting is more beneficial, along with managed fallows or cover-cropping.

483 Bolivia: the agricultural sector report.

La Paz: British Embassy Commercial Section; London: British Trade International, December 1998. 75p. map.

This is a carefully researched and detailed report on Bolivia's agriculture and agro-industries. After outlining the chief characteristics of the Santa Cruz, Cochabamba, and La Paz agricultural and processing regions, the report provides information on all the major agricultural, livestock and forest products, processed materials, output, and export destinations where appropriate. Lists of Bolivian importers of agricultural machinery and equipment, spare parts, and agrochemicals offer valuable supporting detail, as do several other nuggets of information. The document clearly identifies the business opportunities for potential British investors or companies in this field. It also reveals the dominance of the Department of Santa Cruz in Bolivia's agriculture sector.

484 Linking with agricultural input suppliers for technology transfer: the adoption of vertical tillage in Bolivia.

Graham Thiele, Richard Barber. *Journal of Soil and Water Conservation*, vol. 53, no. 1 (1998), p. 51-56. bibliog.

Around Santa Cruz, many large-scale mechanized farms face the problem of severely compacted soil. The authors describe the attempts made to tackle the problem through the introduction of vertical tillage, known in the United States as mulch or conservation tillage, since it is also designed to reduce wind and water erosion, and improve soil fertility. The value of this paper is its detailed account of how local farmers were persuaded to adopt or adapt the complex new technology by soil researchers, field demonstrations and, most of all, through frequent visits by the specialists to individual farmers over a long period of time to assist and encourage the continued use of the new style of cultivation.

485 Grains of truth.

The Geographical Magazine, vol. 71, no. 10 (1999), p. 68-69.

Four reports on food production are presented in an article to mark World Food Day, one of them by Ilario Caricari, a Bolivian peasant farmer in the village of Calacala, Department of Potosí. He describes a non-governmental organization project, funded by Christian Aid UK, which introduced greenhouse cultivation into the village in 1997 in order to grow a wide range of vegetables and animal fodder. A recycling system sustains these crops, as well as providing organic fertilizer for the outside potato plots, and for general soil recovery from contamination caused by mining pollution. Originally dismissed as wildly impractical, the project has proved so far to be a great success. It employs fifteen families, provides surplus for market, and illustrates the contribution that small, specialized enterprises can make to struggling farming communities.

486 Informal potato seed systems in the Andes: why are they important and what should we do with them?

Graham Thiele. *World Development*, vol. 27, no. 1 (January 1999), p. 83-99. map. bibliog.

In a well-researched study which includes Bolivia, Peru and Ecuador, Thiele observes that informal potato seed systems employed by peasant farmers using tubers (once assumed to be of poor quality) are in fact much more important than formal systems using true botanical seed. Governments now recognize complementarity and seek to link the relative strengths of both. Seed from the higher Andean regions is normally of superior quality and is slower to degenerate than that from the lowlands. In Bolivia, some peasant farmers have become specialist potato-seed producers; women play a central role in seed management, and in seed distribution, both to local and more distant farmers. But while the vigorous informal potato seed system is more effective in selecting and diffusing the best varieties, the formal system is more successful at developing new ones.

487   Origins of domestication and polyploidy in the Andean tuber crop *Oxalis tuberosa* Molina (Oxalidaceae).
Eve A. Emshwiller.   PhD thesis, Cornell University, Ithaca, New York, 1999. 341p. bibliog.

Oxalis tuberosa, commonly known as oca, is one of the most important tuber crops to have been domesticated in the central Andes. This study sets out to clarify the origins of domesticated oca through phylogenetic analyses of molecular and morphological data, drawn both from cultivated oca and wild *Oxalis*, in Bolivia and Peru. Emshwiller widens her research into the crop's origins with an investigation of its traditional uses and earlier cultivation based on archaeological and historical evidence. Two wild tuber-bearing *Oxalis* taxa are identified here as possible progenitors.

488   Overlapping patchworks of mountain agriculture in Peru and Bolivia: toward a regional-global landscape model.
Karl S. Zimmerer.   *Human Ecology*, vol. 27, no. 1 (1999), p. 135-65. maps. bibliog.

Overlap and patchiness, rather than sharp zonal boundaries, are distinctive traits of mountain agriculture in the author's two case-study regions of Paucartambo (Peru) and Cochabamba (Bolivia). While a tiered 'stacking' of belts of farm and land use have been identified by several fieldworkers in the valleys of Bolivia and Peru, Zimmerer finds this to be of limited application, examining instead the local topographical, cultural, and commercial features which influence peasants' decision-making and produce a much more complex pattern of multiple cropping in any given area.

Ranching and forestry in eastern Bolivia

489   The introduction of legumes into degraded tropical pastures in Bolivia.
R. T. Paterson.   PhD thesis, University of Reading, England, 1988. 338p. bibliog.

Sets out in detail and discusses various procedures for introducing pasture legumes to improve the carrying capacity and productivity of pastures which have been degraded by extensive cattle-ranching in eastern Bolivia.

490 The grasses of Chiquitania, Santa Cruz, Bolivia.
Timothy J. Killeen. PhD thesis, Iowa State University, Ames, Iowa, 1989. 146p. bibliog.

This study presents an annotated checklist of grasses (*Gramineae*) in a portion of eastern Bolivia which is underlain by the Brazilian Shield. Killeen includes keys to the 276 species of tropical grasses listed, with notes on their geographical and habitat distributions, their cytology, phenology, and palatability. Six new taxa are also described.

491 Conservation of tropical forests through the sustainable production of forest products: the case of mahogany in the Chimanes Forest, Beni, Bolivia.
Raymond Edward Gullison. PhD thesis, Princeton University, Princeton, New Jersey, 1995. 192p. bibliog.

Mahogany (*Swietenia macrophylla*) is a difficult species for sustainable development because of the special conditions it requires for regeneration. The author contends that with the current lack of management control in the Chimanes Forest, supplies of mahogany there are almost exhausted. Under efficient management, however, the search for, and harvesting of, lesser known but commercially viable timber species could help to achieve sustainable silviculture in this region.

492 The economics of sustainable development in the Gran Chaco of South America.
Tomas Carlos Miller-Sanabria. PhD thesis, Colorado State University, Fort Collins, Colorado, 1996. 141p. bibliog.

A study of land use in the Gran Chaco, emphasizing the continuing decline of agricultural and ranching production, and proposing methods of achieving sustainable development in parts of the region.

493 Development: reflections from Bolivia.
James C. Jones. *Human Organization*, vol. 56, no. 1 (1997), p. 111-20. bibliog.

Concentrating on the Department of Beni, Jones examines the reasons for what he regards as the failure or partial failure of recent development programmes in this region, with particular reference to ranching and forestry. He acknowledges that improvements are difficult to achieve given the isolation of the Beni, conflicting interests, and the complexity of the various national and international organizations involved. This is a personal essay, recommended as a concise overview for the general reader.

494 The effects of markets on neotropical deforestation: a comparative study of four Amerindian societies.
Ricardo Godoy, David Wilkie, Jeffrey Franks. *Current Anthropology*, vol. 38, no. 5 (1997), p. 875-78. bibliog.

One Honduran (the Tawahka) and three Bolivian societies (the Mojeño, Yuracaré, and Chimane) are studied here, all of them having varying degrees and types of contact with their markets. In considering the factors that influence the cutting of secondary forest by these different communities, the authors conclude that integration into the market through the sale of annual crops increases deforestation, while integration into the market through wage labour (e.g. for ranchers, loggers, and others) reduces it.

495 Effects of liana cutting on trees and tree seedlings in a tropical forest in Bolivia.
Diego Rafael Pérez-Salicrup. PhD thesis, University of Missouri, St. Louis, Missouri, 1999. 130p. bibliog.

The author investigates the relationship between lianas (tree creepers and climbers) and trees in the Oquiriquia tropical forest concession in Bolivia, particularly whether liana cutting benefits tree growth. Liana density and infestation at Oquiriquia is the highest in Bolivia, and research indicates that liana cutting resulted in increased water availability (significant in the drier season), and in increased growth among particular species. As a regular silvicultural practice, liana cutting proved effective in reducing the density and infestation of the forest by 95 per cent, and is therefore generally recommended despite its high cost.

496 The effects of structural adjustment on deforestation and forest degradation in lowland Bolivia.
David Kaimowitz, Graham Thiele, Pablo Pacheco. *World Development*, vol. 27, no. 3 (March 1999), p. 505-20. map. bibliog.

A brisk, well-balanced paper which measures the effects of Bolivia's structural economic reforms since 1985 on two types of rural land use in lowland Bolivia. The authors find that apart from coca planting in the Chapare, the reforms did not trigger any significant increase in forest clearance by small-scale peasant farmers for their annual crops, but that the structural adjustment did contribute to large-scale forest clearance for export-led soybean production, and, to a lesser extent, to forest degradation by lumber companies. The economic benefits from both may well have outweighed the environmental costs, but alternative policies might have reduced those costs and encouraged a wider distribution of the benefits. Given the country's economic collapse in the mid-1980s, however, neither the Bolivian government nor the international agencies were prepared to implement alternative policies on the necessary scale. Despite this, the authors note that Bolivia's loggers extract only a small volume of timber per hectare compared with most other parts of the world, and that environmental problems in the Bolivian lowlands are still relatively small compared with many other tropical countries.

Rubber production

497 The empire builders: a history of the Bolivian rubber boom and the rise of the House of Suárez.
J. Valerie Fifer. *Journal of Latin American Studies*, vol. 2, no. 2 (1970), p. 113-46. map. bibliog.

The Bolivian 'rubber baron' Nicolás Suárez dominated much of the upper Amazon region during the wild rubber boom in the late-19th and early-20th centuries. Born in Santa Cruz in 1851, Suárez was to control rubber production within a huge sector of the northern rainforest, as well as ranching on a grand scale farther south around Trinidad and Santa Cruz. With skilled management, the House of Suárez survived the collapse of the Amazon rubber boom and remained a going concern until Nicolás Suárez' death in 1940 at Cachuela Esperanza, the company headquarters on the lower Beni river. Based on original sources, this comprehensive study remains the only major history of the Bolivian rubber boom and of the House of Suárez – its organization, infrastructure and business interests, both in Bolivia and in London and Paris.

498 Food and debt among rubber tappers in the Bolivian Amazon.
Steven Romanoff. *Human Organization*, vol. 51, no. 2 (1992),
p. 122-35. map. bibliog.

This study of the present-day economy in the far northeast of Bolivia focuses on parts of the Beni, but excludes the Department of Pando. Little has changed in well over a century. Tapping wild rubber and gathering Brazil nuts still form the economic basis of the region, supplemented locally by the commercial and service activities in the towns of Riberalta and Guayaramerin, and by small-scale farming close to these two riverine settlements. Chronic food shortages continue to afflict the most isolated areas, where rubber tappers remain in a permanent state of debt to their *patrón* on whom they still rely for food and other supplies in the age-old manner. Indeed, the author suggests that the uncertainty, and often the lack, of regular food supplies underlies the region's social stratification, which is dominated by the relative security of those living in Riberalta and Guayaramerin, but represented elsewhere by a lower class scattered throughout the rubber forests, facing poverty, food shortage, and little prospect of anything better.

Alpaca, llama and vicuña herding

499 Vicuñas and llamas: parallels in behavioral ecology and implications for the domestication of Andean camelids.
Steve A. Tomka. *Human Ecology*, vol. 20, no. 4 (1992), p. 407-33.
maps. bibliog.

A detailed analysis of the llama herds owned by a small altiplano community in southwest Bolivia. The author demonstrates that management of the domesticated herds is greatly assisted by the villagers' knowledge of wild camelid behaviour, and goes on to examine in detail how the application of this knowledge to the care of their own animals makes the best use of available labour, and improves the productivity and control of the herds. An extensive bibliography adds to the value of this scholarly, specialized study.

500 The survival and shearing assets of Bolivia's vicuña.
Mike Ceaser. *Américas*, vol. 52, no. 1 (2000), p. 6-13.

By the 1960s, poachers had killed so many thousands of vicuña that this wild Andean camelid had become one of the world's endangered species. As their numbers increase now in the Ulla Ulla National Fauna Reserve, a new experimental vicuña-shearing programme is under way whereby Aymara alpaca herders will be able to obtain a much-needed additional source of income. The wild vicuña's fine, lightweight, heat-retaining wool commands high prices on the world markets. To capture the animals, the Aymara are using a catch-and-release method based on the ancient Inca technique known as *chaku*, and combining it with health checks on the vicuña herds. This article, strikingly illustrated with colour photographs, will be of particular interest to those promoting a system of sustainable development in the wild that also assists the very poorest high-altitude Aymara.

Land reform and colonization

501 Change in the altiplano.
Richard W. Patch. Hanover, New Hampshire: American Universities Field Staff, 1966. 13p. (West Coast South America Series, vol. 13, no. 1).

A success story of land reform and technological innovation in a Bolivian village. Pairumani represents such a remarkable achievement because the reforms have produced changes in attitudes which make innovation and initiative possible. These changes, unimpressive to the statistical economist, are fundamental for the transformation of a dependent, passive population into an independent and active one.

502 Bolivia's pioneer fringe.
J. Valerie Fifer. *The Geographical Review*, vol. 57, no. 1 (1967), p. 1-23. maps. bibliog.

Discusses Bolivia's long-standing struggle to improve internal communications and develop an integrated national transport system by road, rail, river and air. One major problem over the years had been the many unsuccessful attempts to link the city of Santa Cruz effectively with the main centres of population in the Andes. Following the social revolution and the agrarian reform of 1952-53, the isolation of Santa Cruz overland was ended with the construction of the paved Cochabamba–Santa Cruz highway in 1954, and this triggered a wave of colonization along the Andes foothill zone in the 1950s and 1960s around Santa Cruz, as well as in the Alto Beni and the Chapare. This paper analyses the prospects for future development along the foothill zone, particularly in the Santa Cruz region, which by the late 1960s had already emerged as the cornerstone of Bolivia's pioneer development in agriculture, urban growth, and in the oil and gas industry.

503 Problems and conflicts over land ownership in Bolivia.
Ronald J. Clark. *Inter-American Economic Affairs*, vol. 22, no. 4 (1969), p. 3-18.

Discusses conflicts over landownership in post-revolutionary Bolivia. The government has been unable to process landownership claims quickly enough and furthermore, behaviour patterns, especially among the older *campesinos*, have remained traditional in nature. The three principal conclusions drawn here are: title distribution could, and should, be done more quickly; all the lands of large landowners should have been confiscated; and the role of the peasant unions are important on a local level.

504 Revolution and land reform in Chuquisaca and Potosí.
Katherine Barnes von Marschall. La Paz: Sociedad Nacional de
Reforma Agraria (SNRA), 1970. 163p. bibliog.
A case-study of agrarian reform in southern Bolivia, and specifically, the Chuquisaca-
Potosí region. The degree of isolation of the *haciendas* and Indian communities is an
important factor in determining how each has been affected by agrarian reform. Problems
develop when former landowners maintain their presence in the area after reform has
taken place.

505 Revolution and land reform in the Bolivian Yungas of La Paz.
Katherine Barnes von Marschall. La Paz: Sociedad Nacional de
Reforma Agraria (SNRA), 1970. 233p. bibliog.
A study of the former *haciendas* of the Yungas area. This volume outlines the pre-reform
land tenure system, traces the reform process, and details the new tenure system
introduced as part of the 1952 revolution. The new land tenure system is studied in its
social, political and community dimensions.

**506 Changes in family and household organization in an overseas
Japanese pioneer community.**
Stephen I. Thompson. *Journal of Comparative Family Studies*,
vol. 2, no. 2 (1971), p. 165-77.
A community study of a Japanese pioneer colony in San Juan Yapacani, Bolivia. It had
been assumed that the availability of large amounts of land would result in the
fragmentation and breakdown of traditional family life. This has not happened and the
traditional Japanese family structure has adapted and survived in frontier conditions.

507 Land reform and economic change in the Yungas.
Madeline B. Leóns. In: *Beyond the revolution: Bolivia since 1952.*
Edited by J. Malloy. Pittsburgh, Pennsylvania: University of
Pittsburgh Press, 1971. 268p. bibliog.
In post-1952 Bolivia the peasant communities of small landholders have replaced the
hacienda as a social unit. At the same time *mestizo* power brokers have replaced the local
hacendado (landowner). Peasants exercise power through their syndicates, through
participation in the local markets, and through their increased supply of cash.

**508 Emigration and remigration of Okinawans settled in the
lowlands of eastern Bolivia in relation to background
characteristics of their place of origin.**
Hiroshi Kashiwazaki, Tsuguyoski Suzuki. *Human Ecology*, vol. 6,
no. 1 (1977), p. 3-14.
Studies Japanese immigration to eastern Bolivia and attempts to determine which settler
is likely to remain in a pioneering area, and why.

509 The search for a series of small successes: frontiers of settlement in eastern Bolivia.
J. Valerie Fifer. *Journal of Latin American Studies*, vol. 14, no. 2 (1982), p. 407-32. maps. bibliog.

Analyses the dynamic nature of true frontiers of settlement, and examines the varying degrees of success achieved in Bolivia's attempts to populate and develop its eastern region by spontaneous, guided, or highly directed colonization. The article includes a discussion of the problems facing the latest pioneer development around San Julián, in the Department of Santa Cruz, at the start of the 1980s.

510 Agricultural practices and household organization in a Japanese pioneer community of lowland Bolivia.
Hiroshi Kashiwazaki. *Human Ecology*, vol. 11, no. 3 (1983), p. 283-319.

Describes the colonization carried out by Japanese pioneers in Bolivia. Tests two hypotheses: that pioneer agriculture stimulates the formation of large family households to cope with an assumed labour shortage; and that variation in household organization produces variations in agricultural practices. Data does not suggest that large family households are formed. It does, however, indicate that changes in household composition influence the amount of land farmed and the level of mechanization in agriculture.

511 Migration among landholdings by Bolivian campesinos.
Connie Weil. *The Geographical Review*, vol. 73, no. 2 (1983), p. 182-97. maps. bibliog.

From a study of a small farming community north of Cochabamba where spontaneous colonization began in 1965, the author demonstrates that the migration process in the Chapare colonization zone is not a simple movement from one place to another but often involves several small shifts within the region, as well as the maintenance of multiple holdings in different ecological environments. As many as one-third of the community's landowners spend time elsewhere in the lowlands and highlands of Cochabamba, managing their other holdings and spreading their risks.

512 Frontier expansion and settlement in lowland Bolivia.
Lesley Gill. *The Journal of Peasant Studies*, vol. 14, no. 3 (1987), p. 380-98. map. bibliog.

Focuses on the expansion of cash-crop production in the frontier north of Santa Cruz during the 1970s and 1980s, and discusses the effects that these large-scale enterprises are having on smaller producers. Extensive land ownership, improved market opportunities, and ready capital distinguish the cash-crop operations, while at the other extreme, the poorest peasants survive on a limited, hand-to-mouth existence, disadvantaged in respect of both the large-scale businesses and the successful small-to-middle-scale peasant farmers. The author sees an increasingly stratified society emerging throughout the region, and a growing political solidarity among the very poor.

513 The forgotten.
The Economist, vol. 320 (17 August 1991), p. 40.
In his state-of-the-nation address on 6 August 1991, President Jaime Paz Zamora had stressed the dire conditions of Bolivia's most abject poverty sector, the one million or so rural poor, with two out of three of their dwellings without a clean water supply, and three out of four without a sewage system. If standards of living were to improve significantly, any long-term solution would have to involve increased migration to the Santa Cruz area in order to help satisfy the growing need for paid wage-labour in that region's prosperous export economy.

514 The displacement of peasant settlers in the Amazon: the case of Santa Cruz, Bolivia.
Graham Thiele. *Human Organization*, vol. 54, no. 3 (1995),
p. 273-82. maps. bibliog.
Under this somewhat misleading title, the author sets out to explain 'the surprising persistence of peasant settlement at the frontier in Santa Cruz', noting the fact that both small-scale peasant farmers and large-scale producers are still found to co-exist in the Santa Cruz region. He should not find this surprising, since the variety, changing characteristics, and remarkable resilience of this dynamic colonization zone have been studied continuously since the 1950s. Thiele provides a useful summary of some of the causes for the region's diversity, but essentially adds nothing new to our knowledge of the continuing development of the frontier in the Department of Santa Cruz.

Coca Cultivation, the Coca/Cocaine Trade, and the Drug War

Production and illegal trafficking

In the 1970s and 1980s

515 Drugs and politics: an unhealthy mix.
Michael Flatte, Alexei J. Cowett. *Harvard International Review*, vol. 8 (1986), p. 29-31.
Discusses the relationships between the Bolivian government and the cocaine barons.

**516 Lowland colonization and coca control in Bolivia:
a development paradox for colonization theory.**
D. A. Eastwood, H. J. Pollard. *Tijdschrift voor economische en sociale geografie*, vol. 77 (1986), p. 258-68.
Discusses the development of colonization in the Chapare, the dramatic increase in coca production throughout the region from the mid-1970s to the mid-1980s, and the attempts to reduce the cultivation of coca by means of crop substitution. See also the same authors' note, 'The accelerating growth of coca and colonisation in Bolivia' (*Geography*, vol. 72 [April 1987], p. 165-66).

517 The cocaine economies: Latin America's killing fields.
The Economist, vol. 309 (8 October 1988), p. 21-24.
Although not acknowledged in the official trade statistics, coca/cocaine export outstrips tin and natural gas in Bolivia, copper in Peru, and is probably second only to coffee in Colombia. Estimates placed retail sales of South American cocaine, mostly to North America and Europe, at US$22 billion in 1987, and the article offers clear explanations of how the money is distributed through the networks of middlemen, and absorbed in business overheads, with relatively little going to the growers. Even so, since one in every three or four jobs in Bolivia depends in some way on the growing, processing, or export

Coca Cultivation, the Coca/Cocaine Trade, and the Drug War. Production and illegal trafficking. In the 1970s and 1980s

of coca, the writer doubts whether even massive foreign aid to assist alternative employment would be able to weaken the economic dominance of cocaine.

518 Drugs, debt and dependency.
Michael J. Gillgannon. *America* (New York: America Press), vol. 159, no. 12 (October 1988), p. 310-14.

Recounts the life-style of the 'Cocaine King' Roberto Suárez Gómez before his capture in the Beni in July 1988, not least his popularity as a local hero among many peasant coca-growers. The author regards attempts at control and overall reduction of the cocaine trade as a hopeless task, noting that repeated international calls for debate on the problem have produced no solutions.

519 Now let's slay the other dragon.
The Economist, vol. 308 (30 July 1988), p. 42-43.

The 'other dragon' after inflation in Bolivia is the cocaine traffic. The piece is prompted by the recent arrest of the 'drug baron' Roberto Suárez at his ranch in the Beni, a risky action on the government's part given Suárez's immense popularity among the coca-growers. But it is a calculated risk. In return for stamping down on the cocaine industry, Bolivia expects generous aid from the United States, the World Bank, the International Monetary Fund, and the Inter-American Development Bank.

520 Choking off the supply.
John Madeley. *World Health* (June 1989), p. 28-29.

The setting is Coroico in the Alto Beni where limited cultivation of the coca plant (*Erythroxylum coca*) is traditional and legal. Madeley concentrates on the efforts under way to reduce the wider, illegal cultivation of coca through increased production of coffee, fruit, and vegetables. But this was written on a generally optimistic note when the prospects for control appeared more favourable than subsequent events were to prove.

521 Coca: an ancient Indian herb turns deadly.
Peter T. White. *National Geographic Magazine*, vol. 175 (January 1989), p. 2-47. map.

A comprehensive, well-written survey which is recommended to those seeking to know more about the extent and impact of coca/cocaine production in Colombia, Peru and Bolivia at the end of the 1980s. White traces the prehistory and history of coca cultivation, its use in the pharmaceutical and soft drink industries during the 19th century, and the details of the explosive growth in the coca/cocaine economy since the mid-20th century. All the major aspects of the trade are vividly illustrated by José Azel's photography.

Coca Cultivation, the Coca/Cocaine Trade, and the Drug War. Production and illegal trafficking. In the 1970s and 1980s

522 Cocaine, informality, and the urban economy in La Paz, Bolivia.
José Blanes Jiménez. In: *The informal economy: studies in advanced and less developed countries.* Edited by Alejandro Portes, Manuel Castells, Lauren A. Benton. Baltimore, Maryland: Johns Hopkins University Press, 1989, p. 135-49. bibliog.

An essay tracing the multiple linkages that developed in the 1980s in La Paz between Bolivia's expanding cocaine-based economy and a rapidly diversifying informal sector which is estimated to have absorbed about half of the city's economically active population in that decade. Increased purchasing power derived from the drug trade boosted imported contraband, and stimulated demand for consumer durables, as well as for housing, trucks and land. While the cocaine-based economy has been 'legitimized' in some quarters through its effect in reducing unemployment, the author contends that key aspects of social and political life have been degraded to a level from which recovery may prove to be impossible.

523 Bolivia: the politics of cocaine.
Melvin Burke. *Current History*, vol. 90 (February 1991), p. 65-68, 90.

This article concentrates on the political and economic trends during the 1970s and 1980s, including the problems of inflation, hyperinflation, the flight of capital out of Bolivia, and devaluation. These were followed by a stabilization programme and with it, increased unemployment. Given the strength of the drug lords and the unrivalled profitability of the drug trade, little had been achieved in reducing drug trafficking in Bolivia, and the writer is pessimistic about seeing any fundamental change in the future.

524 Political ascent of Bolivia's peasant coca leaf producers.
Kevin Healy. *Journal of Interamerican Studies and World Affairs*, vol. 33, no. 1 (1991), p. 87-121. bibliog.

During the coca/cocaine boom in the 1980s, the peasant *sindicatos* (unions) in the Chapare became a major force within Bolivia's political system. They focused regional opposition to the US–Bolivian coca eradication policies, forged new alliances within Bolivia, and emerged as a form of local government in the Chapare itself, organizing public works, schools and clinics. This is a detailed, well-balanced article of interest both to the specialist and the general reader. See also the same author's article, 'Coca, the state, and the peasantry in Bolivia, 1982-1988' (*Journal of Interamerican Studies and World Affairs*, vol. 30, nos. 2/3 [1988], p. 105-26. bibliog.).

525 Troops, not talks, in Bolivia.
Jo Ann Kawell. *The Progressive*, vol. 55 (July 1991), p. 27-29.

Reviews the varying roles of the United States and the Bolivian military in the 1980s in confronting the increase of cocaine production, together with the use and misuse of American aid designed to control the drug traffic. The article appears to conclude, despite its obscure title, that neither troops nor talks can provide a viable solution to the problem of finding an acceptable alternative cash crop.

In the 1990s

526   Dependence on drugs: unemployment, migration, and an alternative path to development in Bolivia.
Alain Labrousse. *International Labour Review*, vol. 129, no. 3
(1990), p. 333-48.
A clear, systematic account of the illegal drug industry in Bolivia, including the history
of coca cultivation, its economy and trade. The author adds to the value of the article by
giving more attention to the problems of crop substitution than many other studies on the
subject at this time.

527   A booming grass-roots business.
Brook Larmer. *Newsweek*, vol. 119 (6 January 1992), p. 23.
The author witnesses a road-side deal in the heart of the Chapare between a coca-grower
and a group of buyers representing the local cocaine producers. Larmer notes that without
lucrative alternative crops already in place, and with widespread abuse of coca
eradication programmes, the current high prices for coca/cocaine guarantee its dominant
role in the Bolivian economy. The article is preceded by a general survey of the problems
faced by the US-backed 'war on drugs' in Latin America.

528   The economic consequences of cocaine production in Bolivia: historical, local, and macroeconomic perspectives.
Mario de Franco, Ricardo Godoy.   *Journal of Latin American
Studies*, vol. 24, no. 2 (1992), p. 375-406. bibliog.
As much a review as a research article, the paper traces the historical background to coca
production, and then measures the present effects of cocaine production in Bolivia on the
exchange rate, imports, exports, and domestic food production. The authors assess the
validity of the claim that the cocaine industry draws labourers away from traditional
agriculture, thus weakening domestic food production. They find this claim to be
groundless, and that in the short run the Bolivian economy benefits from the drug
industry. The damage this does to Bolivia lies not in the economic sphere but in its
potential for eroding the country's judicial and political system, and in undermining
foreign relations – a point already widely acknowledged.

529   Snowfields: the war on cocaine in the Andes.
Clare Hargreaves.   London: Zed Books; New York: Holmes and
Meier, 1992. 202p. maps. bibliog.
As one of the many studies examining the different aspects of the illegal coca/cocaine
economy in Bolivia, this volume again illustrates how much easier it is to catalogue the
problems than to propose workable solutions. Nevertheless, Hargreaves offers a lively,
wide-ranging account of the cocaine industry based on personal interviews and on
contemporary newspaper and magazine reports, including graphic descriptions of the
varying roles of the drug barons, the police, and the military in the promotion, or
attempted control, of the business.

530 Coca and cocaine: an Andean perspective.
Edited by Felipe E. MacGregor, translated by Jonathan Cavanagh, Rosemary Underhay. Westport, Connecticut; London: Greenwood Press, 1993. 155p. bibliog.

Reviews the history and the economic and social impact of the coca/cocaine industry in Bolivia, Colombia, and Peru. The point is well made that this illegal activity is not an isolated problem but part of a much wider picture of rural poverty and underdevelopment. However, some of the remedies suggested here for Bolivia are surprisingly impractical, e.g. the resettlement of 'surplus' population from the Chapare's coca/cocaine region to other parts of the country.

531 The coca boom and rural social change in Bolivia.
Harry Sanabria. Ann Arbor, Michigan: University of Michigan Press, 1993. 277p. maps. bibliog. (Linking Levels of Analysis Series).

This is a study of coca production in the Chapare region of Cochabamba Department that gives relatively little attention to drug trafficking and other illegal activities, but concentrates instead on the social effects of rapid migration into the area, the colonization patterns, land tenure, and wider agricultural peasant economy of which coca forms a part. The rural community of Pampa provides the basis for Sanabria's analysis which records a comprehensive and detailed anthropological investigation that can be recommended to the specialist reader.

532 Risk and opportunity in the coca/cocaine economy of the Bolivian Yungas.
Madeline Barbara Léons. *Journal of Latin American Studies*, vol. 25, no. 1 (1993), p. 121-57. bibliog.

An anthropological study set in the North and South Yungas region of the Department of La Paz where, unlike the more recent development in the Chapare, coca is a traditional crop, the long-standing source of supply for the miners and *campesinos* (peasant farmers) on the altiplano. The article traces the historical background of coca production in this region and offers a clear analysis of the political and economic strategies adopted by the local population to maintain coca-growing and resist crop substitution. The region is still legally permitted to grow coca but not to process cocaine.

533 Bolivia and coca: a study in dependency.
James Painter. Boulder, Colorado; London: Lynne Rienner Publishers, 1994. 194p. maps. bibliog.

One of the best book-length studies on the subject. The author traces the events leading to the coca boom, its impact on the economy, and the various methods so far adopted to reduce Bolivia's coca/cocaine industry: legislation, interdiction, eradication, and the military option. Focusing on the Chapare, Painter reviews the bleak prospects for alternative development, noting that lack of market, poor planning, and inadequate transport have consistently undermined the policies of crop substitution. In a book to interest both the general reader and the specialist, Painter can foresee no significant structural changes to the present state of affairs in either the immediate or the more distant future.

534 The coca growers.
The Economist, vol. 331 (4 June 1994), p. 45-46.
Examines the nature and extent of crop substitution in the Chapare as the Bolivian government redoubles its efforts in the 1990s to reduce coca cultivation. Given limited local markets, however, and high transport costs, money earned from legal crops can never compare with the income from coca. Moreover, coca is an easy crop to grow and therefore the first choice among ex-miners and other migrating into the region who have never farmed in their lives before.

535 The impact of rainfall frequency on coca (*Erythroxylum coca*) production in the Chapare region of Bolivia.
Michael S. McGlade, Ray Henkel, Randall S. Cerveny. *Yearbook*, Conference of Latin Americanist Geographers, vol. 20 (1994), p. 97-105.
By examining the relationship between climate and coca production in the Chapare (which accounts for about 90 per cent of Bolivia's coca and cocaine output), the authors conclude that in addition to the general temperature and rainfall requirements, a major determinant is the occurrence of days without rain. Coca leaf production is significantly linked to a sufficient number of rainless days to allow for efficient harvest and drying procedures to be completed, which in turn control supply and market price. See also the same authors' note, 'Climate and cocaine' (*Nature*, vol. 361 [1993], p. 25).

536 Coca cultivation, drug traffic, and regional development in Cochabamba, Bolivia.
Robert Laserna. PhD thesis, University of California, Berkeley, 1995. 293p. bibliog.
By analysing family incomes, job opportunities, and the long-term prospects of many coca-growers and small-scale traffickers in the Chapare, the author considers the effects of coca cultivation on regional development, or lack of it, in the Cochabamba area.

537 Economic development, restructuring and the illicit drug sector in Bolivia and Peru: current policies.
Elena H. Alvarez. *Journal of Interamerican Studies and World Affairs*, vol. 37, no. 3 (1995), p. 125-49. bibliog.
Assesses the extent to which by the mid-1990s the restructuring of the Bolivian and Peruvian economies has been helped or hindered by the illegal drug trade. In the case of Bolivia, private investment is found to have been more sluggish than Sánchez de Lozada had earlier hoped for in his structural reforms; the country remains much more dependent on foreign assistance than Peru, and less successful in attracting it. In these circumstances, Bolivia's illegal drug trade has helped to finance the cost of restructuring, although it may have made longer-term economic adjustment more difficult.

Coca Cultivation, the Coca/Cocaine Trade, and the Drug War. Production and illegal trafficking. In the 1990s

538 Coca, cocaine, and the Bolivian reality.
Edited by Madeline Barbara Léons, Harry Sanabria. Albany, New York: State University Press, 1997. 310p. maps. bibliog.

Twelve essays range over the social, economic, political, and environmental aspects of the topic, providing between them a clear and scholarly account of conditions in the late 1990s, including the chronic problems of trying to make the cultivation of alternative crops popular and workable. Coca/cocaine production has stimulated commerce, transport, construction, and the service industries, and enabled large segments of the population to survive the economic crises. Indeed, the ways in which the coca/cocaine industry affects the peasants' everyday lives is a major theme throughout this well-presented study.

539 Alternative development and supply side control in the drug industry: the Bolivian experience.
Menno L. Vellinga. *European Review of Latin American and Caribbean Studies*, no. 64 (June 1998), p. 7-26. bibliog.

With the continued lack of any lasting solution to the problems of the coca/cocaine industry in Bolivia, the endless flow of commentary on the subject becomes, in essence, no more than a repetition of what has been written before. Vellinga reviews the background, the current conditions, and the overall failure of crop substitution and of strategies for alternative development, when only massive long-term programmes for integrated rural development in the coca-producing regions are likely to have any positive effect. The author argues that in Bolivia and Peru the coca/cocaine industry is no longer a threat to the stability and integrity of the state; indeed, as others have noted, continued illegal cultivation of coca pumps revenue into the economy, while maintaining the need for access to international sources of funding for new development projects. When all is said and done by outside observers, however, Bolivian *campesinos* (peasant farmers) involved in the trade know that, so far, growing coca earns them more money with less effort than any alternative crop on offer – an unassailable argument, surely, for the very poor.

540 Bolivia goes to war against coca.
The Economist, vol. 348 (19 September 1998), p. 43-44. map.

Although President Banzer's declared aim is to wipe out illegal coca-growing by the year 2002, ten years of effort under different administrations have had negligible results so far. Eradication is matched by more illicit planting. A new 'Community Compensation' scheme reworks earlier strategies, but the advantages to be gained by alternative crops and improved infrastructure take time. The immediate results of such programmes have so far led to increased migration to urban areas to swell the numbers of unemployed, or to the spread of illegal coca cultivation into more remote areas of Bolivia.

541 The economic and political impact of the drug trade and drug control policies in Bolivia.

Andy Atkins. In: *Latin America and the multinational drug trade.* Edited by Elizabeth Joyce, Carlos Malamud. Basingstoke, England: Macmillan; New York: St Martin's Press, 1998, p. 97-115. bibliog.

The volume as a whole comprises contributions that were originally presented at a conference in 1995 in Toledo, Spain. The author acknowledges that his piece draws heavily on James Painter's book of 1994 (item no. 533). As a result, Atkins's chapter is basically no more than a summary of known events up to 1994, without any updating of the text or the references. Given the book's publication date, the opportunity to rewrite should have been taken. While some chapters in this collection are more illuminating, that on Bolivia compares unfavourably with the many other studies available on the drug trade, and its impact on the country's economy and politics.

542 Economic development and the origins of the Bolivian cocaine industry.

Michael D. Painter. In: *The third wave of modernization in Latin America.* Edited by Lynne Phillips. Wilmington, Delaware: Scholarly Resources, 1998, p. 29-49. bibliog. (Jaguar Books on Latin America, No. 16).

In this perceptive study of Cochabamba's Chapare region, Painter reaches back before the 1980s to the basic tenets of the 1952 revolution's development model. That model, he argues, with its failure to invest in highland agriculture and its reliance on subsidized food imports, maintained a large rural population unable to earn a decent living through farming and unable to survive without it. Early efforts to diversify production foundered on the small size of the domestic market; the Chapare's geographical location, topography and climate, on the other hand, were to favour the more rewarding international market for coca/cocaine. The author notes that it is the coca-growers rather than the cocaine traffickers who continue to bear the brunt of the punitive measures in the drug war, an issue that has energized the growth of worker movements and peasant union resistance in the Chapare. Painter's concise, well-written chapter should be read for its discussion of the long-term historical factors which have contributed to the stagnation of sectors of Cochabamba's agro-economy. While the development of the cocaine industry was not inevitable, the foundations, he contends, had been laid at an earlier stage for the industry to take root and grow.

543 Leaf in the lurch.

Sue Wheat, Philip Withers Green. *The Geographical Magazine,* vol. 71, no. 9 (1999), p. 42-48. map.

Apart from its fatuous title, the article provides a clear résumé for the general reader of the intractable problems of coca/cocaine production in Bolivia. The authors set out President Banzer's current 'Dignity Plan' for the total eradication of illegal coca cultivation by the year 2002, and the resistance to the Plan's enforcement which is regularly organized by the *cocaleros sindicatos* (coca-growers' unions), including mass protest marches, hunger strikes, and road blocks. The government's shift from individual to community compensation for the eradication of illegal coca cultivation is showing some results, but for all the reasons catalogued in the literature over many years, the nub of the problem so far remains unsolved.

544 The Andean coca wars.
The Economist, vol. 354 (4 March 2000), p. 25-27. map.
A comprehensive review of the latest trends in illegal coca cultivation in Bolivia, Colombia, and Peru. In its annual certification process, the US government reported an overall fall of 15 per cent in illegal coca production since 1995 in these three states, although the scale of the decline is challenged by some field experts. The cultivation of opium poppies has risen in Colombia and begun in Peru. Conditions in Bolivia are examined here in some detail. The Banzer administration's clampdown on the coca-growers' unions, the new measures introduced to reduce the import of chemicals needed for cocaine processing, and the public weariness with the violence and corruption that riddle the cocaine industry are all having an effect. The progress made so far in coca substitution and alternative development is well summarized here, including new crops, new roads and market access, and new packaging and storage plants. But coca is still easier to grow and to transport, and new smuggling routes are soon established. Possibly no more than 20 per cent of the Chapare's illegal coca-growers will ever become successful farmers unless alternative development programmes are given price-support and subsidized credit by the government.

Relations with the United States on the drugs issue

545 Drug policy and agriculture: US trade impacts of alternative crops to Andean coca: report to Congressional requesters.
United States General Accounting Office. Washington, DC: Superintendent of Documents, US General Accounting Office, 1991. 58p. map.
A crisp, well-written report to the House of Representatives on how possible competition with US agricultural exports has affected US policy in assisting the introduction of alternative crops to coca in Bolivia and Peru, and what possible impact alternative crops, particularly soybeans and citrus, would have on US agricultural trade. The government's purpose is to prevent giving aid that would significantly and adversely affect US producers and exporters. The report deals mainly with Bolivia, and concludes that even if Bolivia reached its full potential in soybean cultivation and soy products, exports would remain relatively very small. This also applies to citrus production in Bolivia and Peru, even though US growers habitually complain about the increasing threat of imported frozen concentrated orange juice. A useful list of alternative crops, old and new, is included, with the comment that none will compete successfully with coca: pineapples, macadamia nuts, black pepper, palm hearts, oranges, juice and marmalade, coffee, cacao, corn, and bananas. No time is wasted on debating the point. The report gives a good summary of the issues involved, with statistical support, and advises that no project to support and extend soybean export in Bolivia should be funded by the USA, although

efforts to increase cultivation for internal consumption should continue to receive aid. The
author also sheds light on the conflicts of interest that have arisen between the US
Overseas Agency for International Development (USAID) fieldworkers in Bolivia, and
the US Department of Agriculture in Washington. The latter rules.

546   Militarising the drug war in Bolivia.
Waltraud Queiser Morales.   *Third World Quarterly*, vol. 13, no. 2
(1992), p. 353-70.

Highlights what is seen as the weaknesses of the United States–Bolivian Anti-Narcotics
Agreement of May 1990, and in a generally adverse and for the most part cynical
appraisal, criticizes the methods of drug control from the perspectives of the military,
the peasantry, and US–Bolivian diplomacy.

547   Smoke and mirrors: the paradox of the drug wars.
Jaime Malamud-Goti.   Boulder, Colorado: Westview Press, 1992.
117p. bibliog.

This account by an Argentine academic focuses on the problems of drug enforcement and
coca eradication programmes in the Chapare region during the late 1980s and early 1990s.
The study traces the changing and often uneasy relationship in practice between the US
and Bolivian authorities, asserting that while joint control and anti-trafficking policies
will continue to be implemented, their success will at best be moderate – the preferred
option in Bolivia, the author contends, if the country's economy is to survive.

548   Alternatives to coca production in Bolivia: a computable general equilibrium approach.
Bill Gibson, Ricardo Godoy.   *World Development*, vol. 21, no. 6
(1993), p. 1007-21. bibliog.

The authors outline and then question the wisdom of the latest US and Bolivian
government plans to eradicate the cultivation of coca used for cocaine production,
calculating that even a 50 per cent reduction would devastate the Bolivian economy. In
recommending a much smaller reduction, they conclude that sugar, cattle, maize, and
forestry are best suited as substitutes for coca, but stress that even these would introduce
practical problems such as soil erosion or market glut in some areas.

549   Free market reform and drug market prohibition: US policies at cross-purposes in Latin America.
Peter Andreas.   *Third World Quarterly*, vol. 16, no. 1 (1995),
p. 75-87.

The drug export industry in certain Latin American countries is a leading market force
and an integral component of the private sector. Here, Andreas concentrates on the
cocaine export sector in Peru and Bolivia, maintaining that the drug trade and the
neoliberal economic policies adopted as part of the official government austerity
programmes actually fuel each other, a point that the United States and others are
reluctant to debate.

Coca Cultivation, the Coca/Cocaine Trade, and the Drug War. Relations with the United States on the drugs issue

550 Fire in the Andes: US foreign policy and cocaine politics in Bolivia and Peru.
Sewall Hamm Menzel. Lanham, Maryland: University Press of America, 1996. 281p. maps. bibliog.

A well-written, objective discussion of the United States anti-drug programme in Bolivia comprises the first half of this book. Menzel traces the background to policy-making in Washington, DC, Congressional ignorance of the complexity of the political and economic issues at work in Bolivia, and the futility of most of the anti-drug policy while international consumer demand remains high. The lessons learned so far are examined in detail, but the author concludes that the drug war in general continues to be lost.

551 The drug war at the supply end: the case of Bolivia.
F. García Argañarás. *Latin American Perspectives*, vol. 24, no. 5 (1997), p. 59-80. bibliog.

Evaluates the social benefit or, conversely, the harm derived from the US and Bolivian governments' pursuit of coca replacement and eradication policies in Bolivia. In a well-written and (on the whole) objective analysis, the writer emphasizes the failure to produce a viable long-term plan of crop substitution, and records a number of good intentions that have gone wrong through failure to co-ordinate the timing of new initiatives on the ground.

552 "The only war we've got": drug enforcement in Latin America.
Coletta Youngers. *NACLA Report on the Americas* (North American Congress on Latin America), vol. 31, no. 2 (September/October 1997), p. 13-18.

A survey covering Colombia, Peru, and Bolivia which examines the problem of drug enforcement from both the Latin American and the United States points of view. Youngers details the lack of consensus in all quarters as to what to do next in the war against the coca/cocaine industry, and provides an incisive commentary on the vested interests involved. This is a measured, realistic assessment of a problem which has no quick or easy solution.

553 Bolivia: clashes to come.
The Economist, vol. 350 (20 February 1999), p. 34-35.

Within a longer article on the United States war on drugs, the writer notes that Bolivia is one of the states included in America's regular listing of those countries it certifies as trustworthy allies in the drug war, and those not. Although it raises anger and irritation in Latin America, annual certification (and all that goes with it) remains a US Congressional requirement. Thus, despite the often violent resistance by the illegal coca-growers and the enormous scale of the task, the Banzer government presses ahead with increasingly stringent coca eradication and replanting controls, encouraged not only by US demands, but by declining support in the country as a whole for illegal coca production, not least because of the damage it does to Bolivia's national and business image abroad.

554 The United States and Bolivia: fighting the drug war.
Eduardo A. Gamarra. In: *The United States and Latin America: the
new agenda.* Edited by Victor Bulmer-Thomas, James Dunkerley.
London: University of London Institute of Latin American Studies;
Cambridge, Massachusetts: David Rockefeller Center for Latin
American Studies, Harvard University, 1999, p. 177-206. bibliog.

The author does a thorough job in this analysis of the anti-drugs war, and of the variously
smooth or strained relationships between the United States and Bolivia that have marked
their attempts to eliminate the illegal coca/cocaine trade. After his detailed chronology of
the ups and downs of the anti-narcotics programme in recent decades, Gamarra considers
the Banzer government's latest initiative for the eradication of illegal coca cultivation by
the year 2002 (the 'Dignity Plan'), and concludes, like most other investigators, that it is
unlikely to be achieved, especially given the lack of an adequately planned and funded
alternative crop programme. While total eradication is the sort of vehement,
uncompromising policy that wins praise from the United States and from international
organizations, there are dangers that the methods of its implementation would lose much
of the government's popular support. As Gamarra concludes: 'The basic dilemma of the
drug war in Bolivia is not whether it is being won or lost. Instead it has to do with its
impact on the still incipient process of democratization.'

Mining

555 The emergence of the tin industry in Bolivia.
John Hillman. *Journal of Latin American Studies*, vol. 16, no. 2
(1984), p. 403-37. bibliog.

A scholarly examination of the development of the tin industry in Bolivia in the 19th century, based on primary research. Hillman first looks at it from a global perspective, and then traces the emergent industry.

556 The economics of tin mining in Bolivia.
Mahmood Ali Ayub, Hideo Hashimoto. Washington, DC: World
Bank, 1985. 106p. bibliog.

This authoritative study brings together reliable and consistent data on the Bolivian tin mining sector and analyses the development of the industry from an historical perspective. It is arranged into eight chapters and addresses such issues as: (1) the impact of tin mining on the Bolivian economy; (2) tin pricing and competitiveness; (3) problems of the national mining corporation, COMIBOL; (4) the smelting process; and (5) the tax structure. The study concludes on a pessimistic note and suggests that the best that can be done is to maintain production at the present level, evaluate the tin-producing potential of the lowlands, and diversify into other metals. [As this study went to press, events took a dramatic downward turn, but the publication remains a valuable source of reference on the subject and on the run-up to the collapse of the world tin market.]

557 Going for gold in Bolivia.
Stewart D. Redwood. *New Scientist*, vol. 115 (20 August 1987),
p. 41-43.

Provides an interesting, comprehensive account of the centuries-old search for gold in the placer deposits along the Tipuani river north of La Paz. The riverbed has been worked for gold since Inca times and today, in addition to large-scale dredging operations, many miners form their own cooperatives and receive help in purchasing basic mining equipment from the World Bank.

558 **The great tin crash: Bolivia and the world tin market.**
John Crabtree, Gavan Duffy, Jenny Pearce. London: Latin America
Bureau, 1987. 103p. map. bibliog.

A succinct account of the great tin crash of October 1985, when the international tin
market collapsed and the world price of tin fell by half. The authors outline the events
leading up to the crash, the workings of the market, the International Tin Council and the
London Metal Exchange, and Bolivia's extreme vulnerability, as one of the world's
highest-cost producers, to competition from cheaper sources and new technology. Long-
overdue restructuring of Bolivia's mining industry, if tackled, will take time. The
commentary is clear and objective, and is interspersed with personal stories of the dire
consequences of the tin crash on miners and their families. This remains valuable
background reading for the understanding of later events.

559 **Bolivia and the International Tin Cartel, 1931-1941.**
John Hillman. *Journal of Latin American Studies*, vol. 20, no. 1
(1988), p. 83-110. bibliog.

As the depression in tin took hold after 1929, the International Tin Cartel was organized
in 1931 in order that individual tin producers would secure greater benefit in the form of
higher prices by agreeing a restriction of output. While the cartel benefited all producing
nations, Bolivia was the main beneficiary since the high prices obtained by the cartel
maintained the productive capacity at the country's high-cost marginal lode mines over
the longer term. Indeed, this detailed study on conditions in the 1930s and early 1940s
concludes that Bolivia benefited the most while contributing the least to the International
Tin Cartel.

560 **Bolivia and British tin policy, 1939-1945.**
John Hillman. *Journal of Latin American Studies*, vol. 22, no. 2
(1990), p. 289-315. bibliog.

During the Second World War, Bolivia became the single most important source of tin for
the Allies. Against this background, the author discusses the relationships between
Britain, Bolivia, and the United States, including wartime controls, pricing, and the
allocation of resources. Patiño remained a key element in these exchanges, playing off the
UK and the USA against each other to his own advantage whenever the opportunity arose.

561 **The El Dragón mine, Potosí, Bolivia.**
Günter Grundmann, Gerhard Lehrberger, Günter Schnorrer-Köhler.
The Mineralogical Record, vol. 21, no. 2 (1990), p. 133-46. maps.
bibliog.

Bolivia's recently discovered El Dragón mine near Potosí has become a new geological
treasure-store. Not only does it contain rare, almost pure, krutaite (nickeloan), the richest
natural selenium concentration in the world, but in analysing the mine's complex
mineralization, the authors identify over fifty mineral species from the primary vein and
cavities, and illustrate their informative paper with clear sketch maps and colour
photographs.

562 Mining and agriculture in highland Bolivia: ecology, history, and commerce among the Jukumanis.

Ricardo A. Godoy. Tucson, Arizona: University of Arizona Press, 1990. 169p. bibliog.

A study of the survival and growth of small-scale mining (notably in this case for antimony) in a mixed mining and farming region of northern Potosí. Godoy argues that mining ventures such as those of the Jukumanis make commercial sense, appear to achieve good recovery rates, are cost-effective, and do not lead to misuse of the nation's mineral wealth. Mining and agriculture link profitably here to stabilize personal incomes and the local economy.

563 Serendipity or economics? Tin and theory of mineral discovery and development, 1800-1920.

Derek Matthews. *Business History*, vol. 32 (1990), p. 15-48. maps.

A comprehensive survey of the sources, trade, and changing technology of tin mining worldwide in the selected time-span, including the effects from the 1870s onwards of the growing demands of the tinplate, and later the automobile industries, on prices and production. Bolivia becomes a significant world producer at a relatively late stage (in and after the 1890s), triggering new railway construction between the Andes and the Pacific ports. The author argues that the development of tin mining can be satisfactorily explained in terms of economic variables, without reference to chance finds, noting, not surprisingly, that deposits long known about become commercially viable only when demand and prices rise.

564 I spent my life in the mines: the story of Juan Rojas, Bolivian tin miner.

Juan Rojas, edited by June Nash. New York: Columbia University Press, 1992. 390p. map. bibliog.

An absorbing autobiographical account of Juan Rojas, a Bolivian tin miner who began more than forty years of work in the mines in 1933, at the age of eight. Rojas, his wife and his children recounted their experiences to Nash at intervals between 1969 and 1986. These edited, taped conversations reveal in historical perspective the suffering, danger, and endurance of the mining community, whose courage is so well depicted in this fine book. Forty photographs enrich the text.

565 The Bolivian tin mining industry in the first half of the 20th century.

Manuel Eduardo Contreras. London: University of London Institute of Latin American Studies, 1993. 45p. bibliog. (Research Paper, No. 32).

Outlining the development of Bolivia's tin-mining industry up to the nationalization of the principal mines in 1952, the author concentrates on the economic and technical aspects of the industry, analysing the performance of the major mining companies and the impact of the changing international framework within which Bolivia operated during these five decades. The paper includes a comprehensive bibliographical essay on the country's mining industry which provides a helpful review of the earlier literature for those wishing to research the topic further.

566 We eat the mines and the mines eat us: dependency and exploitation in Bolivian tin mines.
June C. Nash.   New York: Columbia University Press, 1979, 1993. 363p. bibliog.
A highly dramatic and moving picture of living conditions and family life in Bolivia's mining areas. This well-illustrated study was based on a year-and-a-half's research and puts flesh on the skeleton of dependency theory. The volume's high quality led to its reissue in 1993, with a new preface, as a Columbia Centennial Classic.

567 Inside the rich mountain.
Isabel Ambler.   *The Geographical Magazine*, vol. 66, no. 5 (1994), p. 26-30.
The Cerro Rico (rich mountain) at Potosí was the site, nearly 500 years ago, of one of the greatest silver strikes of all time, a legendary source of wealth for the Spanish empire. In the 1990s, in what was to become one of the poorest regions of Bolivia, some 10,000 freelance miners have sought a livelihood by tunnelling into the mountain to extract low-grade silver ores. The conditions are appalling and life expectancy short, but there is fierce local resistance to the possibility of large mining companies moving in and introducing opencast working. Most of the article consists of a series of excellent colour photographs taken by Jürgen Bindrim.

568 Competitiveness, environmental performance and technical change: the case of the Bolivian mining industry.
I. F. Loayza.   DPhil thesis, University of Sussex, England, 1995.
This research was carried out at four Bolivian mining companies and seven mining operations, its main purpose being to model the economic relationship between competitiveness and pollution. Competitiveness was estimated by the mining firm's market share of world production, pollution per unit of output by its metal recovery rates, reagent consumption, water management and waste disposal systems. As suggested here, the beneficial link between the two reflects a firm's dynamic efficiency, basically its internal capacity for technological innovation.

569 I am rich Potosí, king of the mountains, envy of kings.
Marguerite Holloway.   *Natural History*, vol. 105 (November 1996), p. 36-43.
Thousands of mine-openings pierce the surface of the historic Cerro Rico, where many individuals or cooperatives continue to work in mines leased from the state. Visiting the Candelaria mine, the author examines the nature and strength of Bolivia's traditional mining culture in an article vividly illustrated with colour photographs by Stephen Ferry.

570 Bolivia: the mining sector.
La Paz: British Embassy Commercial Section, April 1997. [not paginated].
A brief report which concentrates on the development potential of the Precambrian region in eastern Bolivia, following the positive findings of the Precambrian Project in the 1970s-1980s (see item no. 58). Also included are notes on the varied deposits at Potosí's Cerro Rico, Llallagua tin, El Mutún iron, Kori Kollo gold, and the huge reserves of

lithium, boron, potassium, chlorine, and magnesium in the *salares* (salt flats) of Uyuni, Coipasa and Empexa. General advice and lists of useful company contacts are appended.

571 Bolivia: jewel of the Andes.
W. G. Prast, Michael Forrest, Jonathan Guy, Austin Wheeler. *Mining Journal*, vol. 331 (3 July 1998), p. 1-8.

A well-illustrated and informative survey of Bolivia's mineral wealth which can be recommended to both the specialist and the general reader. After a concise summary of the country's geology, mining legislation and taxation system, particular attention is given to the huge investment project at the US-based Apex Silver Mines' San Cristobal site southeast of Uyuni, discovered in 1995 and now recognized as one of the largest silver reserves in the western hemisphere. A low-cost operation, San Cristobal is forecast to become the world's largest opencast silver mine in 2001. In addition, the authors discuss the Kori Kollo (gold) and San José (lead-silver) mines near Oruro; the Cerro Rico (tin-silver) at Potosí; the El Mutún iron ore deposits in southeast Bolivia; and the future commercial possibilities of exploiting the richest of the old mine tailings.

572 Mining in Latin America: the new boom.
Latin American Special Report, August 1998. London: Latin American Newsletters. 12p.

A survey which focuses specifically on the current growth points in Latin America's mining industry. While acknowledging mining's susceptibility to fluctuating world prices, the report notes that Bolivia's gold output trebled in the 1990s. Zinc output rose spectacularly in the same period, while silver production also revived strongly, along with zinc and lead, in the Potosí region. The report is clearly illustrated with charts and diagrams of Latin American mining output on an internal comparative basis, as well as in relation to total world production.

573 An environmental study of artisanal, small and medium mining in Bolivia, Chile, and Peru.
Gary McMahon, José Luis Evia, Alberto Pascó-Font, José Miguel Sánchez. Washington, DC: World Bank, 1999. 61p. bibliog. (World Bank Technical Paper, No. 429).

The main thrust of this investigation is to decide whether or not artisanal and small mines are economically viable when environmental costs are taken into account. The authors' recommendation is that each case should be judged on its merits, since these mines form a very heterogeneous group. If on balance the mine is economically viable, encourage it. If not, do not subsidize the mine in order to sustain or create more employment. Instead, put the money swiftly into alleviating poverty and easing the other dire consequences of mine closure. There is also a need to clarify property rights among small miners, and to overhaul the tax system. Regarding medium and large mines, age was found to be more important than size when assessing environmental costs.

574 I am rich Potosí, the mountain that eats men.
Stephen Ferry. New York: Monacelli Press, 1999. 155p.

An outstanding collection of colour photographs of Potosí's miners at work, below and above ground, and of the mining landscape developed for centuries around the dark, legendary mountain of Cerro Rico. Men, women, and children are pictured here with great skill and sensitivity as they go about their daily routines. Above all, Ferry presents a superb gallery of faces, unforgettable images of endurance, pain, death, and survival.

575 **The alchemy of modernity. Alonso Barba's copper cauldrons and the independence of Bolivian metallurgy (1790-1890).**
Tristan Platt. *Journal of Latin American Studies*, vol. 32, no. 1 (2000), p. 1-54. bibliog.

Between the 16th and 19th centuries, the two main methods of refining silver ores in Europe and America were by smelting and by amalgamation with mercury. After a broad review of silver production, labour and transport in the Potosí region, Platt concentrates on Alvaro Alonso Barba's method of silver refining which involved boiling the pulverized ore in water, together with mercury and salt. This copper-cauldron method had been invented in the *audiencia* of Charcas/Upper Peru as early as 1609, but it was not widely adopted at the time; successful reintroduction into Bolivia came in the 19th century. The topic is interesting and well researched, but the article is too long, and Platt's writing style needs a sharper edge.

Transport

Rail, sea and air

576 From the Pacific to La Paz: the Antofagasta (Chili) and Bolivia Railway Company, 1888-1988.
Harold Blakemore. London: Antofagasta Holdings PLC/Lester Crook Academic Publishing, 1990. 334p. maps. bibliog.

Commissioned to celebrate the company's centenary, this well-illustrated study traces the early development of the railway in Chile, its extension into Bolivia in the late 19th century, its changing fortunes in and after the 1930s, and its subsequent incorporation into the diversified Antofagasta Holdings group in the 1980s. Enlivened by vivid accounts of the individual personalities who built and operated the railway, the book is nevertheless much more than a company history. Its strength also lies in the perceptive commentary on contemporary events, on the political background in both Chile and Bolivia, and on the shifting economic relationship between Britain and Latin America over the last 100 years.

577 The Mad Mary: all aboard to nowhere.
Louis Werner. *Américas*, vol. 42, no. 4 (1990), p. 6-17. map.

After two costly failures in the early and late 1870s, construction of the ill-fated, 228-mile Madeira–Mamoré Railway around the rivers' eighteen sets of falls was eventually completed in 1909-12, at the height of the rubber boom. But the line was dogged to the end by disaster. The year 1912 also marked the collapse of South America's rubber boom and the astronomically high prices being paid for wild rubber; large quantities of cheap plantation rubber from the Far East had entered the world market for the first time. The Madeira–Mamoré Railway (from Pôrto Velho to Guajará Mirim) survived on reduced traffic and subsidy until 1972, when it was replaced by a highway alongside. Remnants of the old track and rolling stock still lie rusting in the jungle, and over the years, travellers have been drawn to this extraordinary line lost in the heart of Amazonia. Werner provides a fascinating account of its final construction, and the hopes of local enthusiasts to re-open about ten miles of track. Photographs of the 1909-12 construction period, and of the present scene by other contributors, add greatly to the interest of Werner's text. See also items 131-133, 137.

578   The Antofagasta (Chili) & Bolivian Railway: the story of the FCAB and its locomotives.
J. M. Turner, R. F. Ellis.   Skipton, England: Locomotives International, 1992. 2nd ed. Skipton, England: Trackside Publications, 1996. 77p. maps.

A gem for the railway historian. Starting in the 1870s, the authors present the early history, consolidation and expansion of the line, accompanying their account of its development with details of the locomotives and other rolling stock that were introduced at each stage. This was a railway carrying close to 2 million tons of freight annually, by narrow gauge, at heights ranging from sea level to more than 4,820 metres (nearly 16,000 feet). Locomotive companies in the United States, Britain, France and Germany all serviced the Antofagasta & Bolivia Railway (in Spanish, the FCAB), but the US engines were found to be the best adapted to local conditions. Like others, the Antofagasta & Bolivia Railway's chief engineer was still reporting at the start of the 20th century that Philadelphia's Baldwin Company locomotives were 'infinitely more suitable for our line than any English engine supplied up to the present... The workmanship of the English engines is far superior to that of the American, and would be preferable if only English makers would construct their engines on American lines.' The authors' detailed, well-written text is copiously illustrated with archive photographs and engineers' drawings, as well as with travellers' accounts. This is a collector's item based on extensive research, and will appeal not only to railway enthusiasts but also to those specializing in the development of locomotive engineering.

579   Aircraft of the Chaco War.
Dan Hagedorn, Antonio Luís Sapienza.   Atglen, Pennsylvania: Schiffer Publishing, 1997. 114p. maps. bibliog.

This piece of aviation history is highly recommended to all those interested in the aircraft, their development, and the strategy and tactics adopted by both Bolivia and Paraguay during the Chaco War. The authors present a skilful blend of technical detail and historical commentary, well supported with drawings and photographs of aircraft, crews, and the Chaco environment. Good use is made of archive material, while the study is soundly researched from primary sources in the United States and South America.

580   William Wheelwright (1798-1873): steamship and railroad pioneer. Early Yankee enterprise in the development of South America.
J. Valerie Fifer.   Newburyport, Massachusetts: The Historical Society of Old Newbury, 1998. 150p. maps. bibliog.

Published to mark the bicentenary of William Wheelwright's birth in 1798 in Newburyport, Massachusetts, the book includes a record of early trade on Bolivia's former Pacific coast by one of the 19th century's most enterprising and successful pioneers. A New England ship's captain by the age of nineteen, Wheelwright concentrated his activities for many years along the west coast of South America developing, among his other services, the trade between Valparaíso and Bolivia's port of Cobija in the Atacama desert. Wheelwright's schooners brought regular supplies of Chilean flour, fruit, vegetables, eggs, poultry, timber, and barrels of drinking water, along with mail and passengers, to the isolated settlements in Bolivia's Litoral province. As return cargo, Wheelwright brought back copper and, even more importantly, silver specie and bullion transported down from Bolivia's mines in the high Andes, whose value at Cobija was recorded by a US government officer during the port's boom years in the late 1830s at between US$800,000 and US$1,000,000 annually. In 1838-40, Wheelwright turned from sail to steam and introduced the first successful commercial steam navigation into the Pacific, the Pacific Steam Navigation Company, which he registered in Britain. This book includes Wheelwright's own unique manuscript map (redrawn) of the west coast of South America on which he plotted and timed the long, circuitous routes out into the Pacific that he had to follow under sail because of dangerous winds and currents, in order to reach the ports between Chile and Panama, and also the new fast coastal steamship routes he introduced, again including Cobija, which were to revolutionize transport and trade along the west coast of South America.

Pipelines and the oil and gas industry

581 Gas-powered integration.
George Hawrylyshyn. *Américas*, vol. 45, no. 3 (1993), p. 3. map.
The construction of the Bolivia–Brazil gas pipeline was the single most ambitious engineering project undertaken in Latin America during the 1990s. Here, at the start of the project, the author sets out the plan to pipe Bolivian natural gas from Santa Cruz over 3,390 km (2,120 miles) to the huge, heavily industrialized market in southern Brazil, first to São Paulo, followed by extensions to Curitiba and Pôrto Alegre.

582 A giant on the doorstep: Bolivia presses ahead.
Power in Latin America (Financial Times special series, London), no. 36 (June 1998), p. 4-5.
The giant is Brazil. Here, the prospects for Bolivia's expansion as a natural gas exporter to Brazil via the new Bolivia–Brazil gas pipeline are analysed with special reference to southern Brazil's vast energy needs, to Bolivia's current plans for the construction of its own new gas-fired electricity plants near the Brazilian border fed by the pipeline, and for new Bolivian hydro-electric plants in the Andes. While Bolivia's gas fields are not, unfortunately, on the doorstep into Brazil, and the investment required is enormous, the programme reflects the fact that Bolivia has its sights on the future export of electricity to Brazil, as well as the export of natural gas.

583 Bolivia gas rush pitfalls.
Power in Latin America (Financial Times special series, London), no. 43 (January 1999), p. 5-6.
The effect of possible future Argentine competition to supply southern Brazil's energy market is considered in this cautionary study, as Argentina, by mutual agreement with Bolivia, ceases to purchase Bolivian natural gas after the inauguration of the new Bolivia–Brazil gas pipeline. Argentina now aims to secure a slice of Brazil's lucrative energy market in the next few years, with increasing gas-field exploration and new pipelines of its own.

584 Bolivia: the upstream oil and gas market. An update report.

Aberdeen; Glasgow: Scottish Enterprise Operations, July 1999. 48p. maps.

An objective and informative survey of Bolivia's oil and gas industry, which begins with a brief introductory section on the country's geography, history, transport, and present political and economic structure. The history of the oil and gas industry is then traced through successive decades towards a detailed examination of the current state of exploration and discovery, exploitation, pipeline transport, and reserves. Listings of companies presently working in Bolivia, contracts already issued, and areas where further investment and automation are required, are matched alongside much practical information on local ground conditions, site access, and the essential support services that are still needed for growth and for pipeline export. While designed as a technical study, this report is crisply written, jargon-free, and valuable not only for the specialist but also for the general reader seeking up-to-date information on the subject.

585 Exploration: opportunity knocks?

Engineering and Mining Journal, vol. 200, no. 10 (1999), p. 8.

Records a wide-ranging and exclusive interview by the New York journal's editor-in-chief with Jorge F. Quiroga, Bolivia's Vice-President and an engineering graduate, in which Quiroga reviews the country's political and economic achievements since the 1980s, and discusses the benefits derived from the modernized Bolivian mining code of 1997, the current structure of the mining industry, and the key role that Bolivia's natural gas export is expected to play in the 21st century. Aside from this interview, the Bolivia–Brazil natural gas pipeline is widely considered to be the cornerstone of the efforts to establish an energy grid in the Southern Cone. Outside estimates, based on known reserves, judge Bolivia's gas production capacity to be sufficient to meet Brazil's requirements, via the pipeline, until at least 2011.

586 Bolivia's sedimentary basins hold large gas, oil potential.

Juan Carlos Pucci.   *Oil and Gas Journal*, vol. 98, no. 20 (15 May 2000), p. 32-38. maps. bibliog.

A concise, informative analysis of Bolivia's existing and potential gas and oil reserves, well supported by clear maps and geological cross-sections in colour. The South sub-Andean, Foothills and Chaco basins are already in commercial production, and also have the best exploration potential for gas and oil. Pucci examines each of them in turn, noting that the Devonian and Carboniferous measures are the main reservoirs in Bolivia. He then moves on to the altiplano, where the best oil reservoirs are probably the fine Upper Cretaceous and Tertiary sandstones. Oil has also been recovered from the Madre de Dios basin, but both this and the altiplano basin are high-risk exploration zones.

Trade and Industry

General

587 Bolivia: Trade Policy Review.
General Agreement on Tariffs and Trade Organization, Geneva,
1993. 2 vols. bibliog.

Provides a well-organized, comprehensive review of every major component of Bolivia's
economic production, trade, tariffs, and new policy initiatives from 1985 when the
stabilization programme was introduced up to the end of 1992. Text, diagrams, and tables
combine to present a mass of factual detail with clarity and authoritative comment.

588 Bolivia: selected issues and statistical annex.
R. Rennhack, B. Clements, M. Cortes, M. Garza, T. Gudec,
G. Peraza. Washington, DC: International Monetary Fund, 1997.
91p. (IMF Staff Country Report, No. 97/99).

A detailed compilation of basic data on Bolivia, including analysis of the gross domestic
product, banks and the banking system, wages, pensions, trade, and taxation. Annual
statistical tables in general cover the period 1992-1996. Trade provides the pivotal factor
here.

589 Structural adjustment and Bolivian industry.
Rhys Jenkins. *The European Journal of Development Research*,
vol. 9, no. 2 (December 1997), p. 107-28. bibliog.

Focuses on the impact of structural adjustment on Bolivia's manufacturing industry, a
sector which had been highly protected before the introduction of the New Economic
Policy in 1985. Jenkins reports where improvements have occurred, but notes that where
increased productivity and international competitiveness have been achieved, this is
largely the result of less favourable working conditions rather than through improved
technology, infrastructure, and organization. He concludes that the reforms have not laid

170

the foundation for dynamic industrial growth in Bolivia, but that Bolivia is not unique in this respect when compared with other underdeveloped countries elsewhere in the world.

590 Trade liberalisation in Latin America: the Bolivian case.
Rhys Jenkins. *Bulletin of Latin American Research*, vol. 16, no. 3 (1997), p. 307-25. bibliog.

Examines the trade liberalization introduced in 1985 as part of Paz Estenssoro's sweeping New Economic Policy reforms and finds its results disappointing. Trade liberalization in a low-income economy like that of Bolivia needs to be accompanied by new investment, new technology, improved infrastructure, and a fundamental restructuring of the economy, if it is to become an effective component in boosting productivity and export performance. Since these other requirements have not been introduced on the necessary scale, if at all in some cases, the writer remains sceptical that a wholesale policy of trade liberalization alone can bring a new dynamism into the Bolivian economy. See also the same author's paper, 'Trade liberalisation and Bolivian manufacturing' (London: University of London Institute of Latin American Studies, 1995. 139p. [Research Paper, No. 39]).

591 Old Bolivian customs.
The Economist, vol. 347 (11 April 1998), p. 27.

Reviews the inefficiency and corruption of the customs control service in Bolivia. The country's own National Chamber of Commerce estimates that Bolivia lost nearly US$450 million in 1997 in uncollected duties and value-added taxes. Contraband trade and the black market are of long standing and continue to flourish. The new administration of 1997 under President Banzer is pledged to tackle the problem, but Bolivia's frontiers are long and often unpopulated, while many customs posts are isolated and ill-equipped.

592 Free trade, economic growth, and income redistribution in Bolivia.
Hugo Toledo Roca. PhD thesis, Auburn University, Alabama, 1999. 176p. bibliog.

Investigates the varying impact of free-trade policies on the Bolivian economy and notes that with increasing economic integration in South America, Bolivia is likely to continue the production and export of primary commodities, in which it has a comparative advantage. The author contends that the mineral, natural gas, and manufacturing sectors will benefit from free trade, while agriculture, the service industries, and those employed in them, will suffer.

Information for foreign companies and investors

593 Bolivia: general information.
London: British Trade International. 28p. maps.

Updated every quarter, this publication provides a concise but comprehensive survey of Bolivia designed primarily for those wishing to export. It includes briefing on the country and its people, politics, the economic reform programme, currency, trade, transport, and common-sense advice for the unwary, as well as useful addresses in the UK, Bolivia, and on the Internet. This is a good starting-point, helping prospective British exporters to pursue more specific lines of enquiry elsewhere.

594 Bolivia: overseas trade services.
London: Foreign and Commonwealth Office & Department of Trade and Industry. 74p. maps. (DTI Export Publications Series).

This regularly updated manual prepared for intending British exporters visiting Bolivia offers helpful advice, first on preliminary planning and then on the basic information that will be required on arrival. Entries, brief and to the point, include facts about Bolivia and its major cities, currency, social customs, language and translation services, import and exchange-control regulations, methods of doing business, and essential local points of contact and assistance.

595 Bolivia: travel advice.
London: Foreign and Commonwealth Office, Consular Division. [pagination varies].

Practical, up-to-the-minute advice and instruction for visitors to Bolivia regarding matters of personal safety, including details on the various types and methods of street crime which require particular vigilance. Details of current dangers in particular areas are also included, along with the risks of arrest and prosecution for any involvement in the use or trafficking of drugs, the need to employ only registered guides and travel agencies, and the extreme vulnerability of those travelling alone overland. Health advice is provided. The information throughout is helpful, not alarmist; the document notes that visits to Bolivia are generally trouble free.

596 Bolivia: fertile land for investment.
Prepared by Müller & Asociados. La Paz: Banco Santa Cruz, 1997. 7th ed. 55p.

An upbeat message to potential foreign investors on the Bolivian economy and financial system. It includes a clear sectoral analysis of the country's agriculture, mining, oil and gas, electricity, tourist, and transport industries, along with details of banking, fiscal, customs, trade, and labour policies. The work is prefaced by a summary of Bolivia's recent reform programmes, including those of capitalization, social security, popular participation, education, and land tenure. This is a stylish publication, well supported by statistics, charts, and diagrams, and by information on the existing foreign investors in Bolivia.

597 Bolivia: export directory.
La Paz: PAP, 1998. 2nd ed. 258p.

A detailed directory, published in English and Spanish, that provides a comprehensive listing of Bolivia's manufacturers, exporters and importers, together with the relevant agencies, air freight and shipping companies, courier services, and insurance companies serving Bolivia. This is an invaluable supplementary source of reference for individuals or companies wishing to develop trade with Bolivia and seeking basic information on the types of commercial and manufacturing opportunities available. The index is clear and well organized.

598 Cámara de Industria y Comercio de Santa Cruz. Directorio 1998. (The Santa Cruz Chamber of Industry and Commerce directory for 1998.)
Santa Cruz de la Sierra: Publimar, 1998. 276p.

Concentrating on the Santa Cruz region, the directory sets out (in English and Spanish) general information on the city and its surroundings, before recording the range of business opportunities in this rapidly expanding area of Bolivia. It lists national and foreign companies, materials produced and commercialized, and the variety of services offered to traders and investors. This is a well-illustrated volume which also offers detail for those seeking contacts in Montero, Camiri, and other centres in the Department of Santa Cruz.

599 Doing business in Bolivia.
Amsterdam: Price Waterhouse World Firm Services BV, 1998. 132p.

A detailed guide for those interested in doing business in Bolivia by one of the world's largest international organizations of accountants and consultants, in this case with offices in La Paz and Santa Cruz. Following a clear and comprehensive profile of Bolivia, a small guidebook in itself, the publication analyses in meticulous detail the business environment, foreign investment and trade opportunities, investment incentives, exchange controls, banking and finance, labour relations, social security, and every major aspect of taxation and audit. This is an excellent source of reference both for companies and individuals entering this field.

600 Bolivia: consumer goods report.
La Paz: British Embassy Commercial Section; London: British Trade International, January 1999. 39p.

Bolivia's internal market for consumer goods is very small, and is dominated by the United States, Chile, and Argentina. Imports from the UK are primarily whisky and other spirits. This report aims to break new ground by providing information and advice, and by identifying a wider range of opportunity in Bolivia to would-be UK exporters.

601 Major companies of Latin America and the Caribbean.
London: Graham & Whiteside, 1999. 4th ed. 1331p.

Nearly eighty major companies operating in Bolivia are listed in this volume of business information. The entries comprise details on each firm's location, principal products or activities, directors and management, date of foundation, status as a state or privately owned enterprise, and the number of employees. This is a useful, well-presented source of reference for foreign companies interested in doing business in Bolivia.

602   Bolivia: background brief.

London: Foreign & Commonwealth Office, January/July/September 2000. [not paginated]. maps.

A clear and comprehensive summary of Bolivia's present government and political coalition, the major components of its economy, trade and investment, and the achievements thus far in the counter-drugs action plan to eliminate illegal coca production by the year 2002. The largest British companies with commercial and investment interests in Bolivia are noted, along with the best current opportunities for UK investment in Bolivian manufacturing and service industries. Concise and objective, this brief is recommended to those seeking regularly updated information on current political and economic conditions in Bolivia, and on UK–Bolivia relations.

Environment and Conservation

603 Beautiful barter in Bolivia.
The Economist, vol. 304 (18 July 1987), p. 26.
Registers the new 'debt-for-land' agreement between Conservation International and the Bolivian government, emphasizing that the former has a pragmatic approach to wilderness areas, and recognizes the need in Third World countries to mix conservation with economic development.

604 Cutting the debt, saving the forest.
Diana Page. *Environment*, vol. 29 (September 1987), p. 4-5.
The author gives a guarded welcome to the 'debt-for-land' agreement of July 1987 by which Bolivia became the first country to negotiate some US$650,000 of debt relief (a tiny fraction of the total debt) in exchange for a commitment to protect about four million acres of Amazonian rainforest. Page's note of caution is based not on intention but on implementation. In practice, neither banking nor environmental groups can dictate the priorities of debtor nations in this respect. Each state makes its own decisions based on the price people are willing to pay to preserve their biological diversity and natural resources for future generations.

605 Debt for easement saves land.
Church Briggs. *American Forests*, vol. 93 (November/December 1987), p. 10.
Noting the innovative move by Conservation International in July 1987 to purchase part of Bolivia's national debt in exchange for environmental protection, the author emphasizes an important follow-up which took place in the US Congress a few days later – the introduction of the Tropical Forest Act 1987. The purpose of this new legislation is to examine the broader issues of tropical forest management, and to devise sustainable methods of combining both forest use and forest protection.

606 Two cheers for the rainforest: the deal is on in Bolivia.

Marisa Gaines. *Sierra*, vol. 72 (November/December 1987), p. 16.

Welcomes the agreement of 13 July 1987 between Bolivia and Conservation International (a non-profit organization based in Washington, DC), to preserve 3.7 million acres of Amazon rainforest in the northern Beni in exchange for a reduction in Bolivia's national debt. The area is adjacent to the existing Beni Biosphere Reserve which already supports thirteen of Bolivia's eighteen endangered animal species.

607 Debt deal stacked against Indians.

Merrill Collett. *The Progressive*, vol. 53 (August 1989), p. 17-18.

Examines complaints by the Moxos Indians regarding the inroads being made into the Beni Forest Reserve established in 1987 in exchange for a reduction of part of Bolivia's national debt. The dispute revives the debate between the concept of untouched wilderness and that of controlled exploitation of the forest as a sustainable resource (the guiding principle of the Conservation International organization). The current world boom in mahogany has, however, hastened cutting, and in some areas reduced the agreed replanting programme, but the logging companies are unlikely to heed any attempt to curtail their activities.

608 Debt for nature: a flawed panacea.

The Geographical Magazine, vol. 62, no. 12 (1990), p. 21.

Another example of the damaging effects of the 1987 'debt-for-land' agreement, this time on the forest homelands of the Chimane and other Indian hunting-and-gathering communities, as sections of the wilderness are opened up by logging companies, new roads, and the arrival of agricultural colonists. Although this is only a brief report, some attention should have been given to the huge practical problems of control faced by the authorities in these remote regions, and to the difficulties of reconciling the often conflicting claims for conservation and exploitation.

609 The river of the Mother of God (río de Madre de Dios).

Aldo Leopold. *Wilderness*, vol. 54 (spring 1991), p. 18-26. map.

After a general introduction to this remote region of Bolivia and Peru by Susan Flader, there follows an early, previously unpublished essay on the area by Aldo Leopold, who was a co-founder of the Wilderness Society in 1935. He called for the preservation of the upper Madre de Dios basin as a wilderness area of outstanding biodiversity, noting that over the years the forest had been exploited by rubber gatherers, gold prospectors, and loggers. The response came many years later, when the Peruvian government established a national park in the Madre de Dios headwater region in the 1970s, which was recognized by UNESCO as the Manu Biosphere Reserve. Further additions to the Reserve were made in 1990, thus prompting the publication of Leopold's original work.

610 Beni: surviving the crosswinds of conservation.

Liliana Campos-Dudley. *Américas*, vol. 44, no. 3 (1992), p. 6-15. maps.

A well-illustrated account by the regional coordinator of Conservation International's various projects in the Andean states. The Beni Biosphere Reserve, created in 1982, was officially recognized by UNESCO in 1986, the year in which the adjacent Forest Reserve was opened to timber extraction. The author examines the effects of the 1986 and the

1987 'debt-for-land' legislation on the Chimane, Moxeño, Yuracaré, and Móvima Indians, as well as on others inhabiting the region. This is a sympathetic but objective report which also includes background on the work of the field staff in Bolivia's own overstretched Beni Regional Forestry Service.

611 Double defeat for Bolivia.
Wilson T. Boots. *The Christian Century*, vol. 111 (October 1994), p. 942-43.

Draws attention to a projected alarming increase in imported toxic waste-dumping in Bolivia and other Third World countries. The author notes the recent dumping of antimony and arsenic waste behind Patacamaya (Dept of La Paz), and its successive shifting by rail to three townships in Oruro as anger mounted among the communities concerned. The future dumping of imported nuclear radioactive waste in abandoned mine shafts near Potosí is also rumoured. The writer calls upon the government to reject the financial incentives involved and instead to join the search for acceptable alternative solutions to a growing environmental crisis, which is likely to become not only local but global in its impact. See also Rojas Velarde and L'Homme, 'Pious intentions', item no. 962.

612 Toxic sludge flows through the Andes.
Rob Edwards. *New Scientist*, vol. 152 (23 November 1996), p. 4. map.

Reports the release of poisonous waste loaded with heavy metals from a zinc mine reservoir at El Porco, near Potosí, following the collapse of a dam in the high Andes. The extent of the environmental damage that resulted is discussed both here and in correspondence from the mining company published the following month (*New Scientist*, vol. 152 [21/28 December 1996], p. 81).

613 Bolivia's outpost of hope.
Steven Hendrix. *International Wildlife*, vol. 27 (January/February 1997), p. 12-19.

A well-illustrated account of a local Indian community's combined project with Conservation International to establish an ecotourist camp within the Madidi National Park of northern Bolivia. Preliminary work on this rainforest tourist facility at Chalalán on the Tuichi river is reported to be well under way, as is the debate on how to balance the expected influx of visitors with the conservation of a particularly rich wildlife habitat.

614 Caring for the rare.
Fiona McWilliam. *The Geographical Magazine*, vol. 70, no. 7 (1997), p. 40-42.

Records an interview with the 1997 winner of the Whitley Award for Animal Conservation, Susanna Paisley, about her work with endangered spectacled bears in the high Andean cloudforest. The spectacled bear (*Tremarctos ornatus*) is the only surviving bear in South America, but with expanding colonization, the bears are increasingly in conflict with farmers who complain of serious damage to crops and livestock. A workable conservation strategy is now under review.

615 Mining waste poisons river basin.

Javier Garcia-Guinea, Maria Huascar. *Nature*, vol. 387 (8 May 1997), p. 118. bibliog.

Reports the widespread and damaging effects of mining waste, especially metallic sulphides, in the Pilcomayo river basin whose headwaters drain the Potosí and Oruro mining areas in the high Andes. Pollution of fish stocks in the low-lying Chaco region of Bolivia, Paraguay, and Argentina has brought increasing problems to scattered communities there who rely heavily on the Pilcomayo river and its seasonal flood basins for their food supply.

616 Setting priorities for environmental management: an application to the mining sector in Bolivia.

Wendy S. Ayres, Kathleen A. Anderson, David Hanrahan. Washington, DC: World Bank, 1998. 108p. 1 folded map of Bolivia's main COMIBOL mines. bibliog. (World Bank Technical Paper/Pollution Management Series).

A clear, coherent study of the many environmental and community problems surrounding the mines owned and operated by COMIBOL, Bolivia's state mining corporation. With limited funding, the task of revitalizing the mining sector and bringing the surviving centres into profitability demands the skill to establish priorities and to select only the most cost-effective programmes with the widest benefits. This inventory of mines and smelters in Bolivia includes their previous history and current ranking by hazard potential, and provides a useful background for any one engaged in a comprehensive study of the country's mining industry. All told, the authors present an excellent scientific and practical approach to environmental management in Bolivia that can be recommended both to the specialist and the general reader.

617 Essays on energy, equity, and the environment in developing countries.

Debra Kim Israel. PhD thesis, University of Wisconsin, Madison, Wisconsin, 1999. 267p. bibliog.

A well-constructed study based on the responses received, mainly in developing countries and particularly in Bolivia, to questions put to households and individuals about fuel, taxes, and environmental protection. These questions sought to discover: (1) Whether there was any willingness to pay somewhat higher taxes to the government if the money were to be spent on environmental protection, including the prevention of land, water, and air pollution; (2) What were the determinants of household fuel choice, particularly firewood, given the damaging effects of deforestation and of indoor air pollution; and (3) What had been the impact of the elimination of fuel subsidies under Bolivia's new economic reform programme in 1985.

618 Forest structure and dynamics in the Beni Biosphere Reserve, Bolivia.

James Andrew Comiskey. PhD thesis, University of London External, England, 1999. 269p. bibliog.

Bolivia established the Estación Biológica del Beni in the Llanos de Mojos in 1982, and by 1986, UNESCO had recognized the Beni Biosphere Reserve, which comprises about

50 per cent grassy savannah, 30 per cent tree savannah, and 20 per cent forest. By 1995, fourteen biodiversity monitoring plots were part of the research programme set up by the Herbario Nacional de Bolivia in La Paz, the Smithsonian Institution in Washington, DC, and the Field Museum in Chicago. Comiskey concentrates on the dynamics of the different forested habitats: their structure, floristic composition, species diversity, and growth rates, relating his findings to their implications for the management and conservation of the forests in the Reserve, where soils and seasonal flooding are the flora's two major determinants. This is a detailed, well-documented study which will interest botanists and environmentalists.

619 Sustainable management of the Gran Chaco of South America: ecological promise and economic constraints.
E. H. Bucher, P. C. Huszar. *Journal of Environmental Management*, vol. 57 (1999), p. 99-108. map. bibliog.
A first-rate paper which makes a significant contribution to a neglected area in the literature. The Gran Chaco extends over parts of Bolivia, Paraguay, Argentina and, marginally, Brazil – a vast, sparsely populated plain of some 1.3 million sq. km (c. 500,000 sq. miles) that suffers both seasonal flooding and seasonal drought. Despite this, poor *campesinos* have increasingly encroached on the Chaco, and this has resulted in severe overgrazing by cattle and goats, deforestation of the wooded savannah for charcoal production, over-hunting and fishing, and rural migration to the cities by some of the most destitute local communities. The authors discuss possible management systems for sustainable development, particularly the system successfully pioneered in the Argentine province of Salta. The obstacles to the Argentine system's wider application are the initial investment, and the time required to achieve land repair and subsequent full productivity. This lucid, comprehensive study is well argued, and will interest agronomists, geographers, and other field researchers.

620 Transnational relations and the politics of species conservation in poor countries: evidence from Costa Rica and Bolivia, 1967-1997.
Paul Frederick Steinberg. PhD thesis, University of California, Santa Cruz, 1999. 344p. bibliog.
Addresses the history of biodiversity policy reforms in Costa Rica and Bolivia, both of which the author contends have emerged as leaders in tropical conservation in recent decades. How so? The formula for success presented here appears to be in the hands of individuals who have established a long-term presence in the country and been able to forge close ties between the appropriate international organization and domestic policy-makers. Positive action is also encouraged when the environmental agency is located in the developing country, since this provides valuable opportunities for foreign and domestic personnel to meet on a regular basis.

621 Bolivia's Nature Lodge.
Mike Ceaser. *Américas*, vol. 52, no. 3 (2000), p. 4-5.
Reports on the encouraging progress being made at the Ecotourist Chalalán Lodge in Bolivia's Madidi National Park. Established in 1997 near the Tuichi river (a tributary of the Beni), with help from the Inter-American Development Bank and Conservation International, the Lodge is run by the local Tacana/Quechua community of San José de

Uchupiamonas. After a slow start, Chalalán is now attracting an increasing number of visitors, 'a mix of young backpackers and senior citizens', all drawn to the lakeside activities, and to the extraordinary biodiversity to be observed with the help of the Indian guides along the twenty miles of jungle trails. Despite future uncertainties, which are mainly linked to the Bala Dam project on the Beni River, the San Josesaños remain hopeful, and are already planning new amenities at the Lodge.

622 Madidi: Bolivia's spectacular new National Park.

Steve Kemper, photography by Joel Sartore. *National Geographic Magazine*, vol. 197 (March 2000), p. 2-23. map.

By the end of the 20th century, Bolivia's new Madidi National Park had been officially enlarged to 4.7 million acres, an enormous sweep that includes Andean glaciers, cloudforest, rainforest, savannah woodland, grassland, scrub and swamp, along with one of the most varied assemblages of flora and fauna in South America. Tourist lodges at Chalalán, Charque, and Caquiahuara have been completed, but plans for the future success of ecotourism have still to gain momentum in the face of limited funding. In a candid overview, Kemper discusses the opportunities and the constraints on trying to speed the development of the Madidi National Park. He also notes the recent threat to part of the area by a proposal to build a hydroelectric plant on the upper Beni River in order to supply electricity to Brazil. Nevertheless, this is still an optimistic analysis of the future of this magnificent National Park which will be of great interest to conservationists and ecotourists. At the same time, Kemper is a realist, and does not hesitate to point out that people struggling to survive, one way or another, do not enjoy the luxury of placing biodiversity and environmental issues at the top of the agenda.

Urban Social Conditions

Town life and urban migration

623 Environments of integration: three groups of Guaraní migrants in Santa Cruz de la Sierra, Bolivia.
C. I. P. Davison. DPhil thesis, University of Oxford, England, 1987. 353p. bibliog.

Follows the fortunes of three groups of Guaraní Indians who migrated to Santa Cruz and settled into three different socio-economic niches within the city's regional society. One group on the city's fringe relies mainly on casual wage labour and self-employment in both the urban and rural sectors. A second group, holding more land, produces sugar-cane and other crops for the urban market. The third group became full-time, waged factory workers. Aspects of their cultural adjustment to their new surroundings provide the focus of the research.

624 The quest for *tranquilidad*: paths to home ownership in Santa Cruz, Bolivia.
Gill Green. *Bulletin of Latin American Research*, vol. 7, no. 1 (1988), p. 1-15. map. bibliog.

Studies the issues of ethnicity and housing tenure in Bolivia's fastest-growing city. Home ownership, not rented accommodation, is the goal of virtually all the newcomers to Santa Cruz, whether they be *Cambas* (people from the tropical lowlands, mainly of Spanish-speaking European stock), *Kollas* (people from the Andes, speaking Quechua or Aymara), or *Vallegrandiños* (a smaller group sharing some of the characteristics of the first two). *Cambas* are the politically dominant ethnic group, a dominance displayed in home ownership, employment, and kinship networks. *Kollas* face a longer route towards home ownership as they adjust to an unfamiliar geographical environment as well as to the realities of ethnic discrimination by *Cambas* in housing and employment opportunities.

625 Household shelter strategies in comparative perspective:
     evidence from low-income groups in Bamako and La Paz.
     Paul Van Lindert, August Van Westen.   *World Development,*
     vol. 19, no. 8 (1991), p. 1007-28. bibliog.

In a comparison between Bamako (Mali) and La Paz, the latter displays much greater
dynamism in the housing market and in the mobility between the inner city, former
periphery, and present peripheral zones. The poor of La Paz on the edges of town build
sturdier dwellings from the start, acquire electricity and water supplies much faster than
their African counterparts, and, most importantly, gain ownership of their homes more
rapidly, so that subsequent home improvement becomes a characteristic feature of many
low-income family dwellings in the Bolivian capital.

626 Moving up or staying down? Migrant–native differential
     mobility in La Paz.
     Paul Van Lindert.   *Urban Studies,* vol. 28, no. 3 (1991), p. 433-64.
     map. bibliog.

The article analyses the variations that occur within low-income housing zones in La Paz,
and compares the housing careers of the city-born poor and the migrant poor in Bolivia's
capital city. Mobility characterizes both groups, but the city-born poor usually move
shorter distances and often remain in the central tenement district, while the migrant poor,
many of them from rural areas on the altiplano, settle on the familiar high plateau country
which forms the periphery of La Paz. On this periphery, most of the migrant poor settle
in the rapidly expanding satellite town of El Alto which, by the early 1990s, contained a
population of over 300,000. There, the migrant poor become homeowners more quickly
than the city-born poor, many of whom give homeownership a lower priority, preferring
to live closer to their workplace in or near the city centre, if necessary in rented
accommodation. This is a detailed, carefully focused study, well supported by diagrams
and tables.

627 Living on the edge: a comparison of two marginal *barrios* in
     Tarija, Bolivia.
     Kathleen Schroeder.   PhD thesis, University of Minnesota,
     Minneapolis, Minnesota, 1995. 213p. bibliog.

Compares the development of two *barrios* (neighbourhoods) on the edge of Tarija which
were settled by migrants from contrasted backgrounds. In one, former miners with well-
developed political and organizational skills made rapid contact with government and
non-governmental bodies and were quickly and generously provided with public services.
In the second *barrio*, former peasant farmers maintained contact with the agricultural
areas they had left, relied on family ties rather than official agencies, and were
consequently much slower in acquiring even basic services.

628 Por las propias/In our own hands: resistance and representation
     on the margins of urban Bolivia.
     Daniel Marc Goldstein.   PhD thesis, University of Arizona, Tucson,
     Arizona, 1997. 394p. bibliog.

Explores the relationship between collective identity and political process within the
migrant community of Villa Pagador, which is situated on the edge of Cochabamba. The

author discusses how the community image is shaped and projected to outsiders, including government and local officials, in order to create a positive impression and encourage funding for improvements to the residents' living and working conditions.

629 Small towns and beyond: rural transformation and small urban centres in Latin America.
Edited by Paul Van Lindert, Otto Verkoren. Amsterdam: Thela Publishers, 1997. 145p. maps. bibliog. (Thela Latin America Series, No. 6).

Many studies of urbanism and urbanization in Latin America concentrate on the largest cities. This collection focuses on the smaller urban centres, and analyses the ways and extent to which they serve their rural hinterlands, and assist the development of these areas. As one example, Tarija in southern Bolivia is examined from the standpoint of the variation between the city-born population and the migrants with respect to their employment in the professional and technical, service, and unskilled or semi-skilled sectors. The authors outline the volume and rhythms of migration into the city from the surrounding region, particularly the influx of thousands of unemployed miners and their families from Potosí since the mid-1980s. Although some of the general findings have been made before, the monograph as a whole provides a series of useful empirical studies across Latin America, with good maps, bibliography, and statistical support. These features, together with the clearly organized chapters, make this a most helpful text for students.

Children in the city

630 Surviving the crisis: Bolivia's children at work.
Erica Polakoff. *Society*, vol. 27, no. 3 (March/April 1990), p. 82-85.

This article offers insights into the role of young children working to provide income for their own families. Examples are drawn from the city of Cochabamba where children regularly work in the markets, in brickworks, on construction sites, and even in slaughterhouses, where officially they are forbidden to work. From an early age, they accompany their elders to learn the basic skills – how to buy produce, select livestock, obtain credit, and not least, how to deal with the unions. Soon many of them are in business for themselves, an extraordinarily robust and resilient section of the economy.

631 The Bolivian mystery.
Kenneth J. Herrmann, Jr. *America* (New York: America Press), vol. 164 (January 1991), p. 36.

A brief report on the problem of homeless street children in Bolivia, and how they try to survive by selling newspapers, shining shoes, cleaning windscreens and other odd jobs, as well as by begging and stealing. Some efforts are made by the authorities and by voluntary organizations to protect them, but these are set against the overwhelming scale of the problem and the limited resources available.

632 Go south, young child.
The Economist, vol. 351 (15 May 1999), p. 38.
Arrests in Argentina have highlighted the growing problem of organized trafficking in Bolivian children, teenagers and young adults across Bolivia's southern border, a migration many of the youngsters have been encouraged to make, with or without their parents' consent, by stories of a new El Dorado down south, and by the promise of payment high enough to enable them to send money home. But recent raids on sweatshops in the La Flores district of Buenos Aires found sixty young Bolivian women, without papers, working in counterfeit clothing factories, in deplorable conditions and for a tiny wage. Still they come. By the late 1990s, thousands of teenagers were thought to be crossing at both official and unknown border points into Argentina – economic migrants desperate to escape the poverty at home. The article highlights this rarely publicized form of cross-border smuggling, and the steps being taken to try to end it.

Water supply problems

633 An emerging logic of urban water management, Cochabamba, Bolivia.
Simon Marvin, Nina Laurie. *Urban Studies*, vol. 36, no. 2 (1999), p. 341-57. bibliog.
Describes the Cochabamba municipal water company's difficulties in trying, unsuccessfully, to keep up with the growth of the city, especially on the periphery. As the company prepares for privatization in cooperation with the World Bank, the 'emerging logic' of the title appears to mean what are the problems that will have to be solved if the project is to work, namely, (1) How can the utility make privatization/capitalization more attractive to international water companies than it is now? (2) How can the company persuade bidders to give a firm assurance that at least ninety per cent of the city's population will be connected to the mains water supply within five years, and at reasonable tariffs? (3) How can the company and the city satisfy demands by local community and voluntary groups to be involved in the extension, construction, and management of the new water system?

634 Globalisation, neoliberalism, and negotiated development in the Andes: water projects and regional identity in Cochabamba, Bolivia.
Nina Laurie, Simon Marvin. *Environment and Planning A*, vol. 31, no. 8 (1999), p. 1401-15. maps. bibliog.
An account of the ambitious Misicuni water project in the Department of Cochabamba which has been the focus of controversy for more than thirty years. Designed to bring vital new supplies of drinking water, irrigation, and hydroelectric power to the city and

surrounding areas, Misicuni faces the problem that expensive megaprojects of this type are less popular now among international investors, although Cochabamba itself regards the delay as evidence of the city's loss of power and influence at national level in relation to La Paz and Santa Cruz. Laurie and Marvin discuss the physical, financial, and political obstacles to progress on the Misicuni development project, together with the wider regional issues that are involved, but the article as a whole is burdened by the authors' tortuous style.

635　Bolivia's wave of protest.

The Economist, vol. 355 (15 April 2000), p. 66. map.

Cochabamba residents remain angry at the proposed new water charges to be levied by Aguas del Tunari, the group of international investors who are faced with developing the costly Misicuni water project if any permanent solution to the region's severe water shortage is to be found. Cochabamba's protest recently became the focus of other strikes across Bolivia, triggered by different grievances but all reflecting the growing resentment over the continuing poverty in rural areas. The protestors were joined by those who have lost their income, albeit illegal, as the government's drive towards coca/cocaine eradication and custom reform bites harder. A state of emergency was applied, lifted within two weeks as further efforts were made to find a peaceful solution.

636　Developers and community officials work to solve wastewater issues and drinking water problems in Santa Cruz, Bolivia.

Water Engineering & Management, vol. 147, no. 3 (2000), p. 12-13, 41. map.

The city of Santa Cruz is designed in eight concentric rings around the city centre, but surging population growth has spread through all these rings, and beyond. Water management has not kept pace. The municipal sewage-treatment plant serves only the three inner rings, while the remaining areas use substandard on-site septic systems for wastewater treatment which are costly, inefficient, and pose a serious risk to the quality of groundwater supplies. The article investigates the ways in which local construction firms and city officials are studying advanced technology and new leaching systems to improve wastewater treatment, while protecting drinking water resources. The problem has become one of the most urgent now faced by this booming city.

637　The politics of water in Bolivia.

The Economist, vol. 354 (12 February 2000), p. 66.

Cochabamba's fertile valley has become an increasingly parched and dusty place. The water-table is falling, the population growing, so that water-rationing is now required in some city districts. This report provides a clear summary of the political aspects of Cochabamba's long-running problem, noting that Aguas del Tunari became the city's newly privatized water company in 1999, raising tariffs sharply by the end of that year, and bringing outraged protestors on to the streets. The national government, city mayor, and local residents are all at loggerheads on the water issue. Aguas del Tunari meanwhile, though agreeing to hold back the increased charges pending negotiation, point out the huge costs that will have to be met on the Misicuni project, with its dam, pipelines, and 19-kilometre (12-mile) tunnel. The solution to the water shortage in Bolivia's old 'garden city' of Cochabamba is not yet in sight.

Urban manufacturing and marketing

638 Market processes in La Paz, Bolivia.
Charles Slater (et al.). East Lansing, Michigan: Latin American
Studies Centre, Michigan State University, 1969. 242p.

A first attempt to describe and evaluate the exchange processes for consumer goods and
food in La Paz. This USAID-related project had a special interest in the food-marketing
system, together with peasants' participation in it.

**639 Conduct and code: an analysis of market syndicates and social
revolutions in La Paz, Bolivia.**
Hans Buechler, Judith-Maria Buechler. In: *Ideology and social
change in Latin America*. Edited by June Nash, Juan Corradi.
New York: Gordon & Breach, 1977. 305p. bibliog.

The formation of market syndicates, or market unions, in La Paz was a consequence of
the agrarian reform decree of 1953. Syndicates mediate between the city government and
the vendors, seeking to prevent graft and abuse. Grouped into federations and into larger
confederations, the leadership is democratically elected. In 1974, the unions' activities
were suspended and leadership was co-opted by the government.

**640 Spatial analysis and regional inequality: some suggestions for
development planning.**
Michael Painter. *Human Organization*, vol. 46, no. 4 (1987),
p. 318-29. bibliog.

Presents two case-studies, one from highland Peru (Puno), the other from lowland Bolivia
(the Santa Cruz-Montero region). The analysis is based on the spatial organization of a
regional system, especially market systems, and the underlying social organization from
which these systems arise. In a well-argued paper, the author emphasizes the need for
coordinated goals among the numerous agencies involved in regional development
projects, along with the need to avoid raising hopes which cannot realistically be fulfilled.

**641 These days to be a Bolivian is to die slowly: women factory
workers in La Paz.**
Valerie Anne Estes. In: *Lucha: the struggles of Latin American
women*. Edited by Connie Weil. Minneapolis: The Prisma
Institute, 1988, p. 141-51. bibliog. (Minnesota Latin American
Series).

A case-study of women in the workplace made during the severe economic crisis of the
mid-1980s. The author reports on conditions in a food-processing factory in La Paz,
noting through interview the tedium and limited prospects for the labour force. This is a
melancholy picture, where the women's hopes are pinned to finding a future by obtaining
better education and greater job opportunities for their children.

642 Manufacturing against the odds: small-scale producers in an Andean city.
Hans C. Buechler, Judith-Maria Buechler.   Boulder, Colorado: Westview Press, 1992. 331p. bibliog. (Conflict and Social Change Series).

An investigation by two experienced anthropologists working in Bolivia into the range of small-scale manufacturing in the cities of La Paz and El Alto where, far from being a marginal sector of the economy, these enterprises supply a significant share of the nation's consumer goods. The authors study industries employing anything between one and fifty workers, examining the ways in which these workers, men and women, acquire their skills and marketing techniques, and obtain credit, tools, and raw materials. Indeed, many were able to survive the economic crises of the 1980s. The Buechlers capture vividly the atmosphere of these small domestic and workshop industries with the aid of oral histories and illustrations, all combining to reveal the resourcefulness of Bolivia's small-scale producers.

643 Marketing systems and national development: the Sucre region of Bolivia.
Janette Sue Rawlings.   PhD thesis, Indiana University, Bloomington, Indiana, 1996. 256p. bibliog.

This study questions whether the Bolivian government's market reforms introduced in the early 1980s have benefited two of the groups they were meant to assist: the peasant producers and the urban retailers. With reference to the Sucre region, the author argues that the aims of economic development and social progress have not been realized due, in part, to the reduction of the role of market intermediaries. These were earlier thought to do no more than rob both the rural producers and the urban consumers, but they now appear in some cases to have had a positive role to play.

644 The world of Sofía Velasquez: the autobiography of a Bolivian market vendor.
Hans C. Buechler, Judith-Maria Buechler.   New York: Columbia University Press, 1996. 256p. maps. bibliog.

A detailed autobiographical study compiled over a thirty-year period (1964-1994) which not only describes Sofía's life as a market trader in an altiplano village and in La Paz, but also throws light on Bolivia's political and economic history during the decades which formed the background to her childhood and middle age. This is a powerful testimony. Social networks and marketing unions helped street vendors to cope with recurring crises, and these are examined in an absorbing, well-illustrated volume which will interest all those concerned with studies of gender, class, and ethnicity.

Women and Gender Issues

645 The maternal kin unit in Bolivian urban adaptation.
Gordon Keller. *International Journal of Women's Studies*, vol. 6,
no. 4 (1983), p. 336-51.

Examines some basic changes in the structure, functions and values of the traditional
peasant family in Cochabamba, Bolivia, which result from rural–urban migration and
urban adaptation. In this process the role of the female is crucial, for, as the family unit
breaks down, she assumes more economic responsibility.

646 Women in Spanish American colonial society.
Asunción Lavrin.   In: *The Cambridge History of Latin America*.
Edited by Leslie Bethell.   Cambridge: Cambridge University Press,
1984, vol. 2, p. 321-55. bibliog.

A scholarly analysis of the social history of women in colonial Spanish America which
examines the values and attitudes of women who emigrated from Spain and of those who
were born in the New World. It includes discussion of their status, occupations and legal
rights, education, male–female relationships, convent life, and the position of Indian
women. In an area of limited recent historical research, this well-balanced contribution
offers constructive background for modern studies of women and gender issues.

**647 The extension of women's political interactions in mature
colonization projects: a case study from Bolivia.**
Susan Hamilton.   East Lansing, Michigan: Michigan State
University, 1988. 12p. map. bibliog. (Michigan State University,
Office of Women in International Development, Working Paper,
No. 174).

This is a brief but useful progress report based on fieldwork at San Julián colony north of
Santa Cruz, an ambitious 'semi-directed' or 'guided' government colonization scheme
which got under way in the late 1970s. The colony's physical layout and self-management
policies were designed to promote socio-political cooperation, and in many respects this

has been a marked success. But as San Julián matures, and an earlier pioneering equality wanes, Hamilton finds that the women's opportunities for political linkages are in decline. Women have little access to landownership, capital and outside income because the formal decision-making structures exclude them. Development projects are planned by, and for, men, and this practice may well become institutionalized. Swift and firm action by the government is called for, notably legal equality as landowners, new extension courses for women in farm management, training as teachers and health workers, and credit schemes for establishing small businesses.

648 Just ordinary feminists: women in Peru and Bolivia face the debt crisis.
Helen O'Connell.   London: War on Want, 1989. 37p. bibliog.
A first-hand account based on interviews of how groups of women from among the poorest in society founded support groups and struggled to survive the economic hardships of the late 1980s.

649 Bartolina Sisa: the Peasant Women's Organization in Bolivia.
Rosario León.   In: *Women and social change in Latin America.* Edited by Elizabeth Jelin.   London; Atlantic Highlands, New Jersey: Zed Books, 1990, p. 135-50. bibliog.
A detailed analysis of the principal organization representing the interests and demands of rural women in Bolivia – an organization, the author notes, 'that has perhaps established and consolidated its own identity to a greater degree than any other women's organization in Bolivia'. Bartolina Sisa was the wife of Tupac Katari, leader of the late-18th-century Aymara rebellion in Upper Peru against Spain. León concentrates on the formation and development of the Peasant Women's Organization between 1979 and 1984, tracing its origins, the alliances forged, and the importance of the *Katarista* movement, which produced a number of the organization's peasant women leaders. The early influence of the altiplano's Aymara *campesinas* is giving way to a more nationally based union, as peasants from other regions are incorporated. Struggle, self-awareness, and the determination to remain a women-only organization are among the many aspects discussed in this illuminating case-study.

650 Indigenous women and community resistance: history and memory.
Andean Oral History Workshop/Silvia Rivera Cusicanqui.   In: *Women and social change in Latin America.*   Edited by Elizabeth Jelin.   London; Atlantic Highlands, New Jersey: Zed Books, 1990, p. 151-83. bibliog.
As part of a wider study on Andean rebellions, 1910-1950, this paper examines the various means adopted by the Bolivian Indians in their struggle to prevent the *ayllu* (indigenous Andean community) from being seized by members of the ruling creole class and incorporated into their large estates. This is an incisive commentary, with excellent use made of the recollections preserved in the Andean Oral History Workshop in La Paz, and smoothly linked here by the compiler's thoughtful and informative text.

651 "Like a veil to cover them": women and the Pentecostal movement in La Paz.

Lesley Gill. *American Ethnologist*, vol. 17, no. 4 (1990), p. 708-21. bibliog.

Organized religion is the most common means whereby many of the poorest and loneliest women in La Paz make new friends in ways that are socially acceptable to the community. Gill examines the connections between class, gender, and the evangelical Christian movement, noting that many Aymara women are drawn to the Pentecostal church, where they receive new hope and support from the congregation and are encouraged to participate actively in the services. This account will interest both the specialist and the general reader.

652 Painted faces: conflict and ambiguity in domestic servant–employer relations in La Paz, 1930-1988.

Lesley Gill. *Latin American Research Review*, vol. 25, no. 1 (1990), p. 119-36. bibliog.

Domestic service has historically been the most important source of employment for women in Bolivian cities and in Latin American urban centres in general. This article explores employer–servant relationships in La Paz both before and after the social revolution of 1952, noting that while certain attitudes and practices show little alteration, new opportunities have developed. Thus the change in domestic service from being regarded as a long-term, often a lifetime occupation, to what is now undertaken sporadically between other jobs has become increasingly evident in recent years.

653 Social differentiation, gender, and ethnicity: urban Indian women in colonial Bolivia, 1640-1725.

Ann Zulawski. *Latin American Research Review*, vol. 25, no. 2 (1990), p. 93-113.

A detailed study based on legal records, civil and criminal court cases, and census returns in Chuquisaca, Oruro, and La Paz, which discusses the varying degrees of advantage or exploitation that Indian women experienced in some of the major colonial cities of Upper Peru.

654 Gender and ethnicity in motion: identity and integration in Andean households.

Susan Paulson. PhD thesis, University of Chicago, Chicago, Illinois, 1992. 450p. bibliog.

An ethnographical study of how women in Mizque, Department of Cochabamba, strive to meet the multiple challenges they now face in their combined roles as farm managers and heads of household, as increasing numbers of men migrate to find waged labour in the towns. The author finds that while Mizque women still encourage the traditional Andean systems of reciprocity and communality, they also now play increasingly crucial roles in initiating and negotiating change. The research is well supported by a variety of examples.

655 "Proper women" and city pleasures: gender, class, and contested meanings in La Paz.
Lesley Gill. *American Ethnologist*, vol. 20, no. 1 (1993), p. 72-88. bibliog.
Images of the ideal woman constantly change as men and women from different class and ethnic backgrounds incorporate these images and transform them. Gill concentrates on the varying choices in female fashion – Western style or traditional indigenous dress – to illustrate the changing outlook and occupation of some of the women in La Paz in recent years.

656 Assessing the gender impact of development projects: case studies from Bolivia, Burkina Faso and India.
Vera Gianotten, Verona Groverman, Edith van Walsum, Lida Zuidberg. London: Intermediate Technology Publications; Amsterdam: Royal Tropical Institute, 1994. 103p. bibliog.
The Bolivian case-study, the longest of the three, considers the effects of development projects on the interests and needs of the women who become involved in the projects once they are in place. Gianotten urges developers to include these aspects in the initial planning stages, rather than wait for the impact to emerge later, as so often occurs. The case-study is centred on a project in the Department of Chuquisaca supervised by CARE, a North American non-governmental organization, and involves assisting women in the better management of land and water resources, farming, and finance. A short survey of women's position in Andean rural society and the peasant economy concludes this perceptive addition to the literature.

657 Community participation in Bolivia: the Danida/UNCHS Training Programme.
Susanna Rance, Irene Vance. La Paz: United Nations Centre for Human Settlements (Habitat), 1994. 60p. map.
A heartening, well-illustrated report on the work of a combined United Nations–Bolivian project originally designed to assist ex-mining communities to build and improve their homes, and to raise domestic living standards. The UN-funded project is directed mainly towards women and female-headed households, with emphasis on manageable targets and small-scale but effective improvements. The project's scope widened during the 1990s as on-going home improvement in differing communities became a way of life, with women's groups selecting priorities and organizing small teams of both men and women to carry the work through.

658 Gender issues associated with labor migration and dependence on off-farm income in rural Bolivia.
María Elena Gisbert, Michael Painter, Mery Quitón. *Human Organization*, vol. 53, no. 2 (1994), p. 110-22. bibliog.
Since the 1980s, many Bolivian farming families have become increasingly dependent on off-farm income to survive, as men migrate seasonally to Argentina and Chile to work on harvesting or in the construction industry. Using case-studies from the Department of Cochabamba, the authors examine the heavy burden this places on the women who are left behind to run the farm in addition to their domestic duties. With

little schooling or ability to understand Spanish, the women are often overlooked by rural training agencies, and the article puts forward some of the ways this isolation might be relieved.

659 House, community, and marketplace: women as managers of exchange relations and resources on the southern Altiplano of Bolivia.
Lynn Louise Sikkink. PhD thesis, University of Minnesota, Minneapolis, Minnesota, 1994. 270p. bibliog.

Examines the multiple roles played by the women of Condo as household managers, local market stallholders, and informal traders of goods and services. A distinct division of labour recognizes men as the main agriculturalists and as seasonal wage-labourers, with women in charge of virtually everything else, including money, and the regional collection and lucrative sale of traditional medicines at the neighbouring fair. The theme running through this research is the complexity of the exchange patterns operating in and around Condo, all dominated by women except for those exchanges shared by both men and women when operating inside the traditional structure of their *ayllu*.

660 Precarious dependencies: gender, class, and domestic service in Bolivia.
Lesley Gill. New York: Columbia University Press, 1994. 175p. map. bibliog.

A brief but informative study which brings together the author's earlier research and publication on domestic employer–servant relationships in La Paz, and the attractions the Protestant evangelical church has for Aymara women in need of friends and assistance. Domestic service here is rooted in inequality but it has remained relatively isolated from the mainstream labour movement in Bolivia, unable to organize itself effectively, and rarely perceived as part of a wider class struggle.

661 Honor, alcohol, and sexuality: women and the creation of ethnic identity in Bolivia, 1870-1930.
Gina L. Hames. PhD thesis, Carnegie-Mellon University, Pittsburgh, Pennsylvania, 1996. 278p. bibliog.

Cholas are urban women workers of mixed indigenous and 'white' backgrounds who often hold considerable status in the community. Hames's study explores the development of a strong Bolivian *chola* culture in Sucre between 1870 and 1930, examining the *cholas'* role as small traders, and the added importance they acquired by owning premises and selling *chicha* (maize beer) – a key method of raising their status in the household, the city, and the regional economy.

662 **Life improvement strategies among rural Aymara women of Bolivia: empowerment, income generation, and reproductive health options.**
Wilma J. Johnson. PhD thesis, University of Utah, Salt Lake City, Utah, 1996. 364p. bibliog.
Records a project developed in 1991-95 that was designed to plan and implement strategies which groups of rural Aymara women believed would improve their health and well-being. Important factors were found to be the need for formal group organization, health and agricultural workshops, access to credit for small enterprise development, and basic literacy.

663 **Urban women's employment trajectories in Ghana and Bolivia.**
Sunita Kishor. Calverton, Maryland: Macro International, Institute for Resource Development, 1996. 53p. bibliog. (Demographic and Health Surveys, No. 5).
A short but useful analysis of urban women's employment for those seeking cross-cultural comparisons and contrasts in two developing countries. The data include details of current employment, numbers of children, child-care facilities, levels of education, and housing standards.

664 **Education, labor supply, and household expenditures in Bolivia.**
Maria Gabriela Inchauste Comboni. PhD thesis, University of Texas at Austin, 1997. 201p. bibliog.
Based on a selection of indigenous Bolivian households, the study examines the restricted educational opportunities for women and girls in general, noting that these opportunities are further reduced among married women who are heads of household, have young children, and who are without any source of unearned income. The role of extended family members is also considered, both in decisions regarding labour distribution and in the allocation of scarce family resources.

665 **Colonial domination and the subordination of the indigenous woman in Bolivia.**
María Eugenia Choque Quispe, translated by Christine Taff, Marcia Stephenson. *Modern Fiction Studies*, vol. 44, no. 1 (1998), p. 10-23. bibliog.
A bitter attack on what is seen as a fundamental intolerance of, and socio-ethnic prejudice against, women's basic human rights, especially those of indigenous women in Bolivia. The author is a member and former director of the Executive Board of the Andean Oral History Workshop in La Paz, and this essay is focused on the Aymara. She argues that although the subordination of women is in part a legacy of the colonial period, the native culture is also responsible. Despite the fact that roles and responsibilities are changing, the writer is not hopeful of seeing any dramatic shift in the underlying discrimination against women, given the power of habit and tradition.

666 Will I return or not?: migrant women in Bolivia negotiate hospital birth.
Barbara Bradby. *Women's Studies International Forum*, vol. 22, no. 3 (1999), p. 287-301. bibliog.

Basing her study on groups of Quechua women migrants living on the edge of Sucre, the author makes the following points: (1) There is more emphasis now on regular ante-natal care and hospital, rather than home, delivery; (2) Women arrange the methods of giving birth in hospital, which increasingly take account of the cultural influences and rituals associated with giving birth at home; and (3) The growth of Mothers' Clubs has strengthened women's ability to negotiate in advance with the hospital staff the kind of birth procedures that they want.

Health, Medical and Welfare Services

General health and disease conditions

667 Man in the Andes: a multidisciplinary study of high-altitude Quechua.
Edited by Paul T. Baker, Michael A. Little.   Stroudsburg,
Pennsylvania: Dowden, Hutchinson & Ross, 1976. 482p. maps.
bibliog.

One of a series of volumes which report the research of US scientists participating in the International Biological Programme. The purpose of the study is to gain a better understanding of the structure and function of major ecological systems. Topics reported on include: physical and biotic environment; child care; genetic history; population movement and gene flow; fertility, morbidity and post-natal mortality; pre-natal and infant growth; growth and morphology at high altitudes; nutrition, pulmonary function and oxygen transport; haematology; work performance of newcomers; drug use; and physiological responses to cold.

668 Altitude and reproduction of the Japanese in Bolivia.
Hiroshi Kashiwazaki, Tsuguyoshi Suzuki, Tai-ichiro Takemoto.
Human Biology (Detroit), vol. 60, no. 6 (December 1988),
p. 833-45. bibliog.

Reproduction among Japanese women living at high altitudes in Bolivia was examined in comparison with their counterparts in the Bolivian lowlands. Both pregnancies and live births were significantly fewer in number among the women living at high altitudes, but the authors found that, contrary to much of the literature, the difference in reproductive performance was explained more as the result of later marriage in the high-altitude women compared with the lowlanders, rather than by high altitude as such.

669 Effect of altitude on the stature, chest depth, and forced vital capacity of low-to-high altitude migrant children of European ancestry.
Lawrence P. Greksa. *Human Biology* (Detroit), vol. 60, no. 1 (February 1988), p. 23-32. bibliog.

Analysing a sample of fifty-six male and fifty-two female children (average age 13-14 years) who were born at low altitudes and whose families had migrated to La Paz, Greksa finds that their growth and development at high altitudes results in a moderate delay in the linear growth of well-nourished children, and a significant increase in chest depth and forced vital capacity (maximum lung capacity). Moreover, the author notes that the effects of hypoxia (oxygen deficiency) appear to be similar at all stages of development, and are not, as supposed, a particular feature of childhood and adolescence.

670 The pulmonary circulation at high altitude.
C. R. Williams. PhD thesis, University of Liverpool, England, 1989.

This study of pulmonary circulation at high altitudes in man and in indigenous animal species included fieldwork in the Bolivian and Peruvian Andes. The research was designed to identify the lungs' protective mechanisms against pulmonary oedema (swollen tissue), and to aid the early recognition and treatment of this often fatal condition among those insufficiently acclimatized to high altitudes, including tourists and climbers who are commonly affected.

671 Maternal and child health in Bolivia: report on the in-depth DHS survey in Bolivia.
A. Elisabeth Sommerfelt, J. Ties Boerma, Luis H. Ochoa, Shea O. Rutstein. Columbia, Maryland: Institute for Resource Development/Macro Systems, 1991. 141p. map. bibliog.

Nearly 8,000 women aged 15-49 were interviewed for this survey by the Demographic and Health Surveys (DHS) Program, which concentrated on the major causes of infant mortality, fertility, family planning, pre-natal care, nutrition, and general maternal and child health. There is a useful introduction to health conditions in Bolivia, followed by a discussion of the project's findings. The questionnaires are collected in an appendix and would repay close study by all health workers in this field.

672 Population movements and cholera spread in Cordillera Province, Santa Cruz Department, Bolivia.
P. Guglielmetti, A. Bartoloni, M. Roselli, H. Gamboa, D. J. Antunez, I. Luzzi, F. Rosmini, F. Paradisi. *The Lancet* (North American edition), vol. 340 (11 July 1992), p. 113.

Reports that the Latin American cholera epidemic, then raging, started on the Pacific coast of Peru in January 1991, reached northern Bolivia seven months later, and spread rapidly throughout the continent. Here, the authors considers the effect of the ceremonial gathering of some 6,000 Guaraní Indians from Argentina, Paraguay and Bolivia in the far south of Santa Cruz Department in January 1992 on the subsequent accelerated spread of cholera across the region.

673 Women and congenital Chagas' disease in Santa Cruz, Bolivia: epidemiological and sociocultural aspects.
Esperanza Azogue. *Social Science and Medicine*, vol. 37, no. 4 (1993), p. 503-11. maps. bibliog.

Chagas' disease is caused by the parasite *Trypanosoma cruzi*, whose vectors are commonly found in rough, bug-infested dwellings built of mud, reeds or straw, with dirt floors. After a brief acute phase which is not usually fatal, Chagas' becomes a chronic condition. It remains a serious health problem in the city of Santa Cruz, where its persistence is related to the movement of migrants from rural areas into the poorest urban districts. The author maps the areas of congenital transmission of Chagas' disease in Santa Cruz, together with the pattern of migrant flows, and analyses the various factors that contribute to the distribution of a disease which eventually leads to death from complete heart block.

674 Bolivian hemorrhagic fever – El Beni department, Bolivia, 1994.
JAMA (The Journal of the American Medical Association), vol. 273, no. 3 (1995), p. 194, 196. bibliog.

This is a viral haemorrhagic fever known to be endemic only in Bolivia. Here, a new outbreak of BHF is recorded at Magdalena in the northeastern region of the Beni, in July and August 1994. Outbreaks occurred in eastern Bolivia throughout the 1960s, and in Cochabamba in 1971. This most painful and debilitating fever, fatal in about one-third of the cases, is caused by the *Mapucho* virus hosted by the wild rodent *Calomys callosus*, but the report notes that much of the investigative work into the disease and its treatment is still at an early stage.

675 Developmental, genetic, and environmental components of aerobic capacity at high altitude.
A. Roberto Frisancho, Hedy G. Frisancho, Mark Milotich, Tom Brutsaert, Rachel Albalak, Hilde Spielvogel, Mercedez Villena, Enrique Vargas, Rudy Soria. *American Journal of Physical Anthropology*, vol. 96, no. 4 (1995), p. 431-42. bibliog.

Reports the results of a study made in La Paz on the aerobic capacity (i.e. work/exercise capacity) of some 270 subjects, male and female. The investigation examined those native Bolivians acclimatized to high altitude since birth, those of foreign ancestry acclimatized during childhood, and those living at high altitude only in adulthood. The authors tested whether differences in acclimatization were based on genetic differences or differences in adaptation based on environmental factors. Among the range of variables analysed by the team, it was found that individuals acclimatized before the age of ten had a higher aerobic capacity than individuals acclimatized after that age.

676 Bolivian entry to Brazilian medicine threatened.
Claudio Csillag. *The Lancet* (North American edition), vol. 348 (14 September 1996), p. 745.

Thousands of Brazilian medical students, unable to meet the entrance requirements and the costs of training in one of Brazil's own eighty or so medical schools, have found an easier and cheaper way to study medicine by enrolling in a Bolivian university, notably in Cochabamba, Sucre, or La Paz. In the past, an agreement between the two countries guaranteed that Bolivian medical diplomas were valid in Brazil, but the influx of Brazilian medical students from Bolivia and the automatic recognition of their qualifications has been severely criticized by the Brazilian Federal Council, which in the mid-1990s began action to cancel this bilateral arrangement.

677   Evidence for a major gene controlling susceptibility to tegumentary leishmaniasis in a recently exposed Bolivian population.
A. Alcaïs, L. Abel, C. David, M. E. Torrez, P. Flandre, J. P. Dedet.
The American Journal of Human Genetics, vol. 61, no. 4 (1997), p. 968-79. bibliog.

Tegumentary leishmaniasis is a parasitic disease caused by an infected sandfly bite which, among other effects, can lead to severe facial deformities. The disease is endemic in the Beni and Alto Beni regions of Bolivia. The authors investigate the genetic and environmental factors involved, comparing the susceptibility of the Chimanes and Mosetenes Indian groups native to the area with recent Aymara and Quechua groups who have migrated into the Alto Beni colonization zone. In this scholarly and informative paper, the different agricultural, social and behavioural practices of the two groups are discussed in terms of the varying susceptibility of the long-established communities and the new arrivals to this disease.

678   Weekly iron supplementation is as effective as 5 day per week iron supplementation in Bolivian school children living at high altitude.
Jacques Berger, Victor M. Aguayo, Wilma Téllez, Carmen Luján, Pierre Traissac, José Luis San Miguel. *European Journal of Clinical Nutrition*, vol. 51, no. 6 (1997), p. 381-86. bibliog.

An investigation into the efficacy of daily vs. weekly iron supplementation carried out on children under nine years old in a poor district of La Paz revealed that a weekly iron supplement was as beneficial as a daily dose. Given that iron-deficiency anaemia adversely affects growth, development and behaviour in young children, the authors support a long-term weekly iron supplement for pre-school and primary school children, since this assists the progressive accumulation of adequate iron reserves in later life.

679   Validity of published prediction equations for body composition in high altitude Bolivian Aymara as evaluated by doubly labeled water.
Hiroshi Kashiwazaki, Yasushi Dejima, José Orias-Rivera, William A. Coward. *American Journal of Human Biology*, vol. 10, no. 3 (1998), p. 371-84. bibliog.

Assessment of body composition provides valuable information in a variety of biomedical contexts. The main purpose of this study was to seek simple and valid prediction equations to estimate the body composition of Aymara men and women living on the Bolivian altiplano, including information on body form, height, weight, body fat, and energy expenditure. This is a detailed and specialized paper, with findings and directions for further research meticulously recorded. The discussion on Bolivia also includes its relationship with prediction equations made for other areas in the world.

680 Effect of developmental and ancestral high-altitude exposure on VO₂ peak of Andean and European/North American natives.
Tom D. Brutsaert, Hilde Spielvogel, Rudy Soria, Esperanza Caceres, Giliane Buzenet, Jere D. Haas. *American Journal of Physical Anthropology*, vol. 110, no. 4 (1999), p. 435-55. bibliog.

An interesting, if controversial, contribution to this topic. Peak oxygen consumption (VO₂ peak) was measured in 150 males (aged 18-35) in Bolivia in order to separate developmental from genetic effects of high-altitude exposure. The authors set out clearly how the research was conducted among natives of Aymara/Quechua ancestry and natives of European or North American ancestry, together with the other variables that were introduced. The VO₂ peak values recorded indicated that those in both groups who had been born, raised, and tested at high altitude had similar VO₂ peak values, indicating no genetic effect, or an effect much smaller than that previously reported in the literature. Thus, the team failed to find any support for the hypothesis that high-altitude Aymara and Quechua males are genetically programmed to possess a greater capacity for physical work in an oxygen-deficient environment.

681 Estimating the prevalence of iron deficiency anemia in populations.
Jennifer Hadary Cohen.   PhD thesis, Cornell University, Ithaca, New York, 1999. 130p. bibliog.

Basing her research in Bolivia and Costa Rica, Cohen examines the existing methods of estimating the prevalence of iron-deficiency anaemia and finds that they are inadequate, whether through the limited resources available or through the theoretical bases of such estimates. In Bolivia, groups of pregnant women from La Paz and El Alto were tested, and here the method of haemoglobin concentration-by-altitude, which is grounded in the biological theory of iron metabolism, provided a more accurate measure of the prevalence of iron-deficiency anaemia in a population of pregnant women living at high altitude, than that obtained by existing methods. This is a useful case-study for the specialist.

682 Percent of oxygen saturation of arterial hemoglobin among Bolivian Aymara at 3,900-4,000 metres.
Cynthia M. Beall (et al.)   *American Journal of Physical Anthropology*, vol. 108, no. 1 (1999), p. 41-51. bibliog.

With increasing altitude above sea level, haemoglobin carries less oxygen. However, a range of variation in the percentage of oxygen saturation of arterial haemoglobin occurs among healthy individuals at high altitudes. In Tibet, this variation is attributable to the influence of a major gene, but among the Bolivian Aymara the research team's analysis detected no significant variance attributable to a genetic factor. Genetic variation in the Tibetan sample and its absence in the Aymara sample indicates a potential for natural selection of this trait in the Tibetan, but not in the Aymara population. The higher percentage of oxygen saturation of arterial haemoglobin among the Aymara suggests that they are better adapted than the Tibetans to altitudes around 4,000 metres (over 13,000 feet).

683 Urbanisation of yellow fever in Santa Cruz, Bolivia.
P. Van der Stuyft, A. Gianella, M. Pirard, J. Cespedes, J. Lora,
C. Peredo, J. L. Pelegrino, V. Vorndam, M. Boelaert. *The Lancet*,
vol. 353 (8 May 1999), p. 1558-62. maps. bibliog.

A clear and informative report by an international team on the increased threat of a major yellow fever outbreak within the city of Santa Cruz. Jungle yellow fever is already endemic in the rural areas around Santa Cruz, but relaxation of the eradication programme in the 1970s was followed by a reinvasion of the mosquito *Aedes aegypti*, the principal vector of urban yellow fever. This led to a number of fatalities from yellow fever in the city itself, mainly on the southern periphery. The authors map and analyse the outbreak on a case-by-case basis, stressing the need for an immediate mass vaccination programme, since the existing immunization coverage is low, and the city's population now approaches 1 million.

684 Hygiene and 'the Indian problem': ethnicity and medicine in Bolivia, 1910-1920.
Ann Zulawski. *Latin American Research Review*, vol. 35, no. 2
(2000), p. 107-29. bibliog.

Unlike Mexico and Peru, *indigenismo* never became the ideological basis for a major political movement in Bolivia. Even so, in the first decades of the 20th century, certain Bolivian intellectuals and politicians debated how the country's Indian population should be incorporated into social and political life. Public health was central to this discussion, partly because of élite fears of contagion due to greater contact, and partly because of the realization that if Indians were to be productive members of society, their physical well-being had to be considered. Zulawski examines the proposals of two Bolivian doctors, Nestor Morales in La Paz and Jaime Mendoza in Sucre, for improving the health of the Indian population in the context of the wider national debate about ethnicity and citizenship. The paper records an interesting episode in Bolivia's social history, and the different ways the two doctors went about their task.

Medical and welfare services

685 Bolivia's health couriers.
Cesar A. Chelala. *World Health* (December 1988), p. 18-19.

A good example of the remarkable capacity among many Bolivians for getting things done at local level. Here, in a typical small altiplano village, the author studies the work of one of Bolivia's volunteer health workers (Responsables Populares de Salud), who are unpaid, part-time, elected by their own communities, and given basic training and medical supplies. By the end of the 1980s, these village health workers had become an established feature in many rural areas.

686 The professional nursing role in Cochabamba, Bolivia: clinical nurses' and physicians' perception about ideal and actual functioning; identified role problems; and leadership recommendations.
Margaret Mary Savino. PhD thesis, Cornell University, Ithaca, New York, 1988. 289p. bibliog.

A sympathetic study carried out in Cochabamba of the way the professional nurse's role is perceived by physicians working alongside. Savino's findings revealed that physicians ascribed a more passive and traditional role to nurses than nurses themselves thought was appropriate to their knowledge and skills. A general level of frustration, however, appeared to be based more on a severe lack of resources which undermined patient treatment and recovery, although it was still often easier for nurses and doctors to blame each other when standards fell short of what they both desired.

687 "Health first" in Bolivia.
Ramon Granados, Angel Valencia, Juan Sotelo. *World Health* (May 1989), p. 14-15.

Following the increased promotion of basic health-care services in Bolivia in the early 1980s, the authors claim that by 1987 such facilities were available to most of the population. They investigate conditions at Caranavi and Sorata in the Department of La Paz, and assess the work of local community health centres in the monitoring, prevention and control of a daunting range of problems, including tuberculosis, respiratory infections, acute diarrhoea, goitre, anaemia, scabies, leishmaniasis, malaria, and malnutrition.

688 Community health workers in Bolivia: adapting to traditional roles in the Andean community.
Joseph William Bastien. *Social Science and Medicine*, vol. 30, no. 3 (1990), p. 281-87. bibliog.

An analysis of the training of community health workers in highland Bolivia by an expert in this field. Although such workers are elected from within their own communities to administer primary health care, they do not automatically fit into a 'leadership role' in either modern or traditional medicine. To be successful in the job of raising health standards, they must find a leadership niche. Bastien discusses a series of case-studies where health workers gradually develop a respected place for themselves within the *ayllu*, and learn to combine traditional Aymara or Quechua ritual treatments with modern medical practice.

689 High lands, low sodium.
Henry Goethals. *Américas*, vol. 42, no. 4 (1990), p. 4.

Some sixty-five per cent of Bolivian schoolchildren suffer from iodine-deficiency goitre, the highest rate in the western hemisphere. This article reports the start of a campaign in 1988 to treat 1.5 million rural Bolivians with oral iodized oil to prevent endemic goitre caused by severe thyroid deficiency. The problem is not the cost of the medication but the extreme isolation and poor distribution facilities afflicting many rural communities.

690 From the fat of our souls: social change, political process, and medical pluralism in Bolivia.
Libbet Crandon-Malamud. Berkeley, California: University of California Press, 1991. 267p. bibliog. (Comparative Studies of Health Systems and Medical Care Series).

This is a detailed case-study of the complexity of medical practices operating side-by-side in a small Aymara town on the Bolivian altiplano. The author examines the roles of the indigenous healers, the Methodist and Catholic churches, and modern 'western' medical practitioners in the interpretations and treatment of illness, and goes on to discuss how ethnicity, ritual, and religion influence local decisions made about medical care.

691 Bolivia's *promotores*. (Community health workers.)
Joseph William Bastien. *World Health* (September/October 1992), p. 26-27.

Examines the development of a training project in the Department of Oruro for community health workers, most of them elected peasant farmers who are given short courses in primary health care, and, where necessary, language instruction in Aymara or Quechua.

692 Dietary beliefs, nutritional patterns and nutritional status of urban Aymara women and children.
Isabel M. Parraga. PhD thesis, Case Western Reserve University, Cleveland, Ohio, 1992. 353p. bibliog.

Examines food consumption patterns and the nutritional status of a group of rural Aymara women and preschool-age children who have migrated to El Alto, on the edge of La Paz. Particular attention is given to protein, calcium, iron, and vitamin intakes, to the adverse effects on growth where deficiencies occur, and to the influence of maternal employment on the various problems encountered.

693 Drum and stethoscope: integrating ethnomedicine and biomedicine in Bolivia.
Joseph William Bastien. Salt Lake City: University of Utah Press, 1992. 266p. bibliog.

A plea to scholars and physicians not to reject native healers out of hand, be they herbalists, ritualists, village shamans or the like, but to investigate the possible benefits of working with them when treating the sick in Bolivia's rural communities. Basing his proposals on fieldwork on the altiplano, Bastien retains an objective approach, examining the weaknesses and dangers of ethnomedicine, but arguing that greater understanding and collaboration between Western-style medical practitioners and indigenous healers can often assist a patient's recovery, and harmonize relationships all round.

694 Brief communication: effect of coca-leaf chewing on salivary progesterone assays.
Virginia J. Vitzthum, Miranda von Dornum, Peter T. Ellison.
American Journal of Physical Anthropology, vol. 92 (December 1993), p. 539-44. bibliog.

This is part of a general study regarding fertility determinants at high altitudes. Although reduced fertility, where this occurs, may be due to hypoxia (oxygen deficiency), poor nutrition and other factors, the authors note that coca-leaf chewing temporarily produces misleading results when recording fertility patterns, since it falsely raises the progesterone readings during saliva sample collection, and can lead to errors in identifying ovulatory cycles. This technical paper advises on the most reliable procedures to avoid mistakes.

695 Rural origin as a risk factor for maternal and child health in periurban Bolivia.
Deborah E. Bender, Tirsa Rivera, Donna Madonna. *Social Science and Medicine*, vol. 37, no. 11 (1993), p. 1345-49. bibliog.

An investigation carried out in Cochabamba that again reminds us that life in Bolivia is generally healthier in the town than in the countryside. In their study of migrant settlements to the north and south of the city, the authors found that urban women of rural origin were more likely to have poorer health prospects for themselves and their children than their lifelong urban counterparts. Through careful sampling, the discrepancy is shown to be linked to a number of factors, including levels of education: three-quarters of the women from rural areas had had no schooling at all, or primary schooling only, whereas half of the urban women had completed secondary school, and this variation was reflected in the neglect or the use of local health-care facilities.

696 Bullying by Bolivian pharmaceutical industry.
Raúl Villanueva. *The Lancet* (North American edition), vol. 343 (12 February 1994), p. 410-11.

Complaints from health officials in Bolivia that the United States pharmaceutical industry is often lax in its control and promotion of medicines in the Third World were supported by the US Office of Technology Assessment, whose report in 1993 concluded that standards of labelling and promotional material provided by US companies in developing countries were much worse than those provided at home. Bolivian health professionals produced additional evidence that obsolete drugs, and drugs with an unfavourable risk–benefit ratio, were also being promoted and sold in Bolivia, and called for stricter regulations. The article is objective, but its title is misleading; this is a not a case of bullying by Bolivia, but a call for free speech and fair trading.

697 Children and women in Bolivia.
La Paz: UNICEF-Bolivia, 1994. 148p. maps. bibliog.

Nearly half of all deaths in Bolivia occur among children under the age of five. This wide-ranging and authoritative report examines women's and children's health conditions, focusing on infant mortality, maternal deaths, poverty, contraception, malnutrition, drinking water, sanitation, and disease. Acknowledging the magnitude of the problem, the study reviews what remedial measures have been taken during the early 1990s under the

National Plan of Action: Goals for Children programme, and what remains to be done. The effective use of radio broadcasts is demonstrated, while the report also describes work done with children in particularly difficult circumstances, including street children and the handicapped. This is a clear and concise account, required reading for all those seeking information on one of Bolivia's most fundamental health needs and services.

698 Rural-to-urban migration in Bolivia and Peru: association with child mortality, breastfeeding cessation, maternal care and contraception.
Luis Tam. Calverton, Maryland: Macro International, 1994. 29p. bibliog. (Demographic and Health Surveys Working Papers, No. 8).
The Bolivian case-studies are based on a series of questionnaires carried out in La Paz and Santa Cruz aimed at helping to design improved maternal and child health programmes among the cities' poorest migrants.

699 Cross cultural communication of tetanus vaccinations in Bolivia.
Joseph William Bastien. *Social Science and Medicine*, vol. 41, no. 1 (1995), p. 77-86.
Tetanus is a primary cause of infant mortality among Bolivia's indigenous population, but because of the terrifying characteristics of the disease, it is widely regarded as having supernatural causes. Basing his findings on work among the Aymara, Quechua, and Tupi-Guaraní, Bastien urges health workers involved in tetanus immunization programmes to become more sensitive to the cultural interpretations of the disease among the Indian communities, and to work with their traditional healers in promoting the need for vaccination. This is a detailed and informative study which touches on many related aspects of Indian life.

700 Ethnographic studies of ARI in Bolivia and their use by the national ARI programme.
Patricia Hudelson, Tomas Huanca, Dolores Charaly, Virginia Cirpa. *Social Sciences and Medicine*, vol. 41, no. 12 (1995), p. 1677-83.
This report on the prevalence and treatment of Acute Respiratory Infections (ARI), especially pneumonia, among infants and young children in Bolivia is based on an Aymara community in the Department of La Paz and a Quechua community in the Department of Cochabamba. In trying to identify the factors that facilitate or deter the seeking of prompt medical care, the authors found that advice from the traditional healer was usually sought before an approach, if any, was made to the trained health worker. The paper sets out clearly, and in detail, how this problem can be tackled so that greater awareness by the mother of the early symptoms, and faster access to professional treatment, can be achieved.

701 New hope for Tupiza.
Mirta Roses Periago. *World Health* (March/April 1995), p. 9.
An interesting case-study in local health care. The Tupiza health district (population c. 125,000) was included in a national programme when Bolivia was selected in 1991 as one of the countries to participate in the World Health Organization's Initiative for Intensive Cooperation with particular states. This involved training personnel in basic

techniques, providing medicines and equipment, and constructing new health centres, new schools, and new community water systems. Its success enabled the district to become part of the government's Popular Participation Law of 1994, where local authorities assumed new responsibilities for education, rural roads, irrigation, and health services.

702 Concepts of disease and their relationship to health-seeking behaviour in Chuquisaca Department, South Bolivia.
D. R. Moore.   DPhil thesis, University of Oxford, England, 1996.
Focusing on the Quechua- and Spanish-speaking peasants and share-croppers in Belisario Boeto province, Department of Chuquisaca, the author analyses the basic religious premises on which ideas of health and illness are perceived. Medical knowledge and health-care practices among the *curanderos* (indigenous healers) receive special attention here, along with the roles that ritual, magic, witchcraft, and symbolism play in individual and group therapy.

703 The demand for medical care: evidence from urban areas in Bolivia.
Ii Masako.   Washington, DC: World Bank, 1996. 49p. bibliog.
(Living Standards Measurement Study Working Paper, No. 123).
From a survey carried out in Bolivia's nine departmental capitals and in selected cities with populations of 10,000 or more, the author seeks to identify the most important social and economic factors that determine the demand for medical care, whether by government facilities, non-governmental organizations, private clinics, or by self-care.

704 Whose clinic is it anyway? Utilization of a primary health care facility in Chilimarca, Bolivia.
Edward Lowe Kinman.   PhD thesis, University of Minnesota, Minneapolis, Minnesota, 1996. 323p. bibliog.
Despite their proximity, health services can remain underused. At the primary health clinic in Chilimarca, established in 1991, Kinman's investigation revealed that outsiders were increasingly using the facility, while only 60 per cent of the consultations were by people whom the clinic was ostensibly meant to serve. Failure to consult and involve the local community in the daily operation of the clinic is suggested here as the main cause of the underuse.

705 Definition and prevalence of anemia in Bolivian women of childbearing age living at high altitudes: the effect of iron-folate supplementation.
Jacques Berger, Victor M. Aguayo, José Luis San Miguel, Carmen Luján, Wilma Téllez, Pierre Traissac. *Nutrition Reviews*, vol. 55, no. 6 (1997), p. 247-56. bibliog.
A specialized study which discusses the effects of high altitude on iron metabolism in Bolivian women, and analyses the results of trials made in two settlements near Potosí using an iron-folate supplement. The authors emphasize that nutritional anaemia is a public health problem in such populations, and that many existing methods of assessing

it lead to an underestimation of its prevalence. They recommend therefore that haemoglobin values for the diagnosis of anaemia should be revised for populations living at high altitudes.

706 A water supply development project in Quiescapa, Bolivia.
Larry D. Yates. *Journal of Environmental Health*, vol. 59 (March 1997), p. 20-22.

Not every improvement project is initially welcomed by the members of a small community. The author describes a joint venture by two non-governmental organizations – Andean Rural Health Care and the US-based Water for People – to bring drinking water to an isolated altiplano village with a poor health record, which had hitherto been wholly dependent on two polluted springs and a few unclean wells. But these at least were familiar. Many villagers soon became anxious at the sight of the gravel-pack filter, the concrete storage-tank and chlorinator, and the piped water system, demanding a return to their traditional ways, and damaging the new equipment. Yates records how progress became a mutual learning experience both for the engineers and the villagers, as each problem was solved with patience and collaboration until the project was completed and a huge celebration marked the event.

707 The kiss of death: Chagas' disease in the Americas.
Joseph William Bastien. Salt Lake City: University of Utah Press, 1998. 301p. maps. bibliog.

A thorough and timely study of Chagas' disease, in which the author concentrates on Bolivia where infection rates are higher than in any other Latin American country. Chagas' is transmitted by the *vinchuca* bug (the 'kissing bug') which infests mud and straw dwellings. The bite normally goes undetected in the early, treatable stages, after which the disease becomes a slow-acting killer. Bastien traces its history, and describes in detail the work of Bolivian doctors and health workers who are fighting the disease, now mainly through simple methods of home improvement and community projects. This is the only comprehensive book-length text in English on Chagas' disease, an illuminating investigation that can be recommended both to the specialist and the general reader.

708 Mass media and interpersonal influence in a reproductive health communication campaign in Bolivia.
Thomas W. Valente, Walter P. Saba. *Communication Research*, no. 1 (1998), p. 96-124. bibliog.

Bolivia's rates of infant mortality, maternal death and unwanted pregnancy are among the highest in South America. This study compares the relative effectiveness of mass media and personal networks in getting a message across, in this case communicating ways of gaining access to, and using, improved methods of contraception. TV and radio spots in Aymara, Quechua and Spanish were broadcast in eight major Bolivian cities. Personal networks involved face-to-face discussion with family, friends, and local advisers. Research results showed that the mass media were effective in promoting awareness and knowledge, but that personal communication was necessary for behavioural change. A combination of both methods led to the highest rates of adoption of modern contraceptives.

709 Attaining health for all through community partnerships: principles of the Census-Based, Impact-Oriented (CBIO) approach to primary health care developed in Bolivia, South America.
Henry Perry, Nathan Robison, Dardo Chávez, Orlando Taja, Carolina Hilari, David Shanklin, John Wyon. *Social Science and Medicine*, vol. 48, no. 8 (1999), p. 1053-67. bibliog.

Describes the programmes developed since the 1980s by Andean Rural Health Care (a non-governmental organization) in poor rural and urban communities on the altiplano, around Cochabamba, and in the Santa Cruz region. Each programme, in consultation with the local people, identifies the worst causes of illness and death in the given programme area, and then involves *everyone* there through regular visits, health monitoring, advice, and treatment. The authors discuss the strengths and weaknesses of this system of individual health delivery, and argue that it is neither as complicated nor as costly as might be imagined. The targeting of those at greatest risk from specific life-threatening conditions, combined with regular general home checks for all, is now under way in seven CBIO programme sites in Bolivia where, by the late 1990s, some 75,000 people were being served.

710 Evaluating health service equity at a primary care clinic in Chilimarca, Bolivia
Edward Lowe Kinman. *Social Science and Medicine*, vol. 49, no. 5 (1999), p. 663-78. maps. bibliog.

Expanding his study of the primary health care clinic in Chilimarca on the outskirts of Cochabamba, Kinman records the heavy immigration that occurred in the settlement during the 1990s by displaced miners, poor farmers, and by Cochabamba city-dwellers in search of cheaper accommodation. He focuses on the current population's place of origin, length of residence, and language, as variables which differentiate users and non-users of the clinic, noting that local non-users' complaints include the cost of consultations and medicines, and the staff's inability to speak Quechua. The clinic is now 'overused' by Spanish or bilingual speakers travelling out and back from Cochabamba's city centre, while the local population show more interest in obtaining a reliable water system than a health clinic. This is an illuminating and well-mapped case-study which highlights the often complex issues involved in providing successful local health care.

Languages

General

711 **Compendio de la gramática kechua y aymara; seguido de un vocabulario completo.** (Textbook of Quechua and Aymara grammar; followed by a complete vocabulary.)
Germán G. Villamor. La Paz: Librería Popular, 1942. 157p.
A dated but still useful textbook, suitable for beginners.

712 **The native tribes of eastern Bolivia and western Matto Grosso.**
Alfred Métraux. Washington, DC: US Government Printing Office, 1942. 182p. map. bibliog. (Smithsonian Institution, Bureau of American Ethnology, Bulletin No. 134).
Métraux follows in the ground-breaking tradition of Alcide d'Orbigny, and especially of Erland Nordenskiöld, in this study of the life, economy, language, myths and religion of many of central South America's indigenous cultures. Here he provides a basic source of information on the following tribes and linguistic groups: the Mojo and Bauré, Chiquitos, Paressí, Yuracares, Mosetene and Chimane, Leco, Apolista (or Lapacu), Tacana, Kamchana, Móvima, Kayuvava, Itonama, Chapakuran, Guarayú and Pauserna, Sirionó, Arawakan, Otukean, Guato, Cariban, Nambikuára, Chirquano, Chane and Tupi-Guaraní.

713 **Bolivian Indian grammars.**
Ester Matteson. Norman, Oklahoma: University of Oklahoma Press, 1967. 2 vols.
Presents ten grammars of Bolivian Indian languages. Volume one contains Bauré, Ignaciano, Tacana, Eseeja and Chacobo. Volume two includes Quechua, Guaraní, Sirionó, Itonama, and Móvima. The grammars were prepared by linguists fluent in the spoken languages, although the coverage is not exhaustive.

714 Bolivian Indian tribes: classification, bibliography and map of present language distribution.
Arnold Key, Mary Key. Norman, Oklahoma: University of Oklahoma Press, 1967. 124p.
Discusses what has been written about Bolivian Indian tribes and native languages of Bolivia. The text covers all native languages except Quechua and Aymara.

715 Classification of South American Indian languages.
Čestmír Loukokka. Los Angeles: University of California Press, 1968. 4th ed. 453p. maps. bibliog.
An introduction to native South American languages and a good starting-place for a new student.

716 Manual práctico ABC del aymara, quechua, y castellano.
(Practical ABC manual of Aymara, Quechua, and Spanish.)
Lima: Ediciones Tiempos Modernos, 1975. 112p.
A modern textbook containing phrases and common expressions in the three languages. They are listed under various headings, such as greetings, family, travel, food, etc.

717 Moderno vocabulario del quechua y del aymara y su correspondencia en castellano. (Modern Quechua and Aymara vocabulary with a corresponding Spanish section.)
Germán G. Villamor. La Paz: Editorial Popular, 1981. 4th ed. 168p.
A standard tool in language teaching in Bolivia.

718 The mutual influences of Spanish and Andean languages.
Martha J. Hardman de Bautista. *Word*, vol. 33, nos. 1-2 (1982), p. 143-57.
Language interaction in the Andes has resulted in changes in grammar, and the Spanish spoken in the region reflects the contributions of indigenous tongues. This article deals with phonology and lexicography in a cultural and historical context and concludes that Spanish, together with Aymara, influences, codifies and reflects the Andean reality.

719 América latina, en sus lenguas indígenas. (Latin America, and its indigenous languages.)
Edited by Bernard Pottier; United Nations Educational, Scientific and Cultural Organization (UNESCO). Caracas: Monte Avila Editores, C. A., 1983. 476p. maps. bibliog.
Part of the UNESCO series entitled 'América latina en su cultura'. Previous volumes dealt with music, literature, etc. Pottier brings together a collection of essays by noted linguists, including Xavier Albó, Víctor Hugo Cárdenas, Yolanda Lastra de Suárez, Bernard Pottier and Louisa R. Stark. The volume is organized into six parts: (1) an historical overview, and the politics of linguistics during the colonial era; (2) multilingualism; (3) native languages and the formation of dialects; (4) linguistic

structures; (5) social linguistics; and (6) an extensive bibliography. The study also includes graphs and illustrations.

720 South American Indian languages: retrospect and prospect.
Harriet E. Manelis Klein, Louisa R. Stark. Austin, Texas: University of Texas Press, 1985. 863p. bibliog.

A book of readings by experts on languages and culture. Part two, entitled 'Indigenous languages of the Andes', deals with the Quechua and Aymara languages. Essays include: Lucy T. Briggs's 'A critical survey of the literature on the Aymara language' (p. 546-94); and 'Dialectical variation in Aymara' (p. 595-616); Martha J. Hardman's 'Aymara and Quechua languages in contact' (p. 617-43); and Bruce Mannheim's 'Contact and Quechua external genetic relationships' (p. 644-90).

Aymara

721 Gramática y diccionario aimara. (Aymara grammar and dictionary.)
Juan Enrique Ebbing. La Paz: Editorial y Librería Don Bosco, 1965. 360p.

In addition to the grammar, there is a pronunciation guide, an Aymara–Spanish, Spanish–Aymara dictionary, an index and a verb table.

722 The Aymara language in its social and cultural context: a collection of essays on aspects of Aymara language and culture.
Martha J. Hardman. Gainesville, Florida: University Presses of Florida, 1981. 317p. bibliog. (University of Florida Social Science Monograph, No. 67).

A collection of twenty-two essays on the Aymara language. Subjects covered include: Aymara grammatical and semantic categories; the Aymara language in contact with other languages; and the implications of Aymara studies for applied anthropological linguistics.

723 Enseñanza del idioma aymara como segundo idioma.
(The teaching of Aymara as a second language.)
Juan de Dios Yapita. La Paz: Instituto de la Lengua y Cultura Aymara, 1981. 292p. bibliog.

Discusses the introduction and development of programmes to teach Aymara as a second language. They represent part of a national effort to produce a bilingual culture in Bolivia.

724 Vocabulario de la lengua aymara. (Vocabulary of the Aymara language.)
Ludovico Bertonio. Cochabamba, Bolivia: Centro de Estudios de la Realidad Económica y Social, 1984. 474p.
A new edition of a vocabulary book which was originally published in a rudimentary form as early as 1612.

725 Aprendizaje del Aymara. (Learning Aymara.)
Basílio Mamani. La Paz: CEMCAL (Centro de Educación 'Multigrado' y Capacitación), 1988. 54p.
A text designed for teaching Aymara through conversation.

726 Curso de Aymara paceño. (A course in Aymara as spoken in the La Paz region.)
Juan de Dios Yapita. St Andrews, Scotland: University of St Andrews Institute of Amerindian Studies, 1988. 170p.
A textbook for the systematic teaching of the Aymara language through everyday conversation.

727 Structure and use of Altiplano Spanish.
Billie Dale Stratford. PhD thesis, University of Florida, Gainesville, Florida, 1989. 299p. bibliog.
After nearly 500 years of language and culture contact, and extensive bilingualism, the variety of Spanish spoken on the altiplano of Bolivia and Peru reflects the influence of the region's indigenous languages. In particular, the author notes that in conversation, Aymara influences on the grammar and syntax of this local Spanish dialect have a strongly personal and cultural base.

728 Morfología y gramática Aymara. (Aymara morphology and grammar.)
Donato Gómez, José Condori Cosme. La Paz: [n.p.], 1992. 153p.
A reference book on Aymara grammar.

729 El idioma Aymara, variantes regionales y sociales. (Regional and social variants in the Aymara language.)
Lucy Therina Briggs. La Paz: Ediciones ILCA, 1993. 453p.
A detailed study of the regional and social variations occurring in the Aymara language.

730 Transcripción del vocabulario de la lengua Aymara.
(A transcription of the Aymara language vocabulary.)
Radio 'San Gabriel' Departamento de Lengua Aymara; P. Ludovico Bertonio. La Paz: Aguila, 1993. 982p.
This edition is written in the Aymara alphabet.

731 Aymara método facil. (An easy way to learn Aymara.)
Juan de Dios Yapita. La Paz: Ediciones ILCA, 1994. 182p.

This is a pocket-book containing short, useful conversations and phrases to aid the learning of Aymara.

732 K'isimira I. Gramática viva de la lengua Aymara. (The grammar of Aymara as a living language.)

K'isimira II. Vocabulario temático Aymara. (A thematic Aymara vocabulary.)
Saturnino Gallego, fsc (jilata Satuku). La Paz: Bruño-Hisbol, 1994. Vol. I, 495p. Vol. II, 166p.

Volume I contains common phrases in Aymara, with Spanish translation.

733 Aprendamos Aymara. (Let's learn Aymara.)
Blanca Patiño de Murillo. La Paz: Impreso en Producciones CIMA, 1997. 65p.

A book well suited to the needs of those who are learning to read both the Aymara and Spanish languages. Appropriate sketches are used to match the two vocabularies in an attractive text which has been written specifically for bilingual teaching.

734 Texto de aprendizaje del idioma Aymara (mimeografiado).
(A text for learning the Aymara language; mimeographed.)
Regina Bautista Quisbert. La Paz: Centro de Entrenamiento Cuerpo de Paz, 1997. 99p.

A text for teaching Aymara to Peace Corps volunteers.

735 Aprendizaje de la lengua Aymara. (Practical training in the Aymara language.)
Silvestre Mamani Mamani. La Paz: Editorial Trasos, 1999. 100p.

This text contains a variety of exercises in the Aymara language, with accompanying cassettes.

736 Vocabulario Aymara del parto y de la vida reproductiva de la mujer. (An Aymara vocabulary dealing with childbirth and women's reproductive life.)
Denise Y. Arnold, Juan de Dios Yapita, with Margarita Tito.
La Paz: Industria Gráfica, Margenta, 1999. 286p.

This vocabulary, the result of more than ten years' anthropological and linguistic study into the methods of childbirth among rural and migrant women of the Bolivian altiplano, includes more than 2,000 Aymara words and phrases.

Quechua

737 Elementos de gramática incana o quechua. (Elements of Inca or
Quechua grammar.)
José Antonio Núñez del Prado.   Cuzco, Peru: Garcilaso, 1960.
162p.
An elementary Quechua grammar textbook.

738 An introduction to spoken Bolivian Quechua.
Garland D. Bills, Bernardo Vallejo C., Rudolphe C. Troike.
Austin, Texas: University of Texas Press, 1969. 449p. map. bibliog.
This text includes conversations, vocabulary, review drills, reading and visual aids to help
memorize dialogues. Companion tapes are also available.

739 Gramática kechwa. (Quechua grammar.)
Cesar Augusto Guardia Mayorga.   Lima: Ediciones los Andes,
1973. 388p.
A basic Quechua grammar textbook.

740 Literatura pre-hispánica y colonial. (Pre-hispanic and colonial
literature.)
Edgar Avila Echazú.   La Paz: Librería y Editorial Gisbert, 1974.
202p. bibliog.
Includes selections from the indigenous literature of the Inca and Spanish colonial periods
originally written in Quechua, but translated into Spanish.

741 Los mil rostros del quechua: sociolingüística de Cochabamba.
(The thousand faces of Quechua: a socio-linguistic study of
Cochabamba.)
Xavier Albó.   Lima: Instituto de Estudios Peruanos, 1974. 268p.
(Serie Lengua y Sociedad, 1).
An anthropological study of language distribution and usage in central Bolivia.

742 El quechua y la historia social andina. (Quechua and Andean
social history.)
Alfredo Torero.   Lima: Universidad Ricardo Palma, Dirección
Universitaria de Investigación, 1974. 240p. map.
An examination and socio-historical evaluation of the Quechua language in the greater
Andean region.

743 Diccionario trí-lingüe: Quechua of Cusco, English, Spanish.
Esteban Hornberger S.   Lima: LCA, 1977. 3 vols.
A Quechua–Spanish–English dictionary.

213

744 Diccionario normalizado y comparativo quechua: Chachapoyas–Lamas. (Standard and comparative Quechuan dictionary: Chachapoyas–Lamas dialect.)
Gerald Taylor. Paris: L'Harmattan, 1979. 248p. (Série ethnolinguistique amérindienne).
A dictionary of regional Quechua.

745 Quechua y aymara lenguas en contacto. (Quechua and Aymara languages in contact.)
Martha J. Hardman. La Paz: *Antropología*, vol. 1 (1979), p. 69-84.
Argues that Quechua enjoys a certain prestige as a language in Andean society because it was originally the language of the Incan conquerors.

746 Expansión del quechua: primeros contactos con el castellano. (Expansion of Quechua: first contacts with the Spanish.)
Ibico Rojas R. Lima: Ediciones Signo, 1980. 131p. bibliog.
Discusses how the Quechua language spread after the arrival of the Spaniards, who communicated with the native populations in their own language.

747 Poesía dramática de los Incas. (Dramatic poetry of the Incas.)
Clements Robert Markham. Buenos Aires: C. Casavalle, 1883. 86p.
A collection of Inca poetry, compiled by a well-known English traveller who began his lifelong fascination with Peru in the 1850s when he was commissioned by the India Office to explore Peru and to collect *Cinchona* seeds (native to this region) in order to lay the foundation for cheap quinine production in Southeast Asia. His interests in Peru ranged widely and included the history and language of the indigenous people. He did pioneering work in recording examples of Quechua poetry and narrative, and also wrote a Quechua grammar and dictionary. Markham later became president of both the Hakluyt Society and the Royal Geographical Society.

748 Sesenta canciones del quechua boliviano. (Sixty songs in Bolivian Quechua.)
Compiled and edited by Max Peter Bauman. Cochabamba, Bolivia: Centro Pedagógico y Cultural de Portales, 1983. 195p.
This song book also includes annotation in Quechua and Spanish.

749 La escritura del quechua: problemática y perspectivas. (Writing Quechua: problems and perspectives.)
Federico Aguiló. La Paz: Editorial 'Los Amigos del Libro', 1987. 174p. bibliog.
Discusses the problems associated with writing Quechua, a language which developed in an exclusively oral tradition.

750 Método facil para el aprendizaje del idioma quechua. (An easy method for learning the Quechua language.)
Donato Gómez B., José Condori C., Edgard Humerez. La Paz: Editora 'Andegráfia', 1987. 84p. (mimeographed).
A basic text for beginners.

751 Chiqa willaykuna. (True Quechua stories for children.)
Nina Llanos Primitivo, Torrez Córdova Mamerto. Sucre, Bolivia: Talleres Gráficos de Imprenta Universitaria, 1992. 38p.
Stories in the Quechua language selected mainly for reading aloud.

752 Quechua: elementos para la normalización oral y escrita. (Ways to standardize oral and written Quechua.)
Eustaquia Terceros Carrasco. La Paz: Talleres Gráficos Hisbol, 1993. 43p.
The text is formally developed to assist the learning of Quechua's basic essentials across the morphological division between the spoken and the written language.

753 Qhiswa, Ruwachixkunamanta T'aqainin. (Quechua: a history in song.)
Víctor Ramírez Anagua. P'utuxsi-Qullasuyu: V. Ramírez Anagua, 1996. 56p.
The text is in Spanish and Quechua and presents a moving account of important events in Quechua history expressed through their songs.

754 Diccionario quechua–castellano, castellano–quechua.
(A Quechua–Spanish, Spanish–Quechua dictionary.)
Teófilo Laime Ajacopa, Efraín Cazazola, Félix Layme Pairumano. La Paz: Ediciones Gráficas EG, 1997. 444p.
This valuable dictionary and work of reference is up to date and comprehensive.

Guaraní

755 Resumen de prehistoria y protohistoria de los paises guaranís; conferencias dades en el colegio nacional de segunda enseñanza de la Asunción dos dias de julio, 8 y 21 de agosto de 1913.
(Summary of the prehistory and proto-history of the Guaraní countries; a conference given in the national secondary school of Asunción on two days in July, and the 8 and 21 of August, 1913.)
Moisés Santiago Bertoni.   Asunción, Paraguay: J. E. O'Leary, 1914. 64p.
An early but still useful study of the evolution of Guaraní culture and language.

756 Hispanismos en el guaraní: estudio sobre la penetración de la cultura española en la guaraní, según se refleja en la lengua.
(Hispanicism in Guaraní, a study of the penetration of Spanish culture into Guaraní as reflected in the language.)
Marcos A. Morínigo.   Buenos Aires: Telleres Casa Jacabo Peuser, 1931. 432p. maps. (Collección de estudios indigenistas, 1).
A detailed linguistic analysis accompanied by maps and diagrams. It also includes a vocabulary section which is arranged by subject headings.

757 El guaraní en la geografía de América. (Guaraní in American geography.)
Anselmo Jover Peralta.   Buenos Aires: Ediciones Tupa, 1950. 272p.
A basic study of the geographical distribution of the Guaraní language.

758 Ayvu Rapyta: textos míticos de los Mybá-Guaraní del Guairá.
(The basis of human language: mythical texts of the Mybá-Guaraní Indians of the Guairá.)
Edited by Leon Cadagan.   São Paulo, Brazil: Universidade de São Paulo, Faculdade de Filosofia, Ciencias e Letra, 1959. 217p. (Boletim no. 227, Antropología, no. 5).
Presents myths and legends in Guaraní and Spanish. A vocabulary is also included.

759 A description of colloquial Guaraní.
Emma Gregores, Jorge A. Suárez.   Paris: Mouton, 1967. 248p.
Gives information on the linguistic classification of Guaraní and reviews the literature and written sources which are available. The text includes grammar, phonology and morphemics.

760 Diccionario castellano–guaraní y guaraní–castellano: sintáctico,
fraseológico, ideológico. (Spanish–Guaraní, Guaraní–Spanish
dictionary; syntax, phraseology and ideology.)
Antonio Guasch. Asunción, Paraguay: Ediciones Loyola, 1980.
4th ed. 789p.
A basic Guaraní–Spanish dictionary and grammar text.

Religion

General

761 Missionary pioneering in Bolivia, with some account of work in Argentina.
Will Payne, Charles T. W. Wilson.   London: H. A. Raymond, [1901]. 148p. maps.

Designed to give Christian workers an outline of the existing state of missionary activity in Latin America at the end of the 19th century, this work also names many of the early missionaries who worked in the region.

762 Church and state in Latin America: a history of politico-ecclesiastical relations.
J. Lloyd Mecham.   Chapel Hill, North Carolina: University of North Carolina Press, 1934. 550p. bibliog.

An early work but one which remains a useful source of reference on Church–state relations after Independence. A section on Bolivia is included (p. 221-46).

763 Today's missions in the Latin American social revolution.
C. Peter Wagner.   *Evangelical Missions Quarterly*, vol. 1, no. 2 (1965), p. 19-29.

Examines the difficult role of the foreign missionary in the revolutionary process. Wagner poses the question: does the missionary become involved in this type of political liberation movement, or does he continue to tend only to parochial matters?

764 The condor of the jungle, pioneer pilot of the Andes.
C. Peter Wagner, Joseph S. McCollough. Westwood, California: Revell, 1966. 158p.

A biography of Wally Hernon of the Andes Evangelical Mission. Hernon was one of the first Protestant missionaries to be successful in the evangelical effort in early 20th-century Bolivia.

765 Missionary moments.
Phyllis Cammack. Newberg, Oregon: Barclay Press, 1966. 134p.

An interesting and well-written history of 13 years spent working as a missionary with Bolivia's Aymara Indians.

766 The Protestant movement in Bolivia.
C. Peter Wagner. South Pasadena, California: William Carey Library, 1970. 240p. maps. bibliog.

A comprehensive study of the evolution and existing state of Protestantism in Bolivia and the various organizations working most effectively there. This is an excellent source of information on active Protestant churches and missions which were working in Bolivia in the 1960s.

767 Cristianismo y revolución en América latina. (Christianity and revolution in Latin America.)
Manuel M. Martínez. *Diogenes* (Summer 1974), 146p.

Examines the relationship between the Church and the revolutionary movements in South America. This work also provides a good introduction to 'Liberation Theology' and to changes in the Roman Catholic Church.

768 Religious life in solidarity.
John F. Talbot. *America* (New York: America Press), vol. 159, no. 5 (August 1988), p. 112-13.

Records the proceedings of the Tenth Assembly of the Confederación Latinoamericana de Religiosos (CLAR), held in Cochabamba shortly after Pope John Paul II's first visit to Bolivia in May 1988. During the conference, a recurring theme in papers and discussions had been the need felt by the younger delegates not merely to visit, but to live among the very poor in the shanty towns, and to share actively in their everyday problems and concerns.

769 Searching minds and questing hearts: Protestantism and social context in Bolivia.
David Clark Knowlton. PhD thesis, University of Texas at Austin, 1988. 489p. bibliog.

A study that investigates the growth of Protestantism among three contrasted groups in the Department of La Paz: the peasants of Huacuyo, the townsmen of Copacabana, and former peasants in the city of La Paz. It asks why these people decided to become Protestants, what the significance of this decision is in terms of the wider social context, and what role these Protestant groups play as agents of change.

770 Tribute to a Latin American martyr.
Michael O'Sullivan. *America* (New York: America Press), vol. 160 (January 1989), p. 8-11, 20-21.

Luís Espinal was a Spanish Jesuit missionary who came to Bolivia in 1968, working as a teacher, journalist, and local broadcaster in and around La Paz. He became increasingly at odds with the government authorities on a variety of issues, and received several death threats which he ignored. He was murdered by persons unknown in March 1980.

771 Tongues of fire: the explosion of Protestantism in Latin America.
David Martin. Oxford, England; Cambridge, Massachusetts: Blackwell, 1990. 352p. bibliog.

An incisive, wide-ranging and well-researched study by a noted scholar on the sociology of religion. Martin analyses the rapid spread of Evangelical Protestantism since the 1960s from its epicentre in the United States, identifying it in some respects as part of the Americanization process in Latin America. Protestant expansion is examined in the context of the region's social and economic changes; the spectacular growth of non-Catholic religious groups in Bolivia, for example, resulted in 200 of them being registered by the mid-1980s. Links are examined between the increase in Protestantism and the increase in rural Aymaran migration to the cities. Catholic responses are also reviewed, while students of the subject will welcome the extensive bibliography. This is a book suited to both the specialist and the general reader.

772 More blessed to give: a Pentecostal mission to Bolivia in anthropological perspective.
Göran Johansson. Stockholm, Sweden: Stockholm University, Department of Social Anthropology, 1992. 254p. map. bibliog.

Johansson begins frankly by admitting that 'My only experience of conversion, that from Pentecostalist to backslider, was a big stumbling-block to my project.' The stated purpose of his study of the Nordic (Swedish) Pentecostal Mission's many centres in Bolivia is not to downplay its acknowledged success there, including its growing number of adherents, and its valuable work in the social and health fields. Instead, Johansson argues that the Mission has become too institutionalized, with more emphasis placed on efficiency and organization in the modern secularized society, than on calling and missionary zeal. The study includes a variety of viewpoints for and against, which, along with the author's opinions, would provide a useful basis for discussion on the evolving role of the mission in society.

773 Bridging cultures and hemispheres: the legacy of Archibald Reekie and Canadian Baptists in Bolivia.
Edited by William H. Brackney. Macon, Georgia: Smyth & Helwys, 1997. 138p. map. bibliog.

This volume of essays by Canadian and Bolivian authors was written to mark the centenary of Archibald Reekie's arrival in 1897 in Oruro. A pioneering Baptist missionary from Ontario, Reekie and a small group of colleagues over time established churches, Sunday Schools, clinics, a radio station and an experimental farm, as they expanded their work with the Aymara and Quechua. Despite difficulties, the Bolivian Baptist Union has continued to grow, led now largely by Bolivian ministers. This is an informative study since it provides considerable background on the social, as well as the religious life in Bolivia during the 20th century.

774 Spiritual journals.

Henri J. M. Nouwen. New York: Continuum Publishing Co., 1997. 448p. map.

This is the diary of a monk from upstate New York which includes (on p. 140-291) the Latin American journal he compiled during his time in Bolivia and Peru in the early 1980s. Nouwen was based in Cochabamba, where the detailed daily account of his ministry, his travels around the region, and his impressions of local and national events are well recorded. Through it all flows the strong personal response to his surroundings, and to the poverty and hardship suffered by so many of the Bolivian men and women with whom he worked.

775 Converting difference: metaculture, missionaries, and the politics of locality.

Andrew Orta. *Ethnology*, vol. 37, no. 2 (1998), p. 165-85. bibliog.

In recent years, Catholic missionaries have initiated a set of pastoral reforms in some of the Aymara communities of Bolivia which are based on a perceived evangelical equivalence between Aymara identity and Christian identity. Working with Aymara religious leaders, the missionaries have endeavoured to codify a set of pan-Aymara traits that are held to reflect Christian values. In a thoughtful, well-argued paper, Orta examines the extent of this ethnic inclusion, and its limits, noting that the dual purpose of the reforms is to cast certain Aymara practices as meaningfully Christian with respect to their values, while retaining authentic images of the Aymaras' traditional beliefs.

776 Contesting hybridity: *Evangelistas* and *Kataristas* in highland Bolivia.

Andrew Canessa. *Journal of Latin American Studies*, vol. 32, no. 1 (2000), p. 115-44. bibliog.

Examines the growth of evangelical Protestantism and Aymara nationalism (*Katarismo*) over the last fifty years, arguing that neither Catholicism nor the idea of cultural mixing (*mestizaje*) continues to provide a unifying basis for the Bolivian nation-state. *Evangelismo* is associated by its supporters with 'Western' progress, modernization, and the market economy. *Kataristas* on the other hand, seek to revitalize Indian culture and religion. While both movements are vehemently opposed to each other in many respects, both join in rejecting Bolivian identity as a hybridized product. They also share common ground in their power base: La Paz and the small towns on the northern altiplano. In a clear, well-structured article, Canessa analyses the development of each movement, before considering what their joint impact might be, though from radically different points of departure, on Bolivia's future self-image.

Jesuit missions in eastern Bolivia

777 Mission culture on the upper Amazon: native tradition, Jesuit enterprise, and secular policy in Moxos, 1660-1880.
David Block.   Lincoln, Nebraska; London: University of Nebraska Press, 1994. 240p. maps. bibliog.

The author provides a vivid picture of life in the Jesuit missions founded between 1682 and 1744 in the eastern plains of Bolivia (Llanos de Moxos) which today form part of the Department of Beni. The Moxos were among the most sophisticated groups of Indians who were settled into missions by the Jesuits. Livestock farming, cacao and sugar production, manufacturing workshops, and a flourishing export trade characterized the mission economy, sustained where necessary by additional funding from Lima. Unlike numerous cases elsewhere, the Moxos Indian missions did not collapse after the Jesuits departed; population increased as did the trade in cotton, tallow, and cacao which, until some years after Bolivia's independence, was channelled through commercial agents based in the city of Santa Cruz. This is a scholarly piece of work, of interest to a wide readership. See also W. Denevan's *The aboriginal cultural geography of the Llanos de Mojos* (item no. 344).

778 Godly purpose, earthly missions.
Alcides Parajas Moreno, translated by Ruth Morales.   *Américas*, vol. 47, no. 2 (1995), p. 22-29.

Between 1691 and 1760, the Jesuits founded eleven missions (*reducciones*) in Chiquitos province among the hills that curve along the northern edge of the Chaco. Today, the ten surviving missions are among Bolivia's greatest architectural treasures, six of them designated by UNESCO in 1991 as World Heritage Sites: San Javier, Concepción, San Miguel, San Rafael, San José, and Santa Ana. The author recounts their historic religious and economic roles, and (unlike most in Paraguay) their survival today in the modern small town communities. Stunning photographs reveal the ornate Baroque style of the mission church interiors, and the dazzling colours of restored exterior decoration.

779 Bolivia's Jesuit missions.
Russell Chamberlin.   *History Today*, vol. 47, no. 7 (July 1997), p. 6-8.

Records a visit to San Javier and Concepción, two of the most important and best-preserved of Bolivia's ten historic Jesuit missions. The author notes that the romantic film *The Mission* in 1986 gave fresh publicity to the surviving Jesuit mission churches in Bolivia, Paraguay and Argentina, and stimulated a modest increase in tourism.

Education

General

780 Estudio de la educación rural boliviana: historia, organización, función y recursos. (A study of rural Bolivian education: history, organization, function and resources.)
Marcelo Sanginés Uriarte. La Paz: CIDA, 1967. 141p. bibliog.
A comprehensive study of the extent of the progress made by the mid-1960s on Bolivia's rural education programme as implemented after the 1952 revolution. Education is seen as playing a vital role in the integration of the rural classes into national life.

781 Mito y realidad de la educación boliviana. (Myth and reality in Bolivian education.)
Eduardo Cortes León. Cochabamba, Bolivia: Editorial 'Serrano', 1973. 227p. bibliog.
Discusses the failure of the government to implement the 1955 educational codes in Bolivia, particularly in the rural zones. As a result, educational opportunities of the most basic sort are still lacking in Bolivia. Illiteracy is an obstacle to national integration and economic development, and effectively marginalizes the majority of the population.

782 The formation of a technical élite in Latin America: mining engineering and the engineering profession in Bolivia, 1900-1954.
Manuel Eduardo Contreras. PhD thesis, Columbia University, New York, 1990. 360p. bibliog.
A sound, wide-ranging discussion of the problems faced by the engineering profession in Bolivia during the first half of the 20th century. The author concentrates on the experience of three Bolivian engineering colleges – the mining schools in Oruro and Potosí, and the civil engineering school in La Paz. In an objective analysis, he examines the relative contributions of domestic and foreign training, the interaction (in the Patiño mines) of

Bolivian and foreign mining engineers, and the extent to which successive governments have relied on foreign engineers for senior positions.

783 Curricular relevancy to community needs: assessing applicability of a community empowerment paradigm in Latin America. A case study of an agricultural school in Bolivia.
Jeffrey Dexter Lansdale. PhD thesis, Cornell University, Ithaca, New York, 1991. 152p. bibliog.

Initially, the author discusses reasons for the generally low standard of rural education in Latin America as a whole before developing a case-study of one agricultural high school in Bolivia. Using observation, questionnaires, and interviews, Lansdale examines the school's curriculum, arguing that in framing their courses, teachers should be more responsive to local community needs. This is a contentious finding which here, in the light of the teachers' own points of view, would have benefited from deeper investigation and evaluation.

784 Socioeconomic and ethnic determinants of grade repetition in Bolivia and Guatemala.
Harry Anthony Patrinos, George Psacharopoulos. Washington, DC: World Bank; Technical Department Latin America and the Caribbean, 1992. 26p. (Policy Research Working Papers, Country Operations, No. 1028).

The Latin America and Caribbean region records the highest incidence of school dropout and grade repetition in the world. In their section on Bolivia, the authors focus on urban areas with populations of over 10,000, sampling 5,600 primary schoolchildren aged 7-14 years, and finding that the poorest children and those from indigenous families are the most likely to repeat a grade. More bilingual education could be helpful, but the authors also note that while the much lower incidence in grade repetition found in Bolivia's private schools may have much to do with the socio-economic background of children attending these schools, different teaching methods and other practices in many private schools compared with public schools may also be a contributory factor.

785 The cost of being indigenous in Bolivia: an empirical analysis of educational attainments and outcomes.
Harry Anthony Patrinos, George Psacharopoulos. *Bulletin of Latin American Research*, vol. 12, no. 3 (1993), p. 293-309. bibliog.

Addresses the problems of ethnic inequalities in societies with large indigenous populations. Using data from a large-scale urban household survey conducted in Bolivia in 1989, the authors find that indigenous workers in general have received fewer years of schooling and that of a more variable quality, and that these disadvantages are largely responsible for their lower earning power. The improvement of the educational levels of the indigenous population is the most important single factor in reducing the earning differentials within society, but it is easier to identify the problem than to solve it.

786 A content analysis of school music in Bolivia.
Benjamin Francis Smeall. PhD thesis, University of South
Carolina, Columbia, South Carolina, 1997. 222p. bibliog.

Examines 256 samples of music collected in the field that are used in Bolivian primary
and secondary schools, giving particular attention to their historical dating and points of
origin. A comparison of United States and Bolivian school music is also included.

787 Distance education and rural development: an experiment in training teachers as community development agents.
Eloy Anello. DEd thesis, University of Massachusetts, 1997. 317p.
bibliog.

Assesses an experimental distance-learning course held in 1995 for training teachers as
community development agents in rural areas of Bolivia. The various course components
are evaluated in terms of their likely success in fostering adult education in the villages,
and in training community leaders.

788 Negotiating independence: children and young people growing up in rural Bolivia.
S. Punch. PhD thesis, University of Exeter, England, 1998.

The setting is Churquiales, a small rural community in the Department of Tarija. The
study concentrates on the ways in which the children, particularly those aged 8-14 years,
adjust and compete with adults and among themselves for recognition and status – at
home, at school, at play, and at work. Punch focuses on how the children make the most
of the limited opportunities available to them. The points made are simple, and in many
cases obvious, but the context is more revealing, so that the thesis provides an interesting
illustration of the realities of rural life in southern Bolivia.

789 Neoliberalism and public education: the relevance of the Bolivian teachers' strike of 1995.
Lesley Gill. In: *The third wave of modernization in Latin America*.
Edited by Lynne Phillips. Wilmington, Delaware: Scholarly
Resources, 1998, p. 125-40. bibliog. (Jaguar Books on Latin
America, No. 16).

Thousands of striking public school teachers gathered in El Alto and La Paz in 1995 to
protest against the Education Reform Law (1994) which transferred much of the
responsibility for public school education to the local municipalities. Existing low
salaries, and the future loss of job security and status fuelled the strike, which called for
the repeal of the Reform Law. The most interesting and illuminating part of Gill's account
records the parents' reaction to the strike. In the sample taken, parents supported the need
for higher salaries, but demanded in return better teacher-training, higher qualifications,
and more reliable teacher attendance and performance in schools. Parents condemned all
teachers' strikes, resenting the interruptions they caused to the children's education; nor
did they support the repeal of the Education Reform Law. The vast majority of the
population cannot afford private school education. After eight weeks, government action
and parent pressure sent the teachers back to work. The report provides a poignant
reminder that the scale of the problem involved in raising even basic standards of

education in Bolivia is matched only by the people's need and longing for it to be achieved.

790 The citizen factory: schooling and cultural production in Bolivia.
Aurolyn Luykx. Albany: State University of New York Press, 1999. 399p. bibliog. (SUNY series: Power, Social Identity and Education).

This is a timely study written as Bolivia embarks on a sweeping educational reform programme under the Popular Participation Law of 1994. Based on the work of a teachers' college (*escuela normal*) on the altiplano, the book examines the training of young Aymara men and women intending to become primary school teachers in rural areas, and discusses the aims and methods adopted to harmonize indigenous ethnic loyalties with the awareness of national citizenship. Luykx offers a comprehensive and ambitious treatment of the subject, and although some of her final general observations on education are more fashionable than sound, the study provides a well-organized and informative account of teacher training among Bolivia's Aymara population in the late 20th century.

Bilingual education

791 Bilingual education in Bolivia.
Lucy T. Briggs. In: *Bilingualism: social issues and policy implications.* Edited by Andrew W. Miracle. Athens: University of Georgia Press, 1983, p. 84-95. 188p.

Briggs, a respected Aymara scholar, reviews Bolivian educational policy which has as one of its objectives the universal teaching of the Spanish language, but which neglects native languages as a result. She argues that a few modest programmes should be introduced to teach local idioms, and for the future, suggests that the government should train large numbers of teachers in bilingual techniques.

792 Quechua/Spanish bilingual education and language policy in Bolivia (1977-1982).
Donald H. Burns. *International Education Journal*, vol. 2, 1984, p. 197-220.

Explains and examines the many problems associated with extending bilingual education throughout Bolivia. A principal impediment was the preference among educators for imposing Spanish on peasants in the name of 'national unity'.

793 **The language of Quechua rural teachers in Bolivia: a study of the bilingualism/interlingualism among rural Quechua native speakers.**
A. M. Yraola-Burgos. PhD thesis, St Andrews University, Scotland, 1995.
A linguistic study carried out among a group of bilingual rural schoolteachers in a Quechua-speaking region of Bolivia. It examines the characteristics of the Spanish dialect spoken there, and the nature and extent of the transference from the Quechua mother-tongue. The author concludes that the type of Spanish spoken by these rural schoolteachers can be dubbed an interlanguage, which is currently evolving into a new language form – a semi-language.

794 **Five languages, one dictionary.**
Mike Ceaser. *Américas*, vol. 51, no. 6 (1999), p. 5.
With funding from UNESCO and support from the Bolivian government, Unión Latina has created a five-language electronic dictionary in Spanish, Portuguese, Aymara, Quechua, and Guaraní. This ambitious project, first proposed by the former Bolivian vice-president Víctor Hugo Cárdenas, has taken five years to complete, and includes 10,000 basic concepts concentrated in the fields of health, biodiversity, food and agriculture. The dictionary is designed primarily to help aid workers, teachers, nurses, and others working in rural areas to establish easy, direct communication with the indigenous communities. It is available on the Internet and CD-Rom, and will, as an added bonus, help to preserve the three most widely spoken indigenous languages in South America.

Literature

General

795 Bolivia and its social literature before and after the Chaco War: a historical study of social and literary revolution.
Murdo MacLeod. PhD dissertation, University of Florida, Gainesville, Florida, 1962. 254p. bibliog.

The Chaco War (1932-35), one of the many causes of the 1952 revolution, also created an intellectual revolution in Bolivia. The young writers of the Chaco generation had three general aims: to discover and explain the nature of Bolivian society; to seek and support the campaigns for social justice; and lastly, to develop in Bolivia an independent culture.

796 Esquema de literatura virreinal en Bolivia. (An outline of viceregal literature in Bolivia.)
Teresa Gisbert. La Paz: Dirección Nacional de Informaciones, 1963. 49p.

Examines 17th- and 18th-century writers and includes chapters on Indian theatre, poetry, religious chronologies, the study of languages, socio-economic studies, and histories and travellers' accounts.

797 Panorama de la literatura boliviana del siglo XX. (Panorama of 20th-century Bolivian literature.)
Augusto Guzmán. Cochabamba, Bolivia; La Paz: Editorial 'Los Amigos del Libro', 1967. 41p.

A concise overview by this distinguished Bolivian scholar of the main characteristics of the country's 20th-century literature up to the mid-1960s. The analysis presents cameos on poetry, the novel and novella, traditional narrative, theatre, biography, social studies, works of criticism, oratory, humour, journalism, and finally bibliography.

798 Letras bolivianas de hoy: Renato Prada y Pedro Shimose.
(Bolivian writing of today: Renato Prada and Pedro Shimose.)
José Ortega. Buenos Aires: Fernando García Cambeiro, 1973.
115p. bibliog. (Colección Estudios Latinoamericanos, No. 5).
Following a good, brief historical introduction to Bolivian national literature, two important younger Bolivian writers are presented: Prada, a writer of short stories, and Shimose, a poet. An excellent bibliography is included.

799 Las cien obras capitales de la literatura boliviana. (One hundred major works of Bolivian literature.)
Juan Siles Guevara. La Paz: Editorial 'Los Amigos del Libro',
1975. 513p. bibliog. (Enciclopedia Boliviana).
Discusses one hundred of the best examples of Bolivian writing. The volume is arranged by author, and includes the following topics: the short story, journalism, biography, the essay, history, poetry and the theatre.

800 Estudios de literatura boliviana. (Studies in Bolivian literature.)
Gabriel René-Moreno. La Paz: Biblioteca de Sesquicentenario de
la República, 1975. 290p. bibliog.
A new edition of a classic study of Bolivian literature written by the notable Bolivian essayist and critic, René-Moreno (1836-1908). It includes the first of his biographies of national writers and his works of literary criticism. Several entries presented here appeared initially in Chilean reviews in the 19th and 20th centuries. Subjects covered include: *poetas bolivianos*, Manuel José Tovar, María Josefa Mujía, Mariano Ramollo, Néstor Galindo, Ricardo José Bustamante, and Daniel Calvo.

801 Modern Latin American literature.
Compiled and edited by David William Foster, Virginia Ramos
Foster. New York: Frederick Ungar, 1975.
Volume I contains material on two outstanding Bolivian literary figures: Alcides Arguedas (1879-1946) and Ricardo Jaimes Freyre (1868-1933). Critical extracts on the writings of Arguedas, novelist and historian, review some of his major works, his themes, style, and philosophy concerning the future of Bolivia. Those on the poet Jaimes Freyre consider his subject matter, style, and the main influences on his work.

802 Jaime Mendoza and the new Bolivia.
Fernando Ortiz Sanz. *Américas*, vol. 28, no. 9 (1976), p. 21-26.
A well-illustrated introduction to the life of one of Bolivia's leading intellectuals in the late 19th and early 20th centuries. Jaime Mendoza (1874-1939) was exceptionally gifted, qualifying first as a physician but going on to establish a reputation also as an academic, musician, artist, poet, writer and reformer. His harrowing experiences as a field surgeon in the rubber forests during the Acre War, and later in the tin mines, made an indelible imprint on his mind and his writing. Mendoza's crusade to lift Bolivia from the chaos of its past was expressed through his novels, and in time he came to be recognized as a key figure in the growth of Bolivian nationalism, a spark for the new 'Chaco Generation'. This is an informed, readable article, written by a Bolivian diplomat who was one of

Mendoza's former students at the University of San Francisco Xavier in Sucre, and who became a family friend.

803 **Gabriel René-Moreno and the intellectual context of late nineteenth-century South America.**
Gertrude M. Yeager. *Social Science Quarterly*, vol. 59, no. 1 (1978), p. 77-92.

Studies the life and intellectual development of the eminent Bolivian scholar, Gabriel René-Moreno, who lived much of his life outside Bolivia and participated actively in the intellectual community which existed in southern South America. His relationship to other South American thinkers is also discussed, together with his place in the context of Bolivian letters.

804 **Biografías de la nueva literatura boliviana.** (Biographies of writers of the new Bolivian literature.)
Augusto Guzmán. Cochabamba, Bolivia; La Paz: Editorial 'Los Amigos del Libro', 1982. 154p. (Enciclopedia Boliviana).

A valuable source of reference which contains short biographies of nearly fifty Bolivian authors born between 1925 and 1950, together with a critique of the main works of each of them.

805 **El cuento modernista en Bolivia: estudio y antología.** (A study and anthology of modernistic narrative in Bolivia.)
Carlos Castañón Barrientos. La Paz: Libreria Editorial 'Juventud', 1984. 2nd ed. 144p. bibliog.

A selection of Bolivian short stories, preceded by a concise history of modernistic literature in Bolivia, its recurrent themes, and short biographies of the seventeen writers chosen to represent the key elements of this literary movement.

806 **Narrativa hispanoamericana, 1816-1981: historia y antología.**
(Hispanic-American narrative, 1816-1981: history and anthology.)
Edited by Angel Flores, introduction by Antonio Skámeta. Mexico City: Siglo XXI, 1985.

An anthology of modern Peruvian, Chilean and Bolivian literature. Volume four entitled 'La generación de 1940-1969' (532p.), gives a general overview of Latin American authors of that period. Volume seven, entitled 'La generación de 1939 en adelante: Bolivia, Chile, Peru' (414p.), deals specifically with the Central Andes. Bolivian authors included are: Pedro Shimose Kawamura, Jaime Nistahua, Raúl Teixido, Félix Salazar González, Ramón Rocha Monroy, Rene Bascopé Aspiazu, and Manuel Vargas. Valuable bio-bibliographical data are presented on each author.

807 Tendencias actuales en la literatura boliviana. (Present trends in Bolivian literature.)
Edited by Jorge Sanjinés. Minneapolis, Minnesota: Institute for the Study of Ideologies and Literature; Instituto de Cine, Radio y Televisión, 1985. 284p.

A book of mainly bibliographical and review essays concerning the status of contemporary literature in Bolivia. Includes: (1) Leonardo García Pabon's 'Aproximación a la crítica literaria en Bolivia 1960-1980'; (2) Wilma A. Torrico's 'Indice bibliográfico de libros de crítica y ensayo literario bolivianos publicado entre 1960-1980'; and (3) 'Indice bibliográfico de libros de poesía bolivianos, 1960-1980'; (4) Luis J. Antezana's 'La novela boliviana en el último cuarto de siglo'; (5) Carlos Mesa Gisbert's 'Bibliográfica de la novela boliviana (1962-1980)'; (6) Ruben Vargas Portugal's 'Indice bibliográfico de libros de poesía bolivianos, 1960-1980'; (7) Ana Rebeca Prada's 'El cuento contemporáneo de la represión en Bolivia'; and (8) Oscar Muñoz C., 'El teatro nacional en busca de un punto de partida: 1967'.

808 Literatura de Bolivia: compendio histórico. (Bolivian literature: an historical summary.)
Carlos Castañón Barrientos. La Paz: Ediciones Signo, 1990. 255p. bibliog.

A study of the major Bolivian writers in the colonial and independence periods in which the author examines the leading literary figures and interprets their works in an historical setting. The result is a scholarly and useful reference book.

809 Nueva historia de la literatura boliviana: literatura de la independencia y del siglo XIX. (A new history of Bolivian literature: the literature of Independence and the 19th century.)
Adolfo Cáceres Romero. Cochabamba, Bolivia; La Paz: Editorial 'Los Amigos del Libro', 1995. 289p. bibliog. (Enciclopedia Boliviana).

This is the third volume in Cáceres' planned four-volume history of Bolivian literature. He presents a discerning, comprehensive examination of the poetry and prose of this turbulent 19th-century period, including books, articles, manifestos, proclamations, memoirs, and plays, together with a thoughtful, fluent commentary on the writers, their philosophies, and their times.

Novels and short stories

810 La nueva narrativa boliviana: aproximación a sus aspectas formales. (The new Bolivian narrative: an approach to its formal aspects.)
Oscar Rivera Rodas.   La Paz: Ediciones Camarlinghi, 1972. 218p.
A good introduction to an important Bolivian literary movement of the late 1960s. The writings of Renato Prada, Gaston Suárez, Jesús Urzagasti, Raúl Teixido, Julio de la Vega and Arturo von Vacano are discussed here.

811 La novela social de Bolivia. (The social novel in Bolivia.)
Evelio Echevarría.   La Paz: Difusión, 1973, 2nd ed. 257p. bibliog.
A good introduction to the Bolivian social protest novel. Each chapter examines a different type of novel. Included here are: the *indigenista* novel, the mining novel, the Chaco War novel, the novel of the tropics, and the *mestizo* and political novels. It contains a good bibliography.

812 Paisaje y novela en Bolivia. (Region and novel in Bolivia.)
Reinaldo Alcázar V.   La Paz: Difusión, 1973. 177p. bibliog.
Studies the role played by regions of Bolivia in the national novel. Each chapter addresses itself to a different locale: the altiplano, the Valles, the Yungas, the jungle and the Chaco areas.

813 Temas sobre la moderna narrativa boliviana. (Themes in the modern Bolivian narrative.)
José Ortega.   Cochabamba, Bolivia: Editorial 'Los Amigos del Libro', 1973. 99p.
This collection of critical essays, by a noted specialist of the Bolivian narrative, examines the major themes presented in the 20th-century Bolivian novel. Subjects discussed include: the Chaco War theme, and the individual careers of Augusto Céspedes, Jesús Lara, Renato Prada, Fernando Vaca Toledo, and others.

814 Antología del cuento boliviano. (Anthology of the Bolivian short story.)
Edited by Armando Soriano Badani.   La Paz: Editorial 'Los Amigos del Libro', 1975. 438p.
This anthology is useful to the literary historian. The coverage of the 1900-50 period is more extensive than that of the post-1950 period.

815 Cuentos. (Stories.)
Ricardo Jaimes Freyre.   La Paz: Instituto Boliviano de Cultura, 1975. 55p.
A collection of the poet's modernist short stories originally published between 1896 and 1907.

816 Bolivia en el cuento. Antología de ayer y de hoy. (Bolivia in story.
Anthology of yesterday and today.)
Edited by Néstor Taboada Terán.   Buenos Aires: Editorial
'Convergencia', 1976. 119p.

This useful summary of the Bolivian short story is arranged by themes: mines, Indians,
war, and politics.

817 Cuentos bolivianos contemporáneos. Antología. (Contemporary
Bolivian stories. Anthology.)
Edited by Hugo Lyeron Alberdi, Ricardo Pastor Poppe.   La Paz:
Ediciones Carmarlinghi, 1976. 201p.

Includes eleven contemporary short stories, each written by a different author.

818 The emergence of the Latin American novel.
Gordon Brotherston.   Cambridge; New York: Cambridge University
Press, 1977. 164p. bibliog.

A good general introduction to the Spanish-American novel. There are eight chapters and
each deals with a different author. There is also a chapter devoted to José María Arguedas,
the Peruvian exponent of Quechua language and literature.

819 Children of the Incas.
David Mangurian.   New York: Four Winds Press, 1979. 73p.

A thirteen-year-old boy, a Quechua Indian, who lives near Lake Titicaca, describes his
family, home and daily activities. The story is written for children, and provides plenty of
talking-points.

820 El minero en el moderno relato boliviano. (The miner in the
modern Bolivian story.)
José Ortega.   *Cuadernos Hispanoamericanos*, vol. 417 (March
1985), p. 26-32. bibliog.

This essay offers an overview of how the miner has been depicted in the modern Bolivian
novel.

821 Coup! A novel.
Alexander M. Grace.   Novato, California: Lyford Books, 1991.
236p. map.

Formerly with the State Department, the author weaves his own experiences into a novel
which follows the activities of the fictional US Deputy Chief of Mission in La Paz, and
the sound working relationship he establishes with his Bolivian colleagues in weathering
the political storms, and in trying to control the narcotics trade. Grace has a good ear and
eye; there is rich local colour, along with numerous sharp barbs poked at embassy life.
The novel is at once readable, hard-bitten, hilarious, and sympathetic. It will appeal
particularly to those who already know Bolivia, for they will get the most out of it.

822 The *mestizo* imaginary: isolation and disunity in Néstor Taboada Terán's vision of Bolivia.
K. J. Richards. PhD thesis, University of London, King's College, England, 1994.

Examines the novels of one of Bolivia's most influential writers in terms of the way they identify and treat many of Bolivia's long-standing problems, including the country's isolation, regional rivalries, poor internal land communications, and ethnic divisions.

823 In reference to the national revolution of Bolivia: three novels by women.
Alice A. Weldon. PhD thesis, University of Maryland, College Park, Maryland, 1996. 190p. bibliog.

Explores the tradition of female narrative in Bolivia in the aftermath of the National Revolution of 1952. The study focuses on three contemporary novels written by women with a strongly feminist approach. *Bajo el oscuro sol* (1971) by Yolanda Bedregal; *¡Hijo de Opa!* (1997) by Gaby Vallejo; and *La Flor de 'La Candelaria'* (1990) by Giancarla Zabalaga de Quiroga. All the authors address different aspects of violence in the day-to-day lives of their characters, be it political, physical, sexual, ethnic, or class-based.

824 Stone cowboy: a novel.
Mark Jacobs. New York: Soho Press, 1997. 292p.

At first glance, this is a rambling adventure story of a young American drop-out just released from a long prison sentence in La Paz for drug addiction, who then drifts through Bolivia from the altiplano to Cochabamba, the Chapare, Santa Cruz and beyond. However, the novel works well on several levels: it is cynically well observed, waspish, brittle, and often funny, but it is also laced with a surreal quality, a dark, macabre sense of cruelty, uncertainty, and ultimate resignation.

825 Fire from the Andes: short fiction by women from Bolivia, Ecuador, and Peru.
Edited and translated by Susan E. Benner, Kathy S. Leonard. Albuquerque: University of New Mexico Press, 1998. 187p. bibliog.

Nine short stories by Bolivian women writers are included in this anthology, all of them reflecting the variety of women's experiences in the city or the mining community. The stories are linked by a common thread, that of the struggle and social injustice faced by women whatever the setting, and the nature of their responses to the realities of the situation.

826 Juan de la Rosa: memoirs of the last soldier of the Independence movement.
Nataniel Aguirre, translated by Sergio Gabriel Waisman. New York: Oxford University Press, 1998. 329p. maps. bibliog. (Library of Latin America Series).

A major novel by Nataniel Aguirre (1843-88) which was first published in 1885 in Cochabamba. It is the fictional autobiography of the narrator, Juan de la Rosa, and includes his childhood in late colonial Upper Peru, and the early uprising in Cochabamba against the Royalist troops. Designed to be the first in a four-part work, this was the only book to be completed. It is a work of deep reflection, written in the immediate aftermath of Bolivia's crushing defeat in the War of the Pacific in which Aguirre, an important figure in the Liberal Party, took part. The novel examines the major political and cultural issues facing Bolivia, and calls for a new cohesive national identity which the country must now create and assert. This is the first English translation of the novel, and is edited, with a good introduction, by Alba María Paz-Soldán.

827 The liberation of little heaven and other stories.
Mark Jacobs. New York: Soho Press, 1999. 231p.
An attractive collection of short stories set in Latin America, including Bolivia, in which contrasts in the lives and customs of people within different sections of society provide the main backdrop to the narrative.

Drama and poetry

828 Indice de la poesía boliviana contemporánea. (Index of contemporary Bolivian poetry.)
Juan Quiroz. La Paz: Librería y Editorial 'Juventud', 1965. 438p.
An index of forty-one Bolivian poets who have made a substantial contribution to Bolivian literature. The listing includes examples of their writings.

829 Teatro virreinal en Bolivia. (Viceregal theatre in Bolivia.)
Teresa Gisbert. La Paz: Dirección Nacional de Informaciones, 1965. 35p.
Examines the 17th-century theatre. The author includes brief discussions on comedies, theatre in Indian languages, the tragedies, the works of Diego Occina, 'miner writers', and Spanish dramatists in Charcas.

830 Behind Spanish American footlights.
Willis Knapp Jones. Austin, Texas: University of Texas Press, 1966. 609p. bibliog.
This substantial volume remains a most valuable source of reference in a neglected field. Jones does not waste words; his book reflects a lifetime of scholarship, insight, and trenchant comment on the development of drama throughout Spanish America from the pre-Columbian period to the twentieth century. His chapters examine five major themes; (1) works written or performed in the colonial viceroyalties; (2) Spanish and New World influences; (3) the subsequent growth of drama in the newly independent states; (4) the world of theatre, actors and actresses, and (5) the contributions of the major playwrights – their strengths, weaknesses, and local constraints. The section on Bolivian drama since Independence illustrates well how each chapter adds to a wider understanding of Spanish American theatre as a whole, while a reading list of plays and an excellent bibliography of books and periodicals round off the study. This volume is an indispensable starting-

point for students and specialists working on the history of drama and the theatre in Spanish America.

831 South America of the poets.
Selden Rodman, illustrated by Bill Negron. New York: Hawthorn Books, 1970. 270p. map. (Reprinted, Carbondale, Edwardsville, Illinois: Southern Illinois University Press: Feffer & Simons, 1972.)

Presents a uniquely informal and interesting portrait of the South America the tourist, salesman or diplomat rarely sees. Indeed, so the argument runs, it is from South American artists and poets that we can learn the most. Poetry is deeply woven into the fabric of society; for example, Rodman finds it 'unusual to meet a political figure who has *not* written poetry, or does not number poets among his friends'. He muses on the nature of South American culture and values, meeting poets and others throughout the region during the 1960s. Chapter four is set in Bolivia.

832 Teatro boliviano. (Bolivian theatre.)
Raúl Salmón. Madrid: Paraninfo, 1972. 213p.

Three Bolivian plays are presented here: 'Viva Belzu', 'Tres Generales' and 'Juana Sánchez'. A brief history of the Bolivian modern theatre precedes the plays.

833 Raúl Salmón: playwright of the Bolivian people.
Maria Teresa Mollinedo. PhD thesis, City University of New York, 1991. 199p. bibliog.

Salmón was a populist playwright who concentrated on indigenous Bolivian themes. He founded his Theatre of Social Protest in 1943. Based on research which includes interviews with Salmón and others, the study provides insights into the influences on Salmón's thinking, and on the principles and techniques he used in writing his plays.

834 Bello and Bolívar: poetry and politics in the Spanish American Revolution.
Antonio Cussen. Cambridge, England: Cambridge University Press, 1992. 208p. bibliog. (Cambridge Studies in Latin American and Iberian Literature, No. 6).

Andrés Bello (1781-1865) is the focus here, beginning with the mission from Venezuela to London in 1810 led by Bolívar, with secretary Bello, to enlist help for the Independence movement. Cussen presents a detailed study of the manuscripts of Bello's unfinished poem 'América', reconstructing Bello's version of the Revolution, and its political and cultural consequences.

835 Oblivion and stone: a selection of contemporary Bolivian poetry and fiction.
Edited by Sandra Reyes, translated by John Du Val, Gastón Fernández-Torriente, Kay Pritchett, Sandra Reyes. Fayetteville: University of Arkansas Press, 1998. 273p.

A major and wide-ranging collection that includes the work of thirty-seven Bolivian writers. The poems present a variety of reflections on individual identity and society, some of them introspective, heavily symbolic, and imbued with the imagery of nature and the land. The fiction comprises an anthology of short stories on Bolivian and other themes. The poetry is in the original Spanish and in English translation; the fiction in translation only.

Folk tales and legends

836 The singing mountaineers: songs and tales of the Quechua people.
José María Arguedas. Edited, with an introduction, by Ruth W. Stephan; illustrated by Donald Weismann. Austin, Texas: University of Texas Press, 1957. 203p. bibliog.

Ignore the unfortunate title; this is not the sound of music. The book contains the words of forty-two Quechua songs, among them: 'The head of the town and the demon'; 'The condor's lover'; 'Miguel Wayapa'; 'The snake's sweetheart'; 'The youth who rose to the sky'; and 'Isicha Puytu'. The author also gives an overview of Andean festivals, together with an examination of the role of songs and tales in native culture. For an analysis of the music included in this study see *La musique des Inca et ses survivances* by Raoul Harcourt. A list of available recordings is also included.

837 Con la muerte a cuestas y otros cuentos. (With death on one's shoulder and other stories.)
Raúl Botelho Gosálvez. La Paz: Difusión, 1975. 195p. (Colección Vereda).

The theme of the encroachment of modernity and development on indigenous Bolivian literature is repeated here in varied settings: the city, the mountains, the jungles, and the Yungas.

838 Fantásticas aventuras del Atoj y el Diguillo. (Fables in the Quechua language.)
Manuel Robles Alarcón. Lima: The author, 1975. 149p.

A collection of ten native folk tales which were collected by the author in the 1940s, and adapted for children's theatre in 1943 (they were first published in 1966). Ideal for children, these tales reflect native values and represent part of a national attempt to rediscover the past.

839 La tradición oral en Bolivia. (Oral tradition in Bolivia.)
Edited by Delina Anibarro de Halushka. La Paz: Instituto Boliviano de Cultura, 1976. 458p.

A collection of over one hundred folk tales from Sucre, Potosí and Cochabamba, grouped by region, language, themes and symbolic content. These tales, in Aymara and Quechua, are stories introduced into the region by the Spanish during the colonial period. This remains one of the best books available on Bolivian folk literature.

840 Las mejores tradiciones y leyendas de Bolivia. (The best folk tales and legends of Bolivia.)
Antonio Peredes Candia.   La Paz: Editorial 'Popular', 1979. 399p.

A collection of well-illustrated folk tales and legends. The author is a recognized expert who has published numerous articles and books on the folk culture of Bolivia.

841 From oral to written expression: the native Andean chronicles of the early colonial period.
Rolena Adorno.   Syracuse, New York: Maxwell School of Citizenship and Public Administration, 1982. 181p. bibliog.

Presents native legends, chronicles and folk tales in Spanish and English texts.

The Arts

General

842 A cultural history of Spanish America: from conquest to Independence.
Mariano Picón-Salas, translated by Irving A. Leonard. Berkeley, California: University of California Press, 1962. 192p. bibliog.
A classic work on the cultural evolution of Latin America. Picón-Salas, a noted Venezuelan scholar, traces the major influences that shaped Hispanic America's colonial culture in the 17th and 18th centuries, with excellent chapters on the Baroque in Spain's New World, and on the role of the Jesuits. The book displays an impressive handling of the subject in an easy but authoritative manner, and here, the author is ably served by a lucid, well-nuanced translation.

843 Museo histórico militar. (Historical military museum.)
Adolfo de Morales. La Paz: Dirección Nacional de Informaciones, 1963. [not paginated]. (Epocas y Museos, No. 6).
Describes and illustrates the special collection of weapons, uniforms, accoutrements, banners, and portraits held in Bolivia's military museum in La Paz. The exhibits include items from the Wars of Independence, and from the War of the Pacific – notably the Bolivian national flag flying in the port of Antofagasta until 1879.

844 Museos de Bolivia: Nacional, Moneda, Charcas, Catedral de Sucre, Murillo. Pintura. (Museums of Bolivia: Nacional, Moneda, Charcas, Sucre Cathedral, Murillo. Painting.)
José de Mesa, Teresa Gisbert. La Paz: Fondo Nacional de Cultura, Ministerio de Información, Cultura y Turismo, 1969. 180p.
An informative guide to the paintings housed in the five most important museums in Bolivia – the Nacional and the Casa de Murillo in La Paz, the Casa de Moneda in Potosí, and the Charcas and Sucre Cathedral collections in Sucre. The volume includes clear

black-and-white photographs and a few colour plates of the most important paintings, many of them dating from the colonial period.

845 Pre-Columbian art history: selected readings.
Jean Stearn, Alana Cordy-Collins. Palo Alto, California: Peck Publications, 1977. 519p.

A general introduction to pre-Columbian art history, which includes eighteen essays on Mesoamerican art and fifteen essays on Andean art.

846 Drawing the line: art and cultural identity in contemporary Latin America.
Oriana Baddeley, Valerie Fraser. London: Verso, 1989. 164p. bibliog. (Critical Studies in Latin American Culture).

An introductory text that provides an overview of art in Latin America in the mid-20th century. Despite the strong symbolism of isolated or grouped figures in Latin American painting and collage, more attention should have been given here to artists who depict the physical environment, particularly those who reveal the power of the Andean landscape *per se* as a source of inspiration and cultural identity at this period. The authors do not provide a comprehensive study, but the themes selected for their survey offer useful insights into particular aspects of the subject.

847 Memory and modernity: popular culture in Latin America.
William Rowe, Vivian Schelling. London: Verso, 1991. 243p. bibliog. (Critical Studies in Latin American Culture).

A splendid *tour de force*, in which the authors skilfully distil a huge amount of material into an illuminating and authoritative text. Rowe and Schelling's comprehensive study traces the development and principal components of Latin America's popular culture, exploring its regional distinctiveness, and its rural or urban roots. Much of the material is analysed within the two disciplinary frameworks of folklore and the idea of mass culture. In the Andean context, the authors examine the blending of an Inca past, an indigenous present, and the lingering influence of Spanish colonialism, particularly the roles played in this subtle interaction by carnival, folk music, ritual, and oral narrative. This is a book that will appeal to the specialist and the general reader.

848 Los cimientos de la Paz. (The origins of La Paz.)
La Paz: Sociedad Boliviana de Cemento, 1995. 239p. bibliog.

An impressive volume that examines the founding and development of the city, with particular attention given in text and illustration to the 20th century. A variety of historic and modern street scenes are an attractive feature of the book.

849 Renaissance man of the Andes.
Daniel Buck. *Américas*, vol. 49, no. 6 (1997), p. 48-53.

For many years, Peter McFarren has been the creative force behind numerous projects promoting the culture of his native Bolivia, where, among other activities, he has worked as a journalist, photographer, publisher, potter, folk-art collector, and textile designer. McFarren's latest project is the ambitious Laikakota Cultural Complex, under construction in the late 1990s on a site overlooking La Paz. When completed, it will house the new Museum of Bolivian Arts and Cultures, a Children's Museum, a Craft Development workshop, research facilities, and a public library. Buck's article provides an inviting, well-illustrated introduction to an outstanding new addition to the museums of La Paz, and to the exciting opportunities it will provide for the study and appreciation of Bolivia's cultural life.

850 Oruro inmortal. (Immortal Oruro.)
Edited by ECCO Publicidad Integral. La Paz: Ferrari Ghezzi, 1998. Vol. 1, 272p. Vol. 2, 274p. maps.

In the past, the history of Oruro has been largely eclipsed by that of Potosí. Aside from its annual carnival, Oruro is not a highlight on the tourist trail. Its academic literature was relatively sparse, but *Oruro inmortal* goes far to change that. These two fine volumes examine all major facets of the city and the Department of Oruro through a series of scholarly essays, and a wealth of colour photographs and old prints. Volume 1 discusses the origin of the mining town, its colonial period, 19th- and 20th-century development, its church history, and the pattern of modern urbanization, mining, and manufacturing. Volume 2 explores the Department's geography, the Sajama National Park, the cult of the llama, hidden prehistoric treasures, traditions and costumes, art, sport, and the rise of the 'tin baron', Simón Patiño. This is an ambitious publication. It will do much to correct the impression that Oruro is little more than a bleak mining and railway centre; together, the volumes depict great landscape variety, as well as some of the strongest centuries-old elements in Bolivian society.

Painting, sculpture and carving

Colonial

851 Escultura virreinal en Bolivia. (Viceregal sculpture in Bolivia.)
José de Mesa, Teresa Gisbert. La Paz: Academia Nacional de Ciencias de Bolivia, 1972. 489p.

An important source on colonial sculpture in Bolivia. Part one addresses: 'Sculpture of the low Renaissance', 'Mannerism', and 'Indian sculptors', which includes such masters as Gaspar de la Cueva. Part two deals with sculpture in wood, *retablos* (high, richly decorated altarpieces), pulpits, and funeral art.

852 Bitti: un pintor manerista en Sud América. (Bitti: a Mannerist painter in South America.)
José de Mesa, Teresa Gisbert. La Paz: División de Extensión Universitaria, Instituto de Estudios Bolivianos, 1974. 116p.

The definitive study of the life and works of an important Jesuit painter, Bernardo Bitti, who worked in Upper Peru in the late 1500s, and became one of the most outstanding exponents of Mannerism in South America.

853 **Holguín y la pintura virreinal en Bolivia.** (Holguín and viceregal painting in Bolivia.)
José de Mesa, Teresa Gisbert.   La Paz: Librería y Editorial 'Juventud', 1977. 358p. bibliog.

An important work on painting in colonial Charcas. This is an updated version of an earlier study and includes extensive research undertaken since 1956. The authors take as their subject the leading painter in colonial Upper Peru, Melchor Pérez Holguín, who was born in Cochabamba in the mid-1660s.

854 **Historia de la pintura cuzqueña.** (History of the Cuzco School of Painting.)
José de Mesa, Teresa Gisbert.   Lima: Fundación Augusto N. Wiese; Banco Wiese LIDO, 1982. 2 vols.

The best available source on the Cuzco School of Painting which dominated religious painting in the colonial period. Volume one discusses 16th-century Mannerism, the Cuzco School, the Jesuits, the transition to the Baroque style, the Flemish School, Indian painters, mural painting, techniques and themes, and iconography. Volume two contains illustrations.

855 **Gloria in excelsis: the Virgin and angels in viceregal painting of Peru and Bolivia.**
Edited by John Stringer. Guest curators: Barbara Duncan, Teresa Gisbert.   New York: Center for Inter-American Relations, 1986. 96p. bibliog.

The two motifs of the Virgin and angels abound in Spanish-American colonial painting. This beautiful exhibition catalogue is a mine of information on 17th- and 18th-century art. Together with the outstanding illustrations in colour and black-and-white, six essays examine selected aspects of the viceroyalty's sacred art: (1) The historical background; (2) The distinctiveness of Andean painting, including the Lima School, Cuzco School, Potosí School, and Collao/Lake Titicaca School; (3) European, Indian, and Baroque styles; (4) Statue paintings; (5) Angels with guns; and (6) The materials and techniques of Andean art. This is a richly rewarding work of reference.

856 **Treasured chests of history.**
Caleb Bach.   *Américas*, vol. 42, no. 5 (1990), p. 36-41.

A colourful, well-illustrated study of the *bargueños* (portable desks) used by Jesuit priests in southeastern Bolivia during the 17th and 18th centuries. The desks in Spanish Baroque style held mission records, accounts and inventories, and were often elaborately carved and embellished with gold leaf. Others were decorated with fine marquetry work depicting local flora and fauna. Surviving examples can still be found in museum and private collections in Bolivia and Argentina.

857 Scars of history etched in the Andes.
Roy Querejazu Lewis, translated by Laura Morales. *Américas*, vol. 44, no. 1 (1992), p. 42-47.
A vivid, well-illustrated account of cave paintings and petroglyphs incised in sandstone that have been found in the Departments of La Paz, Oruro, Cochabamba and Santa Cruz, a form of narrative rock art which ranges from pre-Columbian and Spanish colonial times to the period of Bolivian independence.

858 Bolivian masterpieces: colonial painting.
Teresa Gisbert, José de Mesa, Pedro Querejazu, Marisabel Alvarez Plata. La Paz: Secretariat of Culture, 1994. 161p. map.
This elegant volume includes treasures from Bolivia's National Museum of Art, the La Paz city and cathedral museums, and from private collections. Scholarly articles are matched by the exquisite colour photographs, which together provide an authoritative introduction to the main components of Upper Peruvian art, and to the outstanding artists who flourished there from the 16th to the 18th centuries. The chapters include analyses of Mannerism; Baroque; the indigenous element; Flemish influence in Andean art; the representation of angels; and the techniques which characterized colonial painting. The authors have produced an absorbing book, a study guide for both the art historian and the general reader.

859 Iconografía y mitos indigenas en el arte. (Indigenous iconography and myths in art.)
Teresa Gisbert. La Paz: Linea Editorial; Fundación BHN, Editorial Gisbert y Cia, 1994. 2nd ed. 250p. bibliog.
Gisbert brings a lifetime of scholarship and her fine eye for detail to this study of indigenous art in Bolivia and Peru. She analyses the dominant themes and influences on Indian art in the pre-hispanic and the colonial periods, including the various expressions of rebellion epitomized by Tupac Amaru and Tupac Katari. The book is based on extensive research in Seville, Cuzco and La Paz, and is beautifully illustrated in colour and black-and-white.

860 Potosí: colonial treasures and the Bolivian City of Silver.
Edited by John Farmer, Regina Smith, Joseph R. Wolin. Curators: Pedro Querejazu, Elizabeth Ferrer. New York: Americas Society Art Gallery, in association with Fundación BHN, La Paz, 1997. 152p. bibliog.
Originally published to accompany an exhibition in New York, this outstanding volume also serves as an excellent source of reference on Potosí's architecture and artistic output in the late-16th, 17th and 18th centuries, when the imperial city's schools of painting, wood sculpture, and silverwork were at their height. Articles by distinguished Bolivian scholars, translated into English, trace the history of Potosí and its spectacular mining boom, before analysing the essential characteristics of each of the art forms. A Spanish version of the text is appended. The superb colour plates illustrating the volume reveal the opulence and the intricacy of the workmanship in all three media, and provide a rich reminder of Potosí's colonial heritage. Readers will find a useful discussion of the Mannerist, Baroque, and *mudéjar* styles, as well as of religious art in general. Word and

picture together offer a social and an artistic panorama of this extraordinary city. The book is a treasure in itself.

19th and 20th centuries

861 Pintores del siglo XIX. (Nineteenth-century painters.)
Mario Chacón Torres. La Paz: Dirección Nacional de
Informaciones, 1963. 58p. bibliog.

An illustrated guide to 19th-century painters and painting. This publication is one of a number of useful small handbooks on Bolivian arts and letters prepared by the Biblioteca de Arte y Cultura Boliviana, and is No. 5 in the Pintores series.

862 La segunda bienal de arte INBO. (The second biennial art
exhibition sponsored by Inversiones Bolivianas.)
La Paz: Inversiones Bolivianas, 1977. [not paginated].

An attractive exhibition catalogue containing some forty photographs in colour and black-and-white of the work of Bolivian artists active in the 1960s and 1970s. The paintings, drawings and engravings selected were designed to illustrate the wide range of styles and subject-matter representative of this period.

863 The abstract landscapes of Pacheco.
Annick Sanjurjo de Casciero. *Américas*, vol. 39, no. 1 (1987),
p. 14-17, 62-63.

A stimulating, well-illustrated article which evaluates the striking abstracts of María Luisa Pacheco, the award-winning Bolivian artist who died in 1982. Although the last part of her life was spent in New York, the landscapes of the Bolivian altiplano were a lifelong influence on her work which was characterized by the muted earth tones, shapes, and wonderful luminosity of the Andes. As one critic observed: 'Cold teeth that jut up out of the immensely high plain; a fusion of warm earth and stony mountain, ... a unique balance in which everything seems miraculously suspended.' Although Pacheco's activities ranged widely, including those of journalist, textile designer, and UN cultural attachée, she remained pre-eminently a painter whose lasting impressions of the Bolivian landscape were memorably captured for an international audience.

864 Ted Carrasco.
Introduction by Pedro Querejazu. La Paz: T. Carrasco, 1988. 36p.

Striking colour photographs illustrate the work of Ted Carrasco, the Bolivian sculptor whose work in stone and bronze has been exhibited in Europe and Latin America. Andean themes are strongly represented. The text is in English, German, and Spanish.

865 Pintura boliviana del siglo XX. (Twentieth-century Bolivian painting.)
Compiled by Fernando Romero, Pedro Querejazu, Silvia Arze.
La Paz: Banco Hipotecario Nacional, 1989. 317p. bibliog.

A major study of Bolivia's modern and contemporary painting in which the skill and vibrancy of the artists is captured by nearly 300 fine coloured photographs. Early chapters provide a critical history of Bolivian painting that identifies significant trends and influences during the 20th century. Religion, portraiture, landscape, townscape, Indian communities, industry, and abstract art are among the themes discussed, along with Bolivian painting in the context of that of Latin America. Biographies of the painters are also included in what is a sumptuous presentation of Bolivian artistic achievement.

866 Bolivian artists' guide.
Teresa de Prada. La Paz: Quipus, 1991. [not paginated].

A modest guide, but one that includes much useful information on 20th-century Bolivian painters, sculptors, potters, and architects. The author concentrates on those who are working in Bolivia, and records the artists' works, training, biographical detail, exhibitions, and publications.

867 Bright colors, deep source.
Jamie Grant. *Américas*, vol. 50, no. 2 (1998), p. 20-24, 41-43.

Records the life and work of one of Bolivia's best-known young Aymara painters, Roberto Mamani Mamani, whose distinctive style of strong colours and swirling patterns is used to interpret both the Andean landscape and his Aymara heritage. The author traces the ways in which indigenous and European symbols are blended to produce the cultural mixture known as *mestizaje*, and in a well-illustrated article, discusses key aspects of Mamani Mamani's personal philosophy as well as his painting techniques.

868 Fernando Montes: obra 1957-1999. (Fernando Montes: his work from 1957 to 1999.)
Fernando Montes. La Paz: Santillana, 1999. 126p. (Aguilar Series: Pintores Bolivianos Contemporáneos).

An outstanding record of the work of Fernando Montes, one of Bolivia's most accomplished artists with a worldwide reputation. Montes' work in recent years is immediately recognizable – silent figures on the bare landscape, ancient ruins linking past and present, all expressed in the soft earth and stone shadings of the altiplano. But the examples of Montes' earlier work included here remind us also of his skill as a portrait painter and his use of blazing colour in other fields. Beneath the arching vault of sky and mountains, Montes' most characteristic paintings capture the light, shapes and shadows of the landscape, and transmit the unspoken messages of the Andes. The text is in Spanish and English, and the publisher's first-class production does full justice to the artist's work. This is a fine book, displaying tradition and innovation, technical skill and unforgettable imagery.

Architecture

869 Colonial architecture and sculpture in Peru.
Harold Edwin Wethey. Cambridge, Massachusetts: Harvard
University Press, 1949; Westport, Connecticut: Greenwood Press,
1971. 330p. map.

Although it concentrates on the area covered by modern-day Peru, Wethey's masterly study of the colonial architecture and sculpture of the Peruvian Viceroyalty includes much material that is relevant to an understanding of Bolivia. The author discusses in fluent, readable style the major themes in the evolution of Spanish colonial architecture in Peru as he follows the transition through the Baroque, Late Baroque, and French Rococo periods. This sweeping perspective is then backed by illuminating details on individual features such as portals, altars, cloisters, choir stalls, pulpits, figure sculpture, and the *mestizo* style. The book is profusely illustrated with floor plans and 343 photographs, half of them by the author. Anyone seeking a wider background on Bolivia's colonial architecture should read this book.

870 *Mestizo* architecture in Bolivia.
Harold Edwin Wethey. *The Art Quarterly* (Detroit), vol. 14, no. 4
(Winter 1951), p. 283-306. bibliog.

Mestizo art and architecture comprised a blend of European and Indian styles, a cultural mixture which in Bolivia reached its climax in the early 18th century, particularly in the church decoration found in Potosí and La Paz. Wethey, an American art historian, was one of the outstanding pioneers in the study of Peruvian and Bolivian colonial architecture, and here he reveals, in word and picture, the exquisite detail of *mestizo* themes and workmanship. In the magnificent portal of San Lorenzo in Potosí, he finds 'a veritable retable [high, richly-decorated altarpiece] in stone, ... the great beauty of its filigree-like carving unequalled in colonial art'. In La Paz, Wethey discusses the dramatic façades of the churches of San Francisco and San Domingo, as well as considering the *mestizo* style apparent in textiles and furniture. Wethey's clarity and eye for detail produce an absorbing article, a pleasure both for the specialist and the general reader.

871 Hispanic colonial architecture in Bolivia.
Harold Edwin Wethey. *Gazette des Beaux-Arts* (New York),
vol. 39 (1952), p. 47-60. bibliog.

Traces the development of Bolivian colonial ecclesiastical architecture from its modest beginnings in the 16th century, through the high points of the Baroque in the 17th and 18th centuries, to the incursion of the French Rococo style after 1750. Wethey illustrates the way in which many 16th-century churches in Bolivia show the strong influence of Andalusia's *mudéjar* churches of the 15th and 16th centuries which combined Gothic and Arabic styles, particularly in plan, and in the Muslim practice of adding highly decorated surfaces to many of Spain's Christian churches and cathedrals. The author examines the structural components of Bolivian church architecture, and the specialized uses made of the different sections and spaces. Considerable attention is also given to the churches in Chuquisaca (Sucre) throughout the colonial period, although these, unlike Potosí and La Paz, by the 18th century emphasized the European styles of architecture and, for the most part, rejected the cultural mixture displayed in *mestizo* decoration. Drawing on archive sources in Seville, Bolivia, and elsewhere in South America, Wethey provides an eloquent and scholarly article which, fifty years on, remains an enticing introduction to Bolivia's colonial architecture. Wethey published further research on the subject in his monograph *Arquitectura virreinal en Bolivia* (Viceregal architecture in Bolivia) (La Paz: Instituto de Investigaciones Artísticas, 1960. 145p. bibliog.). This includes both civil and ecclesiastical architecture from the 16th to the 19th century.

872 **Iglesias con atrio y posas en Bolivia.** (Bolivian churches with a walled enclosure [atrium] and corner chapels.)
José de Mesa, Teresa Gisbert. La Paz: Academia Nacional de Ciencias, 1961. 24p. bibliog. (Ciencias de la Cultura Series).
A monograph which illustrates admirably how the selection of one or two special architectural features can provide insights into the significance of the structure and its period. Here, the authors concentrate on the walled enclosure and its four small corner structures, known as *posas*, which are found around certain Bolivian churches constructed between the 16th and 18th centuries. After Mexico, Bolivia is the only Spanish American country where these combined features occur. The decorative enclosure, or atrium, was used to provide an assembly area for the instruction of large crowds of Indians, with Mass frequently said in the open air. The atrium was also used for other celebrations, for funeral processions, and occasionally for defence in rural areas. The *posas*, open altars and chapels with their own distinctive architectural styles, were used as stations during religious processions. Such features are found in churches in the Departments of La Paz, Oruro, Potosí, and Chuquisaca; plans and photographs of these lend excellent support to the text.

873 **Bolivia: monumentos históricos arquelógicos.** (Bolivia: historical and archaeological monuments.)
José de Mesa, Teresa Gisbert. Mexico City: Instituto Panamericano de Geografía y Historia, 1970. 146p.
A comprehensive survey of Bolivian colonial architecture. The study includes an excellent bibliography, 110 photographs, details of Bolivian legislation on artistic patrimony, and a list of national monuments.

874 **Arquitectura andina, historia y análisis.** (Andean architecture: history and analysis.)
José de Mesa, Teresa Gisbert. La Paz: Colección Arsanz y Vela, Embajada de España en Bolivia, 1985. 376p. maps. bibliog.
This remains a stimulating survey of colonial architecture, the product of more than twenty years' research by Mesa and Gisbert. Subjects covered include: the architecture of humanism; the Jesuits; the Baroque style, *mestizo* style and late colonial styles of architecture, along with an analysis of all the major styles and movements from the 1530s to 1800. An excellent work which is of use to both art historians and social historians.

875 **Sucre's colonial tapestry.**
Veronica Gould Stoddart, A. R. Williams. *Américas*, vol. 38, no. 1 (1986), p. 8-15.
A gentle, leisurely-paced article, like the city itself. Sucre is the old capital of colonial Upper Peru and the first capital of Bolivia – 'the city of four names': Charcas, La Plata,

Chuquisaca, and finally Sucre. The authors wander around the magnificent colonial buildings, the rich Baroque interior architecture, the church treasures of gold, silver, and jewel-encrusted relics, and the fine city museums. The result? An attractively illustrated introduction to one of the most striking examples of Spain's city-building flair to be found anywhere in the Andes.

876 History of South American colonial art and architecture.
Damián Bayón, Murillo Marx, translated by Jennifer A. Blankley, Angela P. Hall, Richard L. Rees. Barcelona, Spain: Ediciones Polígrafa, 1989. 442p. map. bibliog.

A stunning work of broad strokes and fine detail. Bayón, author of the volume's Hispanic American section, provides a masterly analysis of Bolivian architecture, painting, and sculpture from the 16th to the early 19th centuries, placing them all within his wider South American framework. Thus, the study includes *mudéjar* decoration and panelling in Sucre and Potosí, and *mestizo* carving in Potosí and La Paz (with a unique late example in Sucre), as well as the dramatic *retablos* (high, richly decorated altarpieces) and pulpits to be found in Sucre, Copacabana, and Oruro. Bayón draws on earlier seminal work by Wethey, Mesa and Gisbert, setting Bolivian art and architecture into a series of period and country-based studies that allow both the artistic similarities and the contrasts within colonial Spanish America to be revealed. Visually breathtaking, the volume contains plans and nearly 900 photographs, some 290 of them in colour. Beauty, clarity, and scholarship are the hallmarks of this book.

877 The architecture of conquest: building in the Viceroyalty of Peru, 1535-1635.
Valerie Fraser. Cambridge, England: Cambridge University Press, 1990. 204p. maps. bibliog.

It has long been acknowledged that in Spain's faraway New World empire, the rapid creation of towns by the *conquistadores* – one of the most spectacular town-planning movements in history – was both a state of mind and a declaration of intent. In this study of the critical first century of conquest and consolidation, early Spanish colonial architecture is examined, not as a consequence but as an integral part of the process, a means whereby the planting of towns of distinctive layout and construction imposed Spanish values and beliefs on the indigenous population, and became an essential part of metropolitan Spain's political and religious conquest. The author presents a thoughtful and well-illustrated analysis of Spain's early empire-building period, using selected church and domestic architectural examples in the Viceroyalty of Peru to develop her theme. The book provides a valuable addition to the literature on Spanish colonial architecture.

878 Potosí.
Photography by Daniel Gluckmann, text by Teresa Gisbert, José de Mesa, Valentín Abecia Baldivieso. Madrid: Agencia Española de Cooperación Internacional, Ediciones de Cultura Hispánica, 1990. 226p. maps. (Colección Ciudades Iberoamericanas).

The city of Potosí has never been more beautifully nor more imaginatively portrayed than in this book – a photographic essay of exceptionally high quality. Gluckmann's hundreds of colour photographs record the life, worship, work, and play to be found in the city and its surroundings today, picturing miners, street vendors, craftsmen and women, indeed *potosiños* of all ages and different occupations, along with images of the city's great art and architectural heritage. The introductory text is in Spanish; the photographs, rightly, speak for themselves.

879 Bolivian beacons.
Catherine Slessor. *Architectural Review*, vol. 191 (1992), p. 36-42.
Illustrates the work of Miguel Angel Roca, the Argentine architect who has created a series of visually dramatic municipal centres in some of the administrative districts of La Paz on strikingly geometrical lines. These centres are designed to house and provide a focus for the political, social, and medical services in the city's poorest peripheral communities that they serve.

880 Oruro: catálogo de su patrimonio arquitectónico urbano y rural.
(Oruro: catalogue of its urban and rural architectural heritage.)
Teresa Gisbert, Juan Carlos Jemio S., Nelson Mostacedo D.
La Paz: Instituto Boliviano de Cultura, 1993. 200p. maps. bibliog.
A detailed photographic and annotated inventory of historic buildings which survive today in the Department of Oruro. This is an important contribution to the architectural history of Bolivia.

Textiles and weaving

881 The cloth of the Quechuas.
Grace Goodell. In: *Man's many ways*. New York: Harper & Row, 1973, p. 160-72.
An excellent, popular introduction to the art of highland weaving in Bolivia and Peru. Designs, techniques and dyes are discussed here.

882 The art of Bolivian highland weaving.
Marjorie Cason, Adele Caholander. New York: Watson-Guptill, 1976. 216p. bibliog.
For those interested in craft weaving, this comprehensive study gives details on how to weave, using techniques common in Bolivia. The techniques described were documented during months of fieldwork in highland villages.

883 Bolivian highland weaving of the eighteenth, nineteenth and twentieth centuries.
Kitty Higgins, David Kenny.   Toronto, Canada: Canadian Museum of Carpets and Textiles, 1978. 29p. bibliog.

A catalogue from an exhibition of folk weavings from Bolivia which were collected by the authors. It contains many valuable photographs and a discussion of weaving techniques.

884 Weaving traditions of highland Bolivia: [exhibition] December 19, 1978 to February 4, 1979.
Guest curators: Laurie Adelson, Bruch Takami.   Los Angeles: Craft and Folk Art Museum, 1978. 65p.

A superbly illustrated catalogue with much information on regional weaving techniques, patterns and motifs.

885 El arte textil en Bolivia. (Textile art in Bolivia.)
Teresa Gisbert, Silvia Arze, Marta Cajias.   La Paz: Universidad Mayor de San Andrés, Instituto de Estudios Bolivianos, 1982. 40p. bibliog.

Identifies and provides a systematic account of seven distinctive textile-producing regions in Bolivia and one in Peru. The notes are detailed and well illustrated, providing information on many aspects of textile design, including styles, colours, and weavers.

886 Aymara weavings: ceremonial textiles of colonial and 19th-century Bolivia.
Laurie Adelson, Arthur Tracht.   Washington, DC: Smithsonian Institution, Travelling Exhibition Service, 1983. 159p.

Asks the reader to imagine a world in which textiles are the most valued and respected products of culture. Aymara weaving is part of a tradition dating back to 2500 BC. Beautiful photographs and illustrations of cloth, garments, mantles, bags and belts are included.

887 Space, time and harmony: symbolic aspects of language in Andean textiles with special reference to those from Bolívar Province (Cochabamba, Bolivia).
L. Crickmay.   PhD thesis, St. Andrews University, Scotland, 1992.

A study of the symbolic language contained in the Andean textiles of Cochabamba's Bolívar Province, which shows how the designs communicate information both about the weavers and their social group. This is a detailed examination of these Aymara and Quechua textiles – their history, iconography, colours, weaving techniques, and the interpretations of their designs.

888   Indians win back sacred art.
John Anner.   *The Progressive*, vol. 57 (January 1993), p. 12.
In noting the return of the valuable sacred weavings to Coroma in Bolivia, Anner concentrates on how the villagers enlisted the help of anthropologists, lawyers and government officials, among others, to produce a highly effective network of assistance to pressure dealers and collectors into giving back the textiles.

889   Sacred Bolivian textiles returned.
Angela M. H. Schuster.   *Archaeology*, vol. 46 (January/February 1993), p. 20-22.
Reports the return by the US Customs Service to the Aymara people of Coroma, Bolivia, of forty-eight sacred ceremonial garments (valued at US$400,000) which had been bought and smuggled out of Bolivia by North American dealers during the 1980s. At the request of the Bolivian government, the United States placed an import ban on such items in 1988, and official pressure for their return was brought to bear on dealers who had acquired any of these textiles at an earlier date.

890   The lost and found art of the Jalq'a.
Ruth Massey.   *Choices* (New York), vol. 3 (March 1994), p. 33-35.
The dying art of weaving by the Jalq'a Indians of Sucre was rediscovered in the mid-1980s by two Chilean anthropologists and this led, with United Nations assistance, to the construction of six textile workshops in the region. By 1991, the UN project had been extended to the Tarabuco area, with training programmes and sales of both Jalq'a and Tarabuco textiles in the city of Sucre. By the mid-1990s, the combined sales were averaging US$3,000 a month, bringing a new source of income to these impoverished local communities, and requests from museums and international organizations in Europe and the United States to exhibit their distinctive traditional textiles.

891   Marketing diversity: global transformations in cloth and identity in highland Peru and Bolivia.
Elayne Lesley Zorn.   PhD thesis, Cornell University, Ithaca, New York, 1997. 594p. bibliog.
The author examines the significance of contemporary textiles in Taquile Island, Puno, Peru and the Sakaka *ayllu* in northern Potosí, Bolivia from two perspectives: first, gender roles and weaving's importance for women's prestige and power; and second, the practice of weaving and how it is learned. She then analyses the influence of increased market participation upon textile weaving in recent decades, matched by the need felt by both indigenous cornmunities to use their textiles as the means of projecting a stronger ethnic identity. The women have made some adjustments in response to the growing global market for handwoven cloth, and this has also been accompanied in the two communities by a new creativity in patterns and styles.

892   The fabric of society.
The Geographical Magazine, vol. 71, no. 7 (1999), p. 88-89.
Retells the story of the lost Aymara textiles of Coloma (see items 888-89). This article marked the presentation of a Rolex Award for Enterprise in 1998 to Cristina Bubba Zamora, a Bolivian social psychologist, for her role in and after 1988 in helping to

retrieve the Coloma and other ancient weavings which had been smuggled earlier into the United States and Canada. In 1992, she accompanied a group of elders from the altiplano village on a flight to California to reclaim the textiles at an official ceremony. The United States banned imports of such items in 1988, and since then, Zamora has continued to press for more bilateral legislation elsewhere in the world forbidding trade in these, and similar, sacred and cultural treasures.

Pottery and other crafts

893   Arts and crafts of South America.
Lucy Davies, Mo Fini.   London: Thames & Hudson, 1994;
San Francisco: Chronicle Books, 1995. 160p. map. bibliog.

Bolivia and the high Andes are well represented in this lavishly illustrated record of South American arts and crafts, which here includes textiles, costume, metalwork, jewellery, wood-carving, basketry, and pottery. Through their text and pictures, the authors emphasize the vitality and colour of the indigenous artistic traditions, while in addition providing notes for further study and a glossary of terms.

894   Pottery's role in the reproduction of Andean society.
W. J. M. Sillar.   PhD thesis, University of Cambridge, England, 1995.

From fieldwork in the Department of Cuzco, Peru, and the Departments of Potosí and Cochabamba, Bolivia, Sillar investigates ways in which the making, ownership, trading, and use of pottery maintains and strengthens social relationships, especially those based on gender, age, and kinship.

Photography

895   Nineteenth-century South America in photographs.
Compiled by H. L. Hoffenberg.   New York: Dover Publications, 1982. 152p. (Dover Photography Collections).

Bolivia is conspicuous by its absence from this collection of more than 200 black-and-white photographs, yet the book is recommended to all those keen to capture the atmosphere of 19th-century South America and to understand many aspects of life relevant to Bolivia in that period. The subjects include urban and rural life, transport, the military, Andean Indians, and some of the region's outstanding landscapes. Nearly all the illustrations are drawn from the original vintage prints and are well captioned. The collection also contains a good general introduction by Hoffenberg to 19th-century photography, and to some of the outstanding photographers working in South America at the time.

896 Yesterday's modern images, today's archival treasures.
Daniel Buck. *Américas*, vol. 46, no. 5 (1994), p. 20-27.
A fascinating introduction to the early days of photography in Bolivia. Recent studies of Bolivia's first photographers and of photographic collections are unveiling a valuable record of some aspects of the country's 19th-century life. Included here, in colour and black-and-white, are examples of small portrait calling-cards and other studio work, and later outdoor photographs of landscapes, street scenes, mining camps, and family entertainment. The illustrations are well supported by a description of the methods used by the photographers of the day.

Music

897 Musical and other sound instruments of the South American Indians: a comparative ethnographical study.

Karl Gustav Izikowitz.   East Ardsley, England: S. R. Publishers, 1970. 433p.

This is a systematic classification of musical instruments, such as drums, clappers, trumpets, and rattles. The author's main objective is to provide a better understanding of civilizations that did not produce written histories.

898 Music in Latin America, an introduction.

Gérard Béhague.   Englewood Cliffs, New Jersey: Prentice-Hall, 1979. 369p. bibliog. (Prentice Hall History of Music Series).

This scholarly analysis examines the major works of the most representative composers of each period, in every country, and identifies significant trends. After his discussion of sacred and secular music in colonial Spanish and Luso-Brazilian America, Béhague devotes six of his ten chapters to the 20th century, reflecting the development and considerable accomplishment of Latin American music in this period. This is a book for the specialist, distinguished by its range, balance, and critical assessments.

899 New currents in *música folklórica* in La Paz, Bolivia.

Gilka Wara Céspedes.   *Latin American Music Review*, vol. 5, no. 2 (fall-winter 1984), p. 217-42. bibliog.

An interesting, readable review of the current scene in folk music, its preservation, performance and innovation. The author presents a lively discussion of the cross-currents in urban and rural music-making. Some urban folk musicians now emphasize concert engagements, solo instruments, and virtuosity; others seek to maintain the rural musical styles of group reciprocity and a less formal approach. There is a good survey here of traditional Indian instruments, contrasted with the *mestizo* influence of brass bands. Wara Céspedes is an excellent communicator. His article bubbles with ideas, information, and new lines of thought.

900 Re-sounding lost Masses.
David Einhorn. *Américas*, vol. 41, no. 2 (1989), p. 4-5.
In 1986, musicologists made a remarkable discovery in the archives of Bolivia's old Jesuit mission at Concepción of about 5,000 sheets of colonial liturgical music dating back to the early 1700s. Many were found to be the work of Doménico Zípoli, an Italian Baroque musician, and the only Jesuit composer associated with the missions in South America during the 18th century whose music has been preserved. Efforts continue in Bolivia to find more of his manuscripts; meanwhile, at least three recordings of Zípoli's work have been released in Italy and the United States.

901 The llama's flute: musical misunderstandings in the Andes.
Henry Stobart. *Early Music*, vol. 24, no. 3 (1996), p. 470-82. bibliog.
Stresses the vitality and durability of Andean culture, including its ability to incorporate external changes without loss of identity. Based on work spread over ten years in a Quechua-speaking community in northern Potosí, the author provides a detailed, illustrated account of the history of the local musical instruments (particularly the *pinkillu* flute), tracing Spanish influences, and surveying the important role of village musicians in the various ceremonies held annually to promote the survival and well-being of the community.

902 Magical flutes: music culture and music groups in a changing Bolivia.
Sari Tuula Hannele. FilD, Lunds Universitet, Lund, Sweden, 1996. 253p. bibliog.
Discusses the changing aspects of popular music and society in Bolivia through an ethnographic study of three music groups: Los Masis, Inkallajta, and Flor Tani Tani. The author analyses the urban music movement in Bolivia, along with the urban–rural connection and the role of the media.

903 Mountains of song: musical constructions of ecology, place, and identity, in the Bolivian Andes.
Thomas James Soloman. PhD thesis, University of Texas at Austin, 1997. 625p. bibliog.
Demonstrates how the timing and varied styles of music-making by the Chayanta, a Quechua community in the Department of Potosí, help them to make sense of the world. Music sustains their collective identity, their sacred rituals, and their relationship to the land and its seasonal changes.

Films and the Film Industry

History and criticism

904 Film as a revolutionary weapon: a Jorge Sanjinés retrospective.
Leon Campbell, Carlos Cortes. *History Teacher*, vol. 12, no. 3
(1979), p. 383-402.

Discusses five full-length films by the Bolivian director Jorge Sanjinés, who used film to document the peasants' revolutionary activity in Bolivia. His films are designed to develop mass consciousness and to bring about a better understanding of popular culture in Bolivia. His first films are more radical than the later ones, but in total they make a powerful statement about national culture and the plight of the masses in Bolivia. The article remains an excellent introduction to this neglected area.

905 Neo-realism in contemporary Bolivian cinema: a case study of Jorge Sanjinés' 'Blood of the Condor' and Antonio Eguino's 'Chuquiago'.
José Sánchez-H. PhD dissertation, University of Michigan,
Ann Arbor, 1983. 325p.

Studies the cinematic approaches of two contemporary Bolivian film-makers, Jorge Sanjinés and Antonio Eguino. The author contends that Sanjinés' film 'Blood of the Condor' was mislabelled 'militant' cinema and that it is neo-realist, while Eguino's 'Chuquiago' is neo-realist in a limited sense – part fiction, part documentary. Both films won international acclaim.

906 Cine boliviano 1953-1983: aproximación a una experiencia.
(Bolivian cinema, 1953-1983: approaching reality.)
Carlos D. Mesa Gisbert.   In: *Tendencias actuales en la literatura boliviana* (Presents trends in Bolivian literature).   Edited by Jorge Sanjinés.   Minneapolis, Minnesota: Institute for the Study of Ideologies and Literature; Instituto de Cine, Radio y Televisión, 1985. 284p.

An excellent introductory study of the Bolivian film industry. For a discussion of the period before 1953, see, among other references, *Historia del cine boliviano* (A history of the Bolivian cinema) by Alfonso Gumucio Dagrón (Mexico City: Filmoteca UNAM, 1983. 327p.). Gumucio Dagrón, film-maker, historian and poet, discusses Luís Castillo González, and provides a comprehensive list of all films and film-makers from 1904 onwards.

907 Magical reels: a history of cinema in Latin America.
John King.   London: Verso, 1990. 266p. bibliog. (Critical Studies in Latin American Culture).

Within a chapter on the Andean states of Bolivia, Peru and Ecuador, King examines the development of modern Bolivian cinema in the aftermath of the National Revolution of 1952-53, discussing the dominant themes, styles and characterization, and setting the work of Jorge Ruiz, Jorge Sanjinés and others in the political context of their times. This is a stimulating, scholarly contribution to the history of cinema, both in Bolivia and in Latin America as a whole.

908 The art and politics of Bolivian cinema.
José Sánchez-H.   Lanham, Maryland; London: Scarecrow Press, 1999. 265p. bibliog.

This is the first book in English entirely devoted to the Bolivian cinema, a long-awaited study whose appearance will be warmly welcomed by scholars of both the Bolivian film industry and the history of international cinema. The author, born and raised in Bolivia and now teaching at California State University, Long Beach, has been researching his subject for over twenty years and here presents a detailed history of the Bolivian cinema throughout the 20th century, beginning with the first motion picture made in Bolivia in 1904. The book includes analyses of the work of several of Bolivia's pioneering film-makers and screen writers, including Jorge Ruiz, Oscar Soria, Jorge Sanjinés, and Antonio Eguino, and Sánchez enriches his text with numerous personal interviews. The seamless fabric of film-making and politics in Bolivia is demonstrated throughout, and researchers will find the complete list of Bolivian feature films and film awards, the production and marketing strategies, and the extensive bibliography all of great value. And what of the spirit and purpose of film-making in Bolivia? As Oscar Soria explains: 'We were searching for our own identity, the recognition of our values, the defense of our resources, and our own realities'. This comprehensive study will deservedly become a standard reference in the literature on Latin American cinema.

Documentary films and video films

Documentary films

909 Blood of the condor.
Directed by Jorge Sanjinés, 1969. 72 mins. Quechua and Spanish dialogue with English subtitles, black-and-white. Available through Unifilm, New York City. Cable: UNIFILM NEW YORK.

The film is a searing reconstruction of traumatic events in a Quechua community in the mid-1960s, but it also demonstrates dramatically the relationship of the Indian communities to the rest of Bolivian society, especially *mestizo* society. Under the Quechua title, *Yawar Mallku* (Blood of the Condor), this was the first film to be made in Quechua and Spanish. Three years earlier, Sanjinés had also directed the first feature film made in Aymara and Spanish, *Ukamau* (That's the way it is). The film won international awards but angered Bolivia's military government under General René Barrientos because of its emphasis on the poverty of Indian life and its negative portrayal of Bolivia. Sanjinés and his production team were dismissed from the Bolivian Film Institute which had been created by the MNR after the 1952-53 revolution. It was closed permanently in 1968 and replaced by a state-owned television station.

910 Andean women.
Faces of Change Series. American Universities Field Staff, 1974. 18 mins., sound, subtitles, colour. Available through Indiana University Audio Visual Center. Catalog number GSC-1390.

An interesting film which shows the position of Aymara women who perform many tasks vital to society and yet who see themselves only as helpers. It also explores the cultural ideal of society, while focusing on the gulf between the perception and reality of the women's role. Although not a recent film, this and others in the same series reveal many traditional aspects of Aymaran rural life that are still relevant today.

911 The children know.
Faces of Change Series. American University Field Staff, 1974. 33 mins., sound, subtitles, colour. Available through Indiana University Audio Visual Center. Catalog number GSC-1388.

Rural education is the theme of this film, which explores the deep division in Andean society between *campesinos* and *mestizos*. Prejudices are seen through the eyes of children. The film illustrates that these begin at birth, are perpetuated by the schools, and continue throughout life.

912 Magic and Catholicism.

Faces of Change Series. American University Field Staff, 1974.
33 mins., sound and colour, English subtitles. Available through
Indiana University Audio Visual Center. Catalog number GSC-1392.

Examines religious syncretism in Vitocota, a village on the altiplano. Syncretic religion characteristically combines elements from two, or more, different perspectives to make a comfortable, tension-free relationship. While a Western viewer observes peasants celebrating a Catholic fiesta and a traditional ceremony for ensuring a good harvest, the *campesinos* perceive the same events as being part of an intensely personal relationship with the supernatural.

913 Potato planters.

Faces of Change Series. American University Field Staff, 1974.
17 mins., sound, subtitles, colour. Available through Indiana
University Audio Visual Center. Catalog number GSC-1389.

Compares the daily life of an Aymara family, which is simple and routine, with the complexity of their belief system. It also studies agriculture in the village of Vitocota, the land tenure system, crops and diet, and the division of labour. This is a thoughtful, well-rounded film which captures several key features of rural Aymaran society.

914 The spirit possession of Alejandro Mamani.

Faces of Change Series. American University Field Staff, 1974.
28 mins., sound and colour, English subtitles. Available through
Indiana University Audio Visual Center. Catalog number GSC-1391.

This film portrays an old man, with property and status, who is nearing the end of his life, but lacks contentment. He believes he is possessed by evil spirits, and the film displays his own misery as well as the sympathy, and the irritation, of those around him about his sad condition.

915 Viracocha: the Aymara of the Bolivian Andes.

Faces of Change Series. American University Field Staff, 1974.
30 mins., sound, subtitles, colour. Available through Indiana
University Audio Visual Center. Catalog number GSC-1387.

Mestizos and *campesinos* in the Andean highlands interact within a new economic system. This documentary examines market days and fiestas as times of interaction between the two groups. *Mestizos* exhibit alternately benign and abusive behaviour to assert their traditional social dominance over the peasantry.

Prospective viewers of items 910-915 will find it helpful to read Murdo J. MacLeod, 'The Aymara of the Bolivian Andes' (*Latin American Research Review*, vol. 11, no. 1 (1976), p. 228-32). This article provides a critical assessment of the six films, including more information about their content. An introductory essay comes with each. A few of the films are simplistic and also tend to moralize; all however could form a basis for discussion on the extent of continuity or change since the 1970s in some of the small towns on the altiplano.

916 Chuquiago.
Directed by Antonio Eguino, 1977. 87 mins., Aymara and Spanish dialogue with English subtitles, colour. Available through Unifilm, New York City. Cable: UNIFILM NEW YORK.

Chuquiago is the Aymara name for La Paz. In four separate, yet overlapping, stories, the film examines the lives of individuals from four different social settings. The characters include an Indian boy hired out to work in the market, an Indian teenager who wants to assimilate into white culture, a government bureaucrat, and Patricia, a university student.

Video films

917 Bolivia: corazón de America. (Bolivia: heart of America.)
La Paz: Praxis-Antara, 1992. 43 mins., sound, English commentary, colour.

A comprehensive and unusually detailed documentary on Bolivia. It presents a systematic record of the country's prehistory and archaeological discoveries, its regional geography, ecology, mining and agriculture, its colonial and modern history, major cities, the Santa Cruz development area, the rural population, and a survey of prehispanic, *mestizo*, and contemporary art. The filming is stylish and imaginative. Overall, this is an accomplished introduction to the country as a whole.

918 Bolivia: on the trail of Butch Cassidy and the Sundance Kid.
Washington, DC: Organization of American States. Directed by Claudia Vargas-Sherwood, Gerard Ranson, 1992. 60 mins., sound, English commentary, colour.

An excellent documentary on Bolivia, since in following the trail of Butch and Sundance the film criss-crosses the country from the altiplano, the mines, the railroads, the Yungas, and the Valles, to Santa Cruz and the ranchlands of the Oriente, before doubling back to San Vicente and what is assumed to be the final shootout with the Bolivian Army in 1908. Parker and Longabaugh had made the fatal mistake of stealing a payroll from the Bolivian 'tin baron' Aramayo, whose power and influence were strong enough to ensure that this robbery would be their last. Old photographs, newspaper reports, and correspondence are linked to modern interviews with local people, and with academics in Bolivia and the United States. History, fact, myth and legend have been combined to make a fascinating and informative film.

919 Tiahuanaco: una cultura milenaria. Una visión completa de una de las culturas mas importantes del mundo Andino. (Tiahuanaco: a millenary culture. A complete picture of one of the most important cultures of the Andean world.)
La Paz: Praxis-Antara, 1992. 15 mins., sound, English commentary, colour.

A general introduction to Tiahuanaco and the region's cultural significance, including its location, history, architecture, ceramics, and metallurgy.

920 Bolivia: donde nace la luz. (Bolivia: the birthplace of light.)
Washington, DC: Organization of American States. Directed by
Gabriel Gross, 1993. 20 mins., sound, Spanish commentary, colour.
An absorbing introduction to the Andean world. The film opens with fine views of the
high cordilleras as the camera hovers over the peaks, snowfields and hidden lakes.
Viewers are then given a well-rounded picture of life on and around the altiplano, from
farming, herding, and work in the mines, to the bustle of business and marketing in La
Paz, Oruro and Potosí. Good use is also made of close-up, particularly of musical
instruments, music-making and dance.

921 Bolivia: horizonte de oportunidades. (Bolivia: horizon of
opportunities.)
United Nations Investment Promotion Program, 1994. 30 mins.,
sound, Spanish commentary, colour.
Essentially this is an economic review, with strong emphasis on transport, power supplies,
and the rapid regional development around Santa Cruz. Production of soybean, sugar cane
and cotton are highlighted, along with agro-industry, ranching and forestry. Coffee and
cacao specialization in the Yungas is also included.

922 The Beni Biosphere Reserve and biological station.
La Paz: Ministerio de Desarrollo Sostenible; Dirección Nacional de
Programa el Hombre y la Biosfera, 1996. 25 mins., sound, English
commentary, colour.
An illuminating introduction to the research and conservation projects being developed at
the biological station set up in 1982, and recognized by UNESCO in 1986. The film
includes extensive views of the wildlife and distinctive vegetation of the Beni, the work
of the Forest Rangers, raised-field agriculture above flood levels, the Indian communities
within the Reserve, and the problem of slash-and-burn cultivation by immigrant farmers
in the Reserve's surrounding buffer zone.

923 Bolivia: new opportunities for wise investment.
La Paz: Ministry of Foreign Affairs; Undersecretariat of Economic
Promotion, 1997. 35 mins., sound, English commentary, colour.
A robust, wide-ranging message concerning the country's many opportunities and
attractions for foreign investment. It includes the mining sector, oil and gas, farming and
ranching, agro-industry, leather and jewellery manufacture, and hotel construction.
Attention is drawn to the enlarged market opportunities created by the Andean
Community and MERCOSUR, as well as to the skills of the Bolivian workforce. The
film's value is also enhanced by a clear explanation of the privatization law, tax structure,
tariffs, and banking. This is an excellent documentary that serves its purpose well; it is
lucid, well organized, and informative.

924 Amboró National Park.

La Paz: Ministerio de Desarrollo Sostenible y Planificación; Dirección de Biodiversidad, 1998. 15 mins., sound, English commentary, colour.

A very good record of the great variety to be found within this well-known Bolivian National Park which will appeal to conservationists and ecotourists. Amboró lies between the old (1954) and the new Cochabamba–Santa Cruz highways, and the film considers the advantages and disadvantages of such accessibility.

925 Andean silver.

La Paz: Apex Silver Corporation, with the assistance of the Bolinvest Foundation, 1998. 11 mins., sound, English commentary, colour.

After outlining the wealth of Bolivia's mineral resources still contained within the Andes, the film concentrates on the spectacular discovery of silver made by Apex at San Cristobal in 1995, describing the background to regional exploration, current exploitation, and future potential.

926 Avaroa National Park Reserve.

La Paz: Ministerio de Desarrollo Sostenible y Planificación; Dirección de Biodiversidad, 1998. 20 mins., sound, English commentary, colour.

The park is named in honour of Eduardo Avaroa (Abaroa), hero of Bolivia's resistance to Chile's military invasion of the Litoral Department in the Atacama Desert in 1879, at the start of the War of the Pacific. The Reserve lies in Sud Lipez province in the extreme south of the Department of Potosí, and contains a stunning range of colour in its rock formations, thermal springs, mineral deposits, salt desert, marshes, and in the Laguna Colorada, which attracts more than forty species of aquatic birds. Fifty Aymara families live in the Park, and there is interesting detail on llama and alpaca herding. The film provides a memorable glimpse of one of Bolivia's most spectacular and remote regions of the altiplano and Western Cordillera.

927 Carrasco National Park.

La Paz: Ministerio de Desarrollo Sostenible y Planificación; Dirección de Biodiversidad, 1998. 15 mins., sound, English commentary, colour.

Carrasco National Park lies in the eastern region of the Department of Cochabamba, where the film emphasizes the Park's great variety of climate, forest and tree ferns. It is the home of the Yuracaré Indians, and several endangered species such as the spectacled bear and jaguar. The film illustrates well the Park's attractions for hikers, climbers, botanists, and entomologists, but also addresses the problem of coping with the growing threat from poachers.

928 The diversity of life.
La Paz: Ministerio de Desarrollo Sostenible y Planificación; Dirección de Biodiversidad, 1998. 12 mins., sound, English commentary, colour.

A short introduction to the general subject of biodiversity, and the reasons why it is important to maintain the balance of the natural environment. The film shows what Bolivia is doing in the field of conservation, both now and for the future.

929 Expo oro. (An exhibition of gold.)
Santa Cruz de la Sierra: EXPO ORO, 1998. 10 mins., sound, English commentary, colour.

A literally dazzling record of the international exhibition of gold jewellery, silverware, watches, precious stones, and specialized equipment held in March 1998 in Santa Cruz, and sponsored by the Bolivian government. It attracted dealers from Asia, Europe, and the Americas. In addition to the exhibits, the film shows scenes of the country's great diversity, providing a short, but well-targeted, promotion for Bolivia and its expanding jewellery industry and export.

930 Kaa-iya National Park of the Gran Chaco.
La Paz: Ministerio de Desarrollo Sostenible y Planificación; Dirección de Biodiversidad, 1998. 15 mins., sound, English commentary, some Spanish commentary and subtitles, colour.

A rare opportunity to see the isolated world of the Gran Chaco. The film contains excellent air and ground shots of that part of the Chaco which lies within the Department of Santa Cruz – the tropical dry forest, thorn scrub, dune fields, seasonal flooding, and the great Izozog swamps. The Guaraní and other indigenous peoples inhabit the area, and the film records their hunting-and-fishing economy along the River Parapetí. Superb close-ups show the jaguar, tapir, puma and other wildlife in their natural habitats. Bolivia's National Park strategy, here as elsewhere, is to involve the local people in the protection of their environment, and how this is done is well demonstrated. The new Bolivia–Brazil natural gas pipeline now crosses the northern sector of the Park, but the greater threat to conservation comes from the encroachment into the Park's buffer zone by migrant farmers and ranchers.

931 Madidi National Park.
La Paz: Ministerio de Desarrollo Sostenible y Planificación; Dirección de Biodiversidad, 1998. 10 mins., sound, English commentary, colour.

A Park already famous for its majestic sweep from the glaciers and snowfields of the Andes, through the cloud forests of the cordilleras, to the Yungas, the savannahs of the Oriente, and the true rainforests of Amazonia. Indeed, the Madidi National Park contains the richest biodiversity of any similarly-sized protected area in the whole of Bolivia. The film takes this as its theme, and provides a striking introduction to the variety that exists within the Park.

932　Mining in Bolivia.
La Paz: Corporación Minera de Bolivia (COMIBOL), 1998.
13 mins., sound, English commentary, colour.

A brief but informative survey by Bolivia's state mining corporation. After sketching the historical background, the emphasis is on modern development. The film locates the major mineral resources in the Andes and the Precambrian Shield before concentrating on each important site in turn, showing its layout and current production from both the mine and its tailings. Finally, the film highlights an important aspect of COMIBOL's work today, that of attracting foreign investment and promoting joint ventures with the private sector.

933　Protected areas in Bolivia.
La Paz: Ministerio de Desarrollo Sostenible y Planificación; Dirección de Biodiversidad, 1998. 20 mins., sound, English commentary, colour.

A most useful general introduction to Bolivia's fourteen Protected Areas which constitute ten per cent of the country's total area, and form part of the National System of Protected Areas established in 1993. The theme is the huge diversity of Bolivia's biosphere, and the ways in which the local people participate in its management.

934　Sajama National Park.
La Paz: Ministerio de Desarrollo Sostenible y Planificación; Dirección de Biodiversidad, 1998. 15 mins., sound, English commentary, colour.

This breathtakingly beautiful National Park includes Bolivia's highest peak and adjoins Chile's Lauca National Park in the Western Cordillera. There are fine views of the landscape, cold-desert vegetation, the native camelids (wild vicuña and guanaco, domesticated llama and alpaca), and details of the everyday lives of the Aymara living within the Park. The main challenges to Park management are overgrazing, and the conflict between tourism and the limited carrying capacity of this fragile environment.

935　Bolivia: Transturin Inbound.
La Paz: Transturin Turismo, 1999. 20 mins., sound, English commentary, colour.

An attractive and informative film advertising the range of services offered by Transturin, the new Bolivian tourist company formed by the amalgamation of four existing firms. 'Inbound' begins by presenting the highlights of three popular packages: (1) A tour of the altiplano from Lake Titicaca to the Uyuni salt flats, including La Paz, Tiwanaku, Chacaltaya ski centre, and the Yungas; (2) A tour based entirely on Sucre and Potosí; and (3) A tour including the Amazon rainforest, the Santa Cruz region and the Jesuit Missions. The film commentary includes much historical and cultural detail. It also publicizes the company's new de-luxe catamaran tour of Lake Titicaca which visits all the major cultural centres on and around the lake in both Bolivia and Peru. The emphasis throughout, whether for a group or an individual tour, is on first-class accommodation and a high level of guide and lecture services, reflecting the determination to develop the top end of the market in Bolivia's expanding tourist industry.

936 South by Potosí.
The World in Focus Series. Directed by John Myers, 1999. 40 mins., sound, English commentary, colour.

An interesting video travel film which is more wide-ranging than the title suggests. The journey begins with a good coverage of La Paz, before moving on to the Chacaltaya ski area, Coroico and the Yungas, and Sucre. Potosí, Uyuni, and the remote southwest complete the route. The film strikes a good balance between urban and rural life, and captures vividly the striking contrasts to be found in the high Andes.

Customs, Festivals and Folklore

937 La cultura nativa en Bolivia, su entronque y sus rasgos principales. (Native culture in Bolivia: its derivation and its principal characteristics.)
Carlos Ponce Sanginés.   La Paz: Instituto Boliviana de Cultura, 1975. 112p. bibliog.
A careful and readable introduction to the indigenous culture of modern Bolivia, which traces its survival, growth and evolution from 1200 to 1970.

938 The masked media: Aymara fiesta and social interaction on the Bolivian highlands.
Hans Buechler.   New York: Mouton, 1980. 399p. bibliog.
An examination of the rituals of the peoples of highland areas of Bolivia as instruments for transmitting information about ongoing social ties among the peoples involved. This information is only partly inherent in the symbolism of fiestas; the meanings are created during the performances. Buechler draws on a lifetime of research in the Andean highlands and concludes that the rituals generate, select, and present information about social ties.

939 The technology of self-respect: cultural projects among Aymara and Quechua Indians.
Patrick Breslin.   *Grassroots Development*, vol. 6, no. 1 (1982), p. 33-37.
Describes two projects in Bolivia. The first is among Aymara Indians in the highlands and is an attempt to save, record and reanimate Aymara folk tales for the rural radio network. The other is located in Sucre and is concerned with reintroducing Quechua musical dance forms.

940 *Ayllu*: the Bolivian highlands.
Photography by Peter McFarren, text by Yolanda Bedregal.
La Paz: Museo National de Etnografía y Folklore, 1984. [not
paginated].
Nearly 100 photographs in colour record the rural and urban life of scattered Aymara and
Quechua communities in the Andes throughout the year, including their music, dance,
rituals, dwellings, crops, cultivation and harvest. The text is in English and Spanish.

941 From the Sun of the Incas to the Virgin of Copacabana.
Sabine G. MacCormack. *Representations*, vol. 8 (1984), p. 30-60.
Examines Inca and Christian pilgrimages to the sacred site of the Temple of the Sun and
the Virgin of Copacabana, Bolivia.

942 The colors of carnival.
Manuel Vargas. *Américas*, vol. 38, no. 6 (1986), p. 32-35, 64-65.
Among the numerous descriptions in English of the Oruro Carnival, none is more detailed
and informative than this by a noted Bolivian author. Accompanied by McFarren's
excellent colour shots, Vargas' text brings each element of the Carnival to life as he
examines the history, meaning, and rich complex of myths and beliefs that combine to
produce one of the most important social and religious annual events in Bolivia.

943 Music of the souls.
Henry Stobart. *The Geographical Magazine*, vol. 60, no. 6 (1988),
p. 52-54.
Illustrates how one small Andean community located between Potosí and Sucre
celebrates All Saints' and All Souls' Days, both to honour the dead and to mark the start
of the rainy season. These annual festivities last for four days in November and the
author's description of the elaborate preparation of food and *chicha* (maize beer), the
processions, the rituals, and the music and dancing, reveals the mixed indigenous,
Spanish and Catholic heritage involved in this wild high spot of the villagers' year.

944 Andean rituals of revolt: the Chayanta rebellion of 1927.
Erick Detlef Langer. *Ethnohistory*, vol. 37, no. 3 (1990), p. 227-53.
bibliog.
Describes two of the ritual ceremonies performed in the Chayanta province of northern
Potosí that were designed to relate some of the events that took place during the Chayanta
peasant rebellion of 1927 to the communities' continuing assertion of their ethnic identity
and land rights. The examples are interesting, but the analysis is uneven and in places too
conjectural.

945 Symbolic arrangement and communication in the 'despacho'.
G. Armstrong. PhD thesis, St. Andrews University, Scotland, 1990.
An investigation into the composition of the *despacho*, the ritual offering used to
propitiate the major earth deities in the Bolivian mining town of Oruro. The *despacho* is
also designed to increase *suerte* (good luck) which is viewed not only in terms of material

fortune, but also personal well-being and harmony with the cosmos, particularly among the Aymara and Quechua Indians.

946 Fiesta Boliviana. (Bolivian fiesta.)
Hugo Boero Rojo. La Paz: Editorial 'Los Amigos del Libro', 1991. 125p. (Colección Bolivia Mágica).

A spectacularly colourful photographic record with supporting text of fiestas and carnivals in Bolivia. The eastern plains are represented by the festivities at San Ignacio de Moxos in the Beni; those in the central valleys at Tarabuco, Torotoro, and Urkupiña; and those in the high Andes at Oruro, and in and around La Paz. The book provides a useful anthropological study of the Bolivian fiesta as well as an artistic source of reference.

947 Blessings of the Virgin in capitalist society: the transformation of a rural Bolivian fiesta.
Libbet Crandon-Malamud. *American Anthropologist*, vol. 95, no. 3 (1993), p. 574-96. bibliog.

A good-humoured but shrewd analysis of the changes that have occurred in the annual fiesta to the Virgin in an altiplano village some one hundred miles from La Paz. Since the mid-1980s, *paceños* living in the capital have become increasingly involved as sponsors of the celebration, developing its business potential, elaborating its display, and, in the process, displacing the former local village organizers who no longer feel part of the proceedings. Indeed, they complain that these urban invaders from La Paz never set foot in the village on any other occasion from one year's end to the next. The author supplies a detailed account of the economic, political and social roles of the religious celebration, and offers both the scholar and the general reader rich insights into the lasting importance of fiestas in Bolivian society.

948 Mascaras de los Andes Bolivianos. (Masks of the Bolivian Andes.)
Edited by Peter McFarren, photography by Peter McFarren, Sixto Choque. La Paz: Editorial Quipus/Banco Mercantil, 1993. 171p.

A feast for the eye, this dazzling book examines Bolivia's distinctive Andean masks both as an art form and as part of an important folk dance tradition. The vivid colour photographs illustrate seven chapters by individual Bolivian scholars and artists on the history and techniques of mask-making in pre-Columbian and colonial times, their symbolism, regional variety, and association with particular festivals. A revealing interview, shortly before he died, with the master mask-maker, Antonio Viscarra, is also included. The text throughout is in Spanish and English. This is an indispensable source of reference on the topic, both for the specialist and the general reader.

949 Simón Bolívar, the sun of justice and the Amerindian virgin. Andean conceptions of the *Patria* in nineteenth-century Potosí.
Tristan Platt. *Journal of Latin American Studies*, vol. 25, no. 1 (1993), p. 159-85. bibliog.

Examines ways in which the Indian communities in the early years of the Bolivian republic interpreted the transformation of the colonial Audiencia of Charcas into an independent state. For the most part, the state's new images such as civic processions, public monuments, and the national flag for example, were given a religious interpretation by the Indians, and were thus absorbed relatively easily into their own sacred symbolism and their perception of homeland.

950 **"We have to learn to ask": hegemony, diverse experiences, and antagonistic meanings in Bolivia.**
Maria L. Lagos. *American Ethnologist*, vol. 20, no. 1 (1993), p. 52-71. bibliog.
Examines the celebration of the Virgin of Urkupiña in Cochabamba, tracing its history and the manner in which the concepts and symbolism have been modified over the years. The cult of the Virgin has changed dramatically from a local peasant and Indian festivity into a multi-class and multi-ethnic national phenomenon. The article is over-long and the writing wordy, but its detail would provide a useful case-study for a specialist in this field.

951 **Wak'a: an Andean religious concept in the context of Aymara social and political life.**
Astvaldur Astvaldsson. PhD thesis, King's College, University of London, England, 1995.
Argues by means of examples drawn from the Jesús de Machaca region of highland Bolivia, that instead of trying to understand Andean religion in terms of an absolute division between the sacred and the profane – an unproductive line of enquiry – it is more realistic to examine Andean religion in terms of the socio-cultural environment from which it emerges, the ritual processes by which deities are honoured, and the discourse used by the Aymara people to make sense of their beliefs.

952 **From Viracocha to the Virgin of Copacabana: representation of the sacred at Lake Titicaca.**
Verónica Salles-Reese. Austin, Texas: University of Texas Press, 1997. 208p. map. bibliog.
An interdisciplinary study which explores how Andean myths of cosmic and ethnic origin centred on Lake Titicaca evolved from pre-Inca times to the year of the enthronement of the Virgin of Copacabana in 1583. Three narrative cycles are examined – pre-Inca, Inca, and Christian, as the author draws on material from the region's history, ethnology, theology, and anthropology. This is an ambitious investigation, and though highly specialized and densely written, it offers a detailed chronology and a valuable source of reference on the continuity of myth and religion at Lake Titicaca.

953 **Water and exchange: the ritual of *yaku cambio* as communal and competitive encounter.**
Lynn Louise Sikkink. *American Ethnologist*, vol. 24, no. 1 (1997), p. 170-89. bibliog.
Selecting the altiplano settlement of Condo near Lake Poopó in southern Bolivia, Sikkink describes the *yaku cambio* (water-exchange) ritual which serves to emphasize community rights and responsibilities in rain-making ceremonies, and which is also imbued with cosmic significance. This is an exhaustive account, of interest to those anthropologists seeking a comparative case-study on the role of ritual in promoting community awareness.

954 Neoliberal ritualists of Urkupiña: bedeviling patrimonial identity in a Bolivian patronal fiesta.
Robert Albro. *Ethnology*, vol. 37, no. 2 (1998), p. 133-64. bibliog.

An interpretation of the various strands which combine to form the fiesta of the Virgin of Urkupiña in Cochabamba, held for the most part in the nearby town of Quillacollo. Albro reviews the messages, ambiguities and tensions it contains, the blend of Christian and pagan practices, its commerce, and the competing attitudes of the highland ritualists and the local valley authorities over the ownership and management of the fiesta.

955 Performing national culture in a Bolivian migrant community.
Daniel Marc Goldstein. *Ethnology*, vol. 37, no. 2 (1998), p. 117-32. bibliog.

The community studied here, Villa Pagador, lies on the edge of the city of Cochabamba and was established in 1977 by migrants from Oruro. Goldstein describes in detail the nature and purpose of their annual Fiesta of San Miguel, which is modelled on the famous Oruro Carnival. Apart from drawing the crowds as a *fiesta folklórica*, the celebration is intended to demonstrate the link between the community's origins in Oruro, their new home in Villa Pagador, and their continuing integration and growing identity with the Bolivian state as a whole.

956 Landscape, gender, and community: Andean mountain stories.
Lynn Louise Sikkink, Braulio Choque M. *Anthropological Quarterly*, vol. 72, no. 4 (1999), p. 167-82. bibliog.

The authors investigate the attitudes of a Bolivian community living on the southern altiplano to the landscapes around them, particularly their reworking of history and gender based on stories of the mythical fight between two peaks, 'male' and 'female', in the high Andes.

Mass Media

Newspapers

957 Bolivia: press and revolution, 1932-1964.
Jerry W. Knudson.   Lanham, Maryland: University Press of
America, 1986. 487p. bibliog.
Starting with the Chaco War, which ushered in a new era of Bolivian journalism, Knudson
examines the role of the press in the years leading to the MNR (Movimiento Nacionalista
Revolucionario) revolution of 1952-53 and beyond, arguing that the press was a crucial
vehicle for social change in the absence of any other comparable means at the time for the
widespread circulation of ideas. The book becomes a history of modern journalism in
Bolivia and, in particular, a history of the creation of the first mass-based newspaper,
El Universal, which served as a training-ground for a generation of writers. While the
study focuses on *El Universal*, it also gives attention to a range of other newspapers,
among them *La Calle*, *En Marcha*, *La Nación*, *La Tarde*, *Los Tiempos*, and *El Diario*.
This is a shrewd and scholarly record with many useful insights, providing a social history
of the interaction between the press and Bolivian society during these three decades.

**958 Bolivia: commentary on freedom of expression and information
issues arising from the initial report of the Government of
Bolivia submitted under Article 40 of the Covenant for
consideration by the Human Rights Committee at its July 1989
session.**
London: International Centre of Censorship, Article 19, 1989. 20p.
A pamphlet which considers an official Bolivian government report on the country's
constitutional provisions for freedom of expression in the press, television, and radio. Set
against these legal provisions, the commentary proceeds to record the violations, or
alleged violations, that occur, and presents the grounds for dissatisfaction among many
Bolivians working in the media in the 1980s, concerning genuine freedom of information
and freedom of speech.

Radio

959 Rural radio in Bolivia – a case study.
Robert J. Gwyn. *Journal of Communication* (Annenberg School of
Communications, University of Pennsylvania), vol. 33, no. 2 (1983),
p. 79-87. bibliog.

Indigenous radio stations have assumed an important role in local communication
networks by adapting to community needs. In the early 1980s, the author notes that 110
Bolivian radio stations were in existence, run variously by the government, the churches,
miners, and local village enterprise. Here, Gwyn reports the results of a successful project
developed in the Punata and Jordán provinces of Cochabamba Department to spread
information about soybeans and to persuade isolated Quechua subsistence farmers to
grow them as a cheap source of protein. The article expands into a description of the
equipment and programming at the local radio stations, and the critical times at which
news, music, and messages are broadcast. This includes the regular practice of reading the
contents of national newspapers to the radio audience in Quechua. Overall, the piece
provides an interesting glimpse of a shoestring operation.

960 Tin miners' radio on the ropes.
Jane Slaughter. *The Progressive*, vol. 53 (February 1989), p. 11.

Reports the struggle for survival of the Bolivian tin miners' own radio stations which
were started in 1946 in defiance of the mine-owners and the government. Several stations
were restored after the 1952 revolution but successive governments found them
subversive, and withdrew their licences. This, together with mine closures, left the
network facing possible extinction by the end of the 1980s.

961 The miners' radio stations in Bolivia: a culture of resistance.
Alan O'Connor. *Journal of Communication* (Annenberg School of
Communications, University of Pennsylvania), vol. 40, no. 1 (1990),
p. 102-10. bibliog.

As mines closed during the 1980s, most of the Bolivian miners' smaller radio stations also
ceased operation, until by June 1988 only nine stations were actively broadcasting. In a
well-researched, informative article, O'Connor examines four of these: La Voz del
Minero, Pio XII, Radio Nacional de Huanuni, and Radio Uncía, including their origins,
politics, staffing and programme content.

962 Pious intentions.
Luís Rojas Velarde, Cristina L'Homme. *Index on Censorship*,
vol. 23, no. 6 (1994), p. 61-62.

Reports the protest by villagers of Patacayama on the altiplano against the government-
approved dumping of imported toxic waste on open ground near their homes. Their case
was taken up by the local Catholic radio station, Radio Pio XII, triggering heated and
well-publicized exchanges between the broadcasters and the government officials
involved.

963 A procedural view of participatory communication: lessons from Bolivian tin miners' radio.
Robert Huesca. *Media, Culture & Society*, vol. 17, no. 1 (1995),
p. 101-19. bibliog.

This is based on a study of the Radio Nacional de Huanuni, and focuses on the daily pattern of programme production. Huesca accompanies the producer around town, collecting live interviews, and noting the ways in which the local inhabitants are encouraged to voice their opinions. The contributions are often interesting, but the article itself is marred by the author's turgid prose.

Encyclopaedias and Reference Works

964 Handbook of South American Indians.
Edited by Julian Haynes Steward. Washington, DC: Smithsonian Institution/Bureau of American Ethnology, 1946-59. 7 vols. maps. bibliog..

This is a monumental work which, although in need of updating, remains an indispensable source of reference. The Indians of western and eastern Bolivia are studied in volumes 2 and 3, although later volumes include much relevant material on cross-cultural investigation: ethnology (vol. 5), and physical anthropology, linguistics, and cultural geography (vol. 6).

965 Enciclopedia del arte en América. (Encyclopaedia of American art.)
Buenos Aires: Editorial Bibliográfico Argentina, 1969. 5 vols.

Volumes one and two provide an introduction to the history of art – painting, sculpture and architecture – for each American republic. For Bolivia, see volume one (p. 93-156).

966 Historical dictionary of Bolivia.
Dwight B. Heath. Metuchen, New Jersey: Scarecrow Press, 1972. 324p. bibliog. (Latin American Historical Dictionaries, No. 4).

This remains a helpful research manual for those beginning to study Bolivian national development. It includes information about people and events of political importance, as well as terms relevant to geographical, ethnographic, linguistic, sociological and intellectual aspects of history. A substantial bibliographical essay, 'Towards understanding Bolivia', is also appended.

967 Encyclopedia of Latin America.
Edited by Helen Delpar.   New York: McGraw-Hill, 1974. 651p.
maps. bibliog..

Presents information concerning all aspects of Latin American society, including the arts, literature, biography, history, geography, agriculture, industry, transport, economics and politics. Although an older work, this encyclopaedia remains a valuable source of reference, with contributions by distinguished scholars in their fields. The emphasis in history is on the national period, with entries that are both succinct and informative, amply cross-referenced, and with their own short bibliographies. The volume as a whole is exceptionally clear and well organized.

968 Nomenclature and hierarchy – basic Latin American legal sources.
Rubens Medina, Cecilia Medina-Quiroga with the editorial assistance of Sandra A. Sawicki.   Washington, DC: Library of Congress, 1979. 123p. bibliog.

Identifies the hierarchy of the legal institutions in place at the end of the 1970s for each Latin American nation, thereby providing valuable legal information relevant to each country up to that time.

969 Archives and manuscripts on microfilm in the Nettie Lee Benson Latin American collection: a checklist.
Jane Garner.   Austin, Texas: University of Texas Press, 1980. 48p.

A listing and guide to 6,300 reels of microfilm.

970 Latin America: a guide to illustrations.
A. Curtis Wilgus.   Metuchen, New Jersey: Scarecrow Press, 1981. 250p.

This guide to illustrations of Latin America has two sections of interest to scholars working on Bolivia. Section four deals with pre-Inca and Inca civilization, and catalogues art, architecture, music, pottery and textiles. There is also a section on colonial coinage. For Bolivia there are references to pictures of town and village life, transport, religion and culture.

971 Political and economic encyclopedia of South America and the Caribbean.
Edited by Peter Calvert.   Harlow, England: Longman, 1991. 363p.

A useful source of reference which consists of three types of entry: by country; by individual personalities and political parties of special note; and by general subjects, i.e. problems and topics that are common to a number of countries or to the region as a whole. The text is well cross-referenced. Information on Bolivia appears in all three categories, and includes material on the country's socio-economic background, its major political figures, and its economic development up to the start of the 1990s.

972 The Cambridge Encyclopedia of Latin America and the Caribbean.
Edited by Simon Collier, Thomas E. Skidmore, Harold Blakemore. Cambridge, England: Cambridge University Press, 1992. 2nd ed. 479p. maps. bibliog.

A wide-ranging and well-illustrated volume on all aspects of Latin American society, including the physical environment, economy, peoples, history, politics, and culture.

973 Latin America and the Caribbean: a critical guide to research sources.
Edited by Paula H. Covington.   New York; Westport, Connecticut: Greenwood Press, 1992. 924p.

Bolivia is well represented in this volume, which offers valuable assistance to any researcher studying the humanities in the Latin American and Caribbean region as a whole. Well-organized entries include history, economics, politics, literature, drama, art and architecture, as well as general introductory essays on a range of topics. The material is clearly indexed, and the selected references are drawn from both English and Spanish-language sources.

974 The United States in Latin America: a historical dictionary.
David Shavit.   Westport, Connecticut; New York: Greenwood Press, 1992. 471p.

An eclectic collection of American individuals, institutions, and events which, between the beginning of the 19th and the end of the 20th centuries, brought the United States into contact with Latin America. Shavit's biographical entries range widely, and include diplomats, businessmen, travellers, engineers, scientists, artists, authors, and military personnel. The business firms and other bodies selected here are those considered to have had the biggest impact on particular countries in Latin America, and on US–Latin American relations. Bolivia is well represented, while thorough indexing adds to the value of this reference work.

975 Enciclopedia Bolivia mágica. (Magical Bolivia.)
Edited by Hugo Boero Rojo.   La Paz: Editorial Vertiente, 1993. 3 vols. Vol. 1, 321p.; Vol. 2, 294p.; Vol. 3, 354p. maps. bibliog.

An outstanding publication whose entries range across every aspect of Bolivia's land, people, culture, and economic activity. From landscape, flora, fauna and the natural world, the volumes move on through studies of the nine departments, cities and villages, archaeology, art, architecture, music, literature, cinema, television, and journalism. Finally, the encyclopaedia focuses on the economy in the 1990s, including mining, agriculture, manufacturing industry, construction, transport, and migration. The production is of a consistently high quality, and all three volumes are profusely illustrated, mainly in colour. The purpose throughout is to present a positive view of the country, its heritage and its achievements. It does this brilliantly, with verve, scholarship, and style.

976 The Cambridge History of Latin America, vol. 10. Latin America since 1930: ideas, culture and society.
Edited by Leslie Bethell.   Cambridge: Cambridge University Press, 1995. 645p. bibliog.

Brief entries for Bolivia covering the period from c.1920 to c.1980 include: Architecture (Damián Bayón), p. 382-83; Art since c.1920 (Damián Bayón), p. 432-34; Cinema (John King), p. 496-97, 502; and Music (Gérard H. Béhague), p. 344, 359-60. These entries, together with other extracts from this series, are reprinted in *A Cultural History of Latin America: literature, music and the visual arts in the 19th and 20th centuries*, edited by Leslie Bethell (Cambridge: Cambridge University Press, 1998. 538p.). No new material is added.

977 Dictionary of twentieth century culture: hispanic culture of South America.
Edited by Peter Standish.   Detroit, Michigan: Gale Research Inc., 1995. 340p.

An authoritative and wide-ranging work. It includes entries on: Indigenism in literature and art; Lyrical abstraction; Weaving, pottery and other crafts; Language and culture; and Dances of the Andean region. In addition, there is background on the Bolivian cinema, the Bolivian Film Institute and the Censorship Board, and on the work of Bolivia's major film-makers, including Jorge Ruiz and Jorge Sanjinés.

978 Encyclopedia of Latin American history and culture.
Edited by Barbara A. Tenenbaum.   New York: Simon & Schuster Macmillan, 1996. 5 vols. 'Bolivia', vol. 1, p. 362-83.

The entry for Bolivia, by several contributors, concentrates exclusively on the country's history, constitutions, selected civic, cultural and labour organizations, and the major political parties, with a note on agrarian reform. Extensive cross-referencing directs readers to additional information elsewhere in the set on people, places, events, institutions and economic affairs.

979 Encyclopedia of Latin American literature.
Edited by Verity Smith.   Chicago; London: Fitzroy Dearborn, 1997. 926p. map. bibliog.

This valuable source of reference contains entries on writers, their works, and selected topics of particular significance in the literature of Latin America. In addition, there are survey articles on all the individual states in the region. The introductory article on Bolivia provides an incisive critical review of the country's 19th- and 20th-century prose and poetry which highlights the dominant genres: e.g. the 'mining novel', the 'Chaco War novel', *Indigenista* and *Mestizaje*, the *novella de cholos*, and the differing expressions of national identity in Bolivia's inseparable social and political literature. With its own bibliography, this article provides an excellent starting-point for students intending to work on the period.

980   The Cambridge History of the Native Peoples of the Americas, vol. 3. South America.
Edited by Frank Salomon, Stuart B. Schwartz.   Cambridge, England: Cambridge University Press, 1999. Part 1, 1054p.; Part 2, 976p. maps. bibliog.

This two-part volume brings together the latest research on the indigenous peoples of South America and provides an indispensable record of recent scholarship, updating, though not replacing, Julian Steward's *Handbook of South American Indians* (item no. 964). There are twenty-six chapters in all which reflect the regional specializations of the authors, and particular historical periods. The essays investigate, among other topics, the impact of the Iberian invasions; the indigenous experience under colonial rule; Indian resistance; 19th-century conditions; and the changing circumstances of both the Andean and the Lowland Indians during the 20th century. There are excellent maps and illustrations. The volumes are not an encyclopaedia in the strict sense, but they are carefully indexed for full and rapid reference, and comprise an outstanding contribution to the anthropological and historical literature.

981   Encyclopedia of Latin American and Caribbean art.
Edited by Jane Turner.   London: Macmillan Reference, 2000. 782p. maps. bibliog. (Grove Encyclopedias of the Arts of the Americas, New York).

An impressive source of reference, distinguished by its scope, the high quality of its entries, and its meticulous editing. Country surveys form the encyclopaedia's basic structure, with the Bolivian material arranged under the major headings of: (1) An introduction to the region and its urban planning; (2) Renaissance Plateresque, and early Baroque (1534-1690); (3) *Mestizo* Baroque to Neo-Classicism (1690-1825); (4) Neo-Classicism to Eclecticism (1826-1952); and (5) Modern to Post-Modern (after 1952). Within each of these divisions are entries on Architecture; Painting and graphic arts; Sculpture; Gold and silver; Textiles; Patronage, collecting and dealing; Museums and photographic collections; and Art education. Thus, the encyclopaedia presents an unusually wide interpretation of its title, with separate entries also for selected cities, schools of painting, and individual artists and architects. Each section has its own bibliography, while the volume is profusely illustrated in colour and black-and-white. With all its detail, the encyclopaedia is nevertheless easy to handle and to enjoy, for this is an authoritative, stimulating addition to the literature that will please both the art historian and the general reader.

982   A reference guide to Latin American history.
Edited by James D. Henderson, Helen Delpar, Maurice P. Brungardt, Richard N. Weldon.   Armonk, New York; London: M. E. Sharpe Publications, 2000. 615p. maps. bibliog.

This guide provides: (1) A chronology of Latin America's prehistory and history to the end of the 20th century; regional grouping places Bolivia in the section on the Bolivarian Republics; (2) A study of major topics, e.g. revolutionary movements, democracy and neoliberalism, society and culture; and (3) Biographical sketches of 300 significant figures in Latin American history. This is a useful general volume, but there is relatively little on Bolivia.

Bibliographies

983   Ensayo de una bibliografía general de los periódicos de Bolivia, 1825-1905. (General bibliographical essay of Bolivian newspapers and periodicals, 1825-1905.)
Gabriel René-Moreno.   Santiago de Chile: Universo, 1905. 344p.

This is a uniquely valuable source of reference on the 19th- and early 20th-century press in Bolivia. It reviews all the major newspapers, and provides information about the publishers, editorial policy and publication dates. The volume brings together a thorough catalogue and an excellent guide which was originally published as separate articles in various Chilean reviews.

984   Bibliografía de la lengua guaraní. (Bibliography of the Guaraní language.)
José T. Medina.   Buenos Aires: Tallares Casa Jacabo Peuser, 1930. 93p.

A basic bibliography of the Guaraní language. It is arranged in chronological order and lists works which appeared between the 1530s and the 1920s. The introductory essay describes the origins of the name 'Guaraní' and gives a history of the study of the Guaraní language.

985   Bibliografía de las lenguas quechua y aymara. (Bibliography of the Quechua and Aymara languages.)
José T. Medina.   New York: Museum of the American Indian, 1930. 117p.

A standard reference source on native languages of the Andean region by a noted Chilean historian and bibliographer.

986 Handbook of Latin American Studies.
Edited by Dolores Moyano Martin, assisted by P. Sue Mundell.
Austin: University of Texas Press, 1936- . annual.

This extensive and invaluable bibliographical source is prepared by a number of scholars for the Hispanic Division of the Library of Congress. The volumes alternate between the humanities and the social sciences, the former including art, history, ethnohistory, literature, music, philosophy, and electronic resources. The social sciences handbook covers anthropology, economics, geography, government, politics, international relations, and sociology.

987 Bibliographie des langues aymara et kičua. (A bibliography of the Aymara and Quechua languages.)
Paul Rivet.   Paris: Institut d'Ethnologie, Université de Paris, 1951-65. 4 vols.

This bibliography is arranged chronologically by century and covers the period 1540-1875. The entries give detailed bibliographical and physical descriptions of the relevant works, while the work also includes a list of maps with their library locations. The introduction is in French.

988 Catálogo de la bibliografía boliviana; libros y folletos, 1900-1963.
(Catalogue of Bolivian bibliographies; books and pamphlets, 1900-63.)
Arturo Costa de la Torre.   La Paz: Universidad Boliviana Mayor de San Andrés, 1966. 2 vols.

An excellent listing of works written in Bolivia.

989 Revolution and structural change in Latin America: a bibliography on ideology, development and the radical Left (1930-1965).
Ronald Chilcote.   Stanford, California: Hoover Institution on War, Revolution and Peace, 1970. 2 vols.

The major headings include agrarian reform, anti-Communism, Christian democracy and economic development. There are also sections on individual countries.

990 Bolivia.
Rosa Quintero Mesa.   New York; London: R. R. Bowker, 1972.
156p. (Latin American Serial Documents, a holdings list, Vol. 6).

An inclusive bibliography of Bolivian serial documents published since Independence, which are held in US and Canadian libraries. This volume remains a uniquely valuable source of information for the researcher.

991 Bibliography of philosophy in the Iberian colonies of America.
Walter B. Redmond. The Hague: Martinus Nijhoff, 1972. 175p.
bibliog. (International Archives of the History of Ideas, No. 51).
A highly useful catalogue of over 800 listings of philosophy manuscripts and essays from the colonial era.

992 Protestantism in Latin America: a bibliographical guide.
Edited by John H. Sinclair. South Pasadena, California: William Carey Library, 1976. 414p.
A comprehensive annotated bibliography of selected references, mainly in English, Spanish and Portuguese.

993 Diccionario de la literatura boliviana. (Dictionary of Bolivian literature.)
José Ortega. La Paz: Editorial 'Los Amigos del Libro', 1977. 337p.
A comprehensive reference guide to Bolivian literature, providing biographical and bibliographical information on some 280 Bolivian writers.

994 Information on music: a handbook of reference sources in European languages. Vol. 2. The Americas.
Guy A. Marco, with the assistance of Sharon Paugh Ferris, Ann Garfield. Littleton, Colorado: Libraries Unlimited, 1977. 296p.
A highly selective bibliographical tool which includes material chosen on the basis of excellence and of accessibility. This is a good starting-point for any researcher dealing with cultural material relating to the Western hemisphere. In the ten items on Bolivia (965-974), the subjects covered include: folk music and folk song, historical studies, musical instruments, and selective and critical guides.

995 Genealogical historical guide to Latin America.
Lyman DePlatt. Detroit, Michigan: Gale Research, 1978. 273p.
An indispensable guide for those interested in genealogy and social history. Each Latin American republic has its own chapter, in addition to several topical chapters which include bibliographical data on specific areas.

996 A critical survey of the literature on the Aymara language.
Lucy Briggs. *Latin American Research Review*, vol. 14, no. 3 (1979), p. 87-105.
Describes major bibliographical sources, together with pre-linguistic and linguistic studies of the Aymara language, from colonial times to the present.

997 **The Béeche, Gutiérrez and René-Moreno 'Bibliotecas Americanas': libraries and intellectual life in the nineteenth-century Andes.**
Gertrude M. Yeager. *Inter-American Review of Bibliography*, vol. 31, no. 4 (1981), p. 507-13.

Examines the formation of libraries in Chile and Bolivia in the 19th century. The careers of José Rosendo Gutiérrez of La Paz and Gabriel René-Moreno, a Bolivian scholar who lived in Santiago, Chile, are discussed.

998 **The Catholic Left in Latin America: a comprehensive bibliography.**
Therrin C. Dahlin, Gary Gillum, Mark Grover.
Boston, Massachusetts: G. K. Hall, 1981. 410p.

An excellent research tool for those interested in the political activities of the Catholic Church in Latin America. The Bolivian section (p. 163-69) contains seventy-two citations of essentially periodical literature in the Catholic press, such as *The Americas* (Academy of American Franciscan History), *Catholic Messenger* and *Commonwealth*, among others.

999 **Travel accounts and descriptions of Latin America and the Caribbean, 1800-1920.**
Compiled by Thomas L. Welch, Myriam Figueras.
Washington, DC: Organization of American States, 1982. 293p.

This carefully selected bibliography includes sixty-eight entries for Bolivia recording impressions and observations of the country made by foreign travellers in the 19th and early 20th centuries (p. 21-29).

1000 **Ecclesiastical archives of the Parroquias de Nuestra Señora de La Paz, Bolivia 1548-1940: description and analysis.**
Nelly S. González. *The Americas* (Academy of American Franciscan History), vol. 40, no. 1 (1983), p. 109-17.

Describes the contents of, and access to, parish archives in La Paz. This study is a valuable guide and bibliographical source for those interested in both social and demographic history.

1001 **The Incas: a bibliography of books and periodical articles.**
Compiled by Thomas L. Welch, Rene L. Gutierrez.
Washington, DC: Organization of American States, 1987. 145p.

Contains citations for 715 books and 401 periodical articles pertaining to all aspects of the Inca empire: its history, organization, trade, and daily life. This is an invaluable source for scholars on the literature published up to the mid-1980s.

1002 The Indians of South America: a bibliography.
Compiled by Thomas L. Welch. Washington, DC: Organization
of American States, 1987. 594p.
A major bibliographical source which includes general works, works by topic, specific
regions and peoples, and languages and dialects.

1003 Research collections of Chile's Instituto Nacional.
Gertrude M. Yeager. *The Americas* (Academy of American
Franciscan History), vol. 46, no. 2 (1989), p. 225-30. bibliog.
During the 19th century and until the 1920s, Chile's Instituto Nacional, a national
secondary school, housed one of the most extensive American libraries in South America.
This note discusses the contents of the contemporary library which has an extensive
section on Bolivia, the result of René-Moreno's long tenure as librarian there.

1004 The Cambridge History of Latin America, vol. 11.
Bibliographical essays.
Edited by Leslie Bethell. Cambridge: Cambridge University
Press, 1995. 1043p.
This final volume comprises the collected bibliographies published earlier in this
distinguished Cambridge history series, all of them revised, updated, and in most cases
expanded. It includes bibliographies on Bolivia, c.1820-c.1870 (p. 287-88); Bolivia,
c.1870-1930 (p. 455-62); and Bolivia, 1930-c.1990 (p. 806-10).

1005 Traveller's literary companion: South and Central America,
including Mexico.
Jason Wilson. Brighton, England: In Print, 1993; Lincolnwood,
Illinois: Passport Books, 1995. 459p. maps
A varied literary anthology which contains over 250 extracts from novels, poems, and
short stories about Latin America, along with concise biographies of the authors
concerned. The volume includes seven brief entries on Bolivia which are selected, like
those on the other countries, to give a glimpse of the various regional contrasts to be
found there. This is good supporting text for the general reader and the armchair traveller.

Indexes

There follow three separate indexes: authors (personal or corporate); titles of publications; and subjects. The Index of Authors also includes editors, translators, and film directors. Title entries are italicized and refer either to the main titles, or to other works cited in the annotations. The numbers refer to the bibliographic entries, not to page numbers.

Index of Authors

Fergerstrom, L. M. 478
Fernandez, H. 14
Fernández-Torriente, G. 835
Ferris, E. G. 319, 321
Ferris, S. P. 994
Ferry, S. 569, 574
Fifer, J. V. 15, 132, 231,
  247, 497, 502, 509,
  580
Figueras, M. 999
Finan, J. J. 305
Fini, M. 893
Finot, E. 207
Fischer, S. 396
Fisher, J. R. 223, 232
Flader, S. 609
Flandre, P. 677
Flatte, M. 515
Fleming, J. E. 462
Flores, A. 806
Flores, W. 64
Forrest, M. 571
Förster, A. 94
Foster, D. W. 801
Foster, V. R. 801
Fournier, D. 328
Fox, A. N. 48
Francis, P. W. 34
Francou, B. 41, 50, 52
Franks, J. 494
Fraser, V. 846, 877
Freyre, R. J. 801, 815
Frisancho, A. R. 675
Frisancho, H. G. 675
Fritz, S. C. 43

G

Gade, D. W. 383
Gaines, M. 606
Gallo, C. 282
Galwey, N. W, 475
Gamarra, E. A. 255, 294,
  407-08, 554
Gamble, B. M. 36
Gamboa, H. 672

García Argañarás, F. 283,
  551
García Fernández, W. 467
García-Guinea, J. 615
García Pabon, L. 807
Garfield, A. 994
Garner, J. 969
Garza, M. 588
Gavin, M. 443
Gelula, M. 124
Ghinsberg, Y. 152
Gianella, A. 683
Gianotten, V. 656
Gibbon, L. 130
Gibbs, B. 82
Gibson, B. 548
Gibson, C, 214
Giese, P. 88
Gilbert, A. 19
Gilderhus, M. T. 318
Gill, L. 377, 512, 651-52,
  655, 660, 789
Gillgannon, M. J. 518
Gillum, G. 998
Gisbert, M. E. 658
Gisbert, T. 796, 829, 844,
  851-54, 858-59, 872-74,
  878, 880, 885
Glick, E. L. 227
Gluckmann, D. 878
Godoy, R. A. 352, 381, 461,
  463, 494, 528, 548, 562
Goethals, H. 689
Goldstein, D. M. 628, 955
Gómez B., D. 728, 750
González, N. S. 1000
Goodell, G. 881
Goodnough, D. 242
Goodspeed, T. H. 155
Gott, R. 153
Gould, J. 158
Grace, A. M. 821
Graffam, G. C. 183
Graham, C. 404
Graham & Whiteside 601
Granados, R. 687

Grant, J. 867
Grassi, D. 451
Green, D. 359
Green, G. 624
Green, H. 82
Green, P. W. 543
Greenfield O. 166
Gregores, E. 759
Gregory-Wodzicki, K. M.
  93
Greksa, L. P. 669
Grey, H. M. 145
Grosh, M. 401
Gross, G. 920
Grover, M. 998
Groverman, V. 656
Grunberg, A. 372
Grundmann, G. 561
Guardia Mayorga, C. A. 739
Guasch, A. 760
Gubbels, T. L. 83
Gudec, T. 422, 588
Guevara, J. S. 799
Guglielmetti, P. 672
Guillermoprieto, A. 285
Guise, A. V. L. 143
Gullison, R. E. 491
Gumucio Dagrón, A. 906
Gutierrez, R. L. 1001
Guy, J. 571
Guyot, J.-L. 53, 103
Guzmán, A. 208, 797, 804
Gwyn, R. J. 959

H

Haas, J. D. 680
Hagedorn, D. 579
Hahn, D. R. 284, 376
Hall, A. P. 876
Hames, G. L. 251, 661
Hamilton, S. 647
Hannele, S. T. 902
Hanrahan, D. 616
Hanrahan, M. S. 480
Hanratty, D. M. 6

288

293

Index of Titles

298

R

S

318

Index of Subjects

A

Agrarian reform
see Land reform;
Colonization
Agriculture
in Andes 456-60, 462-68,
478, 481-83, 485-88
in eastern Bolivia 459-60,
471, 483-84, 921-22
colonial period 217, 225-
26, 470, 475, 777
crops
amaranth 470
cacao 545, 921
coffee 921, 520, 545
cotton 921
lupin 972
oca (oxalis) 487
peanut (groundnut)
460, 471
potato 456-58, 462-63,
467, 474, 476, 485-86
quinoa 462, 470, 475
soya 463, 496, 545,
921, 959
large-scale farming 188,
375, 512, 514
mechanization 459, 483-84
small-scale farming 457,
468, 496, 498, 512, 514
subsistence farming 148,
188, 498, 512, 959
see also Camelids; Coca;
Colonization;
Hacienda system;
Prehistory and
archaeology; Soil
erosion, conservation,
and productivity

Air transport 579
Altiplano
settlement 12, 141, 144,
149, 201, 345, 368,
920, 926
geology and structural
formation 33, 35-36,
84-85, 90-91, 96,
926
potential oil reserves
586
saline lakes and salt pans
(*salares*) 171, 570,
935-36
see also Agriculture;
Titicaca; Tiwanaku
Amazon (river) 131-33,
140
Andean Community (Pact,
Group) *see* Foreign
relations
Andes
geography and geology
33, 35-36, 47-52, 79-
83, 86-95
mountaineering 112, 118,
136, 138
travellers' accounts 127,
130, 133, 135, 139,
149
see also Agriculture;
Altiplano
Andrade, Víctor 308, 310
Arab immigration 390
Archaeology *see*
Prehistory and
archaeology
Architecture
colonial 860, 869-78,
880-81

Baroque 842, 869, 874-
75, 981
mestizo 869-70, 874,
876, 981
mudéjar 871, 876
Rococo 869
20th century 848, 979,
981
Argentina 48, 86, 145,
269, 310, 327-28, 354,
402, 439, 451, 600,
615, 658, 672
Bolivian migrant labour
in 354, 449, 479
fossil hunting in 73
see also Salta,
Argentina
Arts
cultural history,
encyclopaedias,
bibliographies 842,
847-48, 850, 965,
970, 976, 981
see also Architecture;
Literature; Museums;
Music; Painting,
sculpture and carving;
Photography; Pottery;
Textiles and weaving
Atlases, general 65-66
ayllus 64
history 63
new municipalities 67
see also Maps;
Gazetteers
Ayllu studies 64, 352, 354,
358, 378-79, 384, 469,
650, 688, 891, 940
Aymara Indians *see*
Indians

321

Map of Bolivia

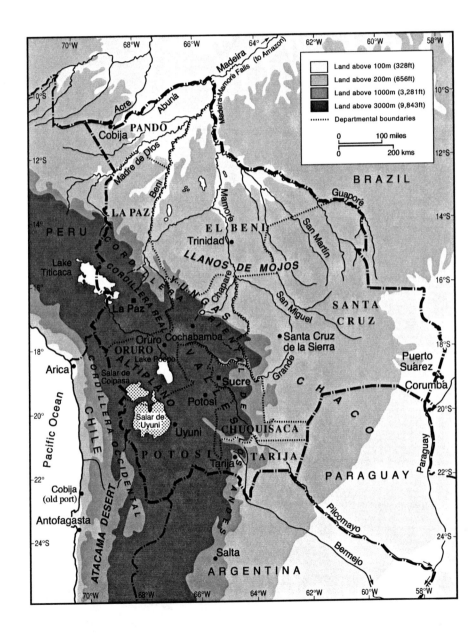

ALSO FROM CLIO PRESS

INTERNATIONAL ORGANIZATIONS SERIES

Each volume in the International Organizations Series is either devoted to one specific organization, or to a number of different organizations operating in a particular region, or engaged in a specific field of activity. The scope of the series is wide ranging and includes intergovernmental organizations, international non-governmental organizations, and national bodies dealing with international issues. The series is aimed mainly at the English-speaker and each volume provides a selective, annotated, critical bibliography of the organization, or organizations, concerned. The bibliographies cover books, articles, pamphlets, directories, databases and theses and, wherever possible, attention is focused on material about the organizations rather than on the organizations' own publications. Notwithstanding this, the most important official publications, and guides to those publications, will be included. The views expressed in individual volumes, however, are not necessarily those of the publishers.

VOLUMES IN THE SERIES